D1766810

Obstetrics and Gynaecology

First edition authors:

Nick Panay

Ruma Dutta

Audrey Ryan

J A Mark Broadbent

Second edition authors:

Maryam Parisaei

Archana Shailendra

Ruma Dutta

J A Mark Broadbent

Third edition authors:

Chidimma Onwere

Hemant N. Vakharia

4th Edition

CRASH COURSE

SERIES EDITORS

Philip Xiu
MA, MB BChir, MRCP
GP Registrar
Yorkshire Deanery
Leeds, UK

Shreelata Datta
MD, MRCOG, LLM, BSC (HONS), MBBS
Honorary Senior Lecturer
Imperial College London
Consultant Obstetrician and Gynaecologist
King's College Hospital
London, UK

FACULTY ADVISORS

Ruma Dutta
BSC, MBBS, MRCOG
Consultant in Obstetrics and Gynaecology
Hillingdon Hospital NHS Foundation Trust
Middlesex, UK

Fevzi Shakir
MBBS, BSC(HONS), MRCOG, MSC
Consultant Obstetrician and Advanced Gynaecological Endoscopic Surgeon
Royal Free London NHS Foundation Trust
London, UK

Obstetrics and Gynaecology

Sophie Eleanor Kay
MBBS BSc(Hons), MRCOG
Registrar in Obstetrics and Gynaecology
University Hospital Lewisham
Lewisham and Greenwich NHS Trust
London, UK

Charlotte Jean Sandhu
MBBS, MRCOG
Specialist Registrar in Obstetrics and Gynaecology, Hillingdon Hospital NHS Trust,
Middlesex UK

For additional online content visit StudentConsult.com

ELSEVIER

ELSEVIER

Content Strategist: Jeremy Bowes
Content Development Specialist: Alexandra Mortimer
Project Manager: Andrew Riley
Design: Christian Bilbow
Illustration Manager: Karen Giacomucci
Illustrator: MPS North America LLC
Marketing Manager: Deborah Watkins

Notices

Practitioners and researchers must always rely on their own experience and knowledge in evaluating and using any information, methods, compounds or experiments described herein. Because of rapid advances in the medical sciences, in particular, independent verification of diagnoses and drug dosages should be made. To the fullest extent of the law, no responsibility is assumed by Elsevier, authors, editors or contributors for any injury and/or damage to persons or property as a matter of products liability, negligence or otherwise, or from any use or operation of any methods, products, instructions, or ideas contained in the material herein.

ISBN: 978-0-7020-7347-2
eISBN: 978-0-7020-7348-9

Printed in Great Britain
Last digit is the print number: 9   8   7   6   5   4   3

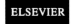

ELSEVIER   your source for books,
journals and multimedia
in the health sciences

www.elsevierhealth.com

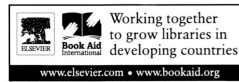

Working together
to grow libraries in
developing countries

www.elsevier.com • www.bookaid.org

The
publisher's
policy is to use
**paper manufactured
from sustainable forests**

Series Editors' Foreword

The *Crash Course* series was conceived by Dr Dan Horton-Szar who as series editor presided over it for more than 15 years – from publication of the first edition in 1997, until publication of the fourth edition in 2011. His inspiration, knowledge and wisdom lives on in the pages of this book. As the new series editors, we are delighted to be able to continue developing each book for the twenty-first century undergraduate curriculum.

The flame of medicine never stands still and keeping this all-new fifth series relevant for today's students is an ongoing process. Each title within this new fifth edition has been re-written to integrate basic medical science and clinical practice, after extensive deliberation and debate. We aim to build on the success of the previous titles by keeping the series up-to-date with current guidelines for best practice, and recent developments in medical research and pharmacology.

We always listen to feedback from our readers, through focus groups and student reviews of the *Crash Course* titles. For the fifth editions we have reviewed and re-written our self-assessment material to reflect today's 'single-best answer' and 'extended matching question' formats. The artwork and layout of the titles has also been largely re-worked and are now in colour, to make it easier on the eye during long sessions of revision. The new on-line materials supplement the learning process.

Despite fully revising the books with each edition, we hold fast to the principles on which we first developed the series. *Crash Course* will always bring you all the information you need to revise in compact, manageable volumes that still maintain the balance between clarity and conciseness, and provide sufficient depth for those aiming at distinction. The authors are junior doctors who have recent experience of the exams you are now facing, and the accuracy of the material is checked by a team of faculty editors from across the UK.

We wish you all the best for your future careers!

Philip Xiu, Shreelata Datta

Preface

As medicine progresses in the 21st century, the specialty of obstetrics and gynaecology continually evolves, combining medical, surgical and practical components which must be grasped by the contemporary medical student. Often in the space of only six to eight weeks, this must seem like an overwhelming task.

As part of the *Crash Course* series, this fourth edition continues to give the essential information in a clear concise manner, combining up-to-date text with tables, figures and algorithms. It gives vital information as well as hints and tips that focus on how important it is to take a good history. Obviously this is necessary in any branch of medicine, but the personal nature of this specialty makes it even more crucial. Similarly, examination of the patient is described in a sensitive manner. After covering management for each topic, the popular self-assessment section has been updated in line with current examination techniques.

In addition to imparting the factual knowledge needed to pass examinations, we hope that this book will give today's students the encouragement to find out more for themselves, to gain clinical experience and not to just learn lists. Although there is a similar basis to both sides of the specialty, actual practice on the shop floor is so diverse that there is something that every student can find to engage them. We hope this textbook is an essential guide to introduce students to a unique and very rewarding specialty, capturing its variety and its challenges.

Sophie Eleanor Kay, Charlotte Jean Sandhu

Dedication

For my extremely supportive family and parents. For my fiancé Rauri – I couldn't have completed this project without your encouragement and patience!

Sophie Eleanor Kay

To my wonderful family. Dad, Mum, James, Lisa and baby nephew Oliver thank you for all your love and support.

Charlotte Jean Sandhu

To my dad, who would have been proud to see my name in print, and to my mum, who is. Also to Paul, Jack and Sadie for all their patience and love.

Ruma Dutta

To my supportive mother, father, brother and family, who have always encouraged and motivated me to work hard to reach my potential and strive for excellence.

Fevzi Shakir

Series Editors' Acknowledgements

We would like to thank the support of our colleagues who have helped in the preparation of this edition, namely the junior doctor contributors who helped write the manuscript as well as the faculty editors who check the veracity of the information.

We are extremely grateful for the support of our publisher, Elsevier, whose staffs' insight and persistence has maintained the quality that Dr Horton-Szar has set-out since the first edition. Jeremy Bowes, our commissioning editor, has been a constant support. Alex Mortimer and Barbara Simmons our development editors have managed the day-to-day work on this edition with extreme patience and unflaggable determination to meet the ever looming deadlines, and we are ever grateful for Kim Benson's contribution to the online editions and additional online supplementary materials.

Philip Xiu and Shreelata Datta

Contents

Contents

Contents

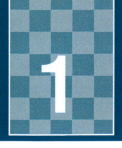

BASIC ANATOMY

An understanding of basic anatomy of the pelvis is important to fully understand the normal structures and identify any pathology. (Figs 1.1–1.4) will provide a good reference when working through the textbook.

GENERAL EXAMINATION

General examination is extremely important for both gynaecology and obstetric patients and is often overlooked. Ensure the patient is comfortable and not unduly exposed. The following general assessment should be made:

- general wellbeing
- body mass index

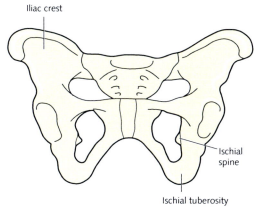

Fig. 1.1 Pelvic bones.

- cardiovascular system, including pulse, blood pressure, cardiac murmurs and clinical signs of anaemia or oedema
- respiratory system
- neurological examination if indicated by history

This should then help to guide your differential diagnosis, and therefore your further investigations.

OBSTETRIC EXAMINATION

As per all examination techniques, the general obstetric examination follows the systemic review by:

- observation
- inspection
- palpation
- auscultation

Observation

Obstetric patients should not be examined flat on their backs because of the risk of postural supine hypotensive syndrome; when lying flat, the pregnant uterus compresses the aorta and reduces blood flow back to the maternal heart which can cause the woman to feel faint.

On general observation you must assess whether she appears comfortable at rest? Is there any indication of pain or distress? Does she look systemically well or unwell? This review should help alert possible immediate cause for concern.

Inspection

- Abdominal mass.
- Stigmata of pregnancy.
- Surgical scars.

Fig. 1.2 Cross section of female pelvic anatomy.

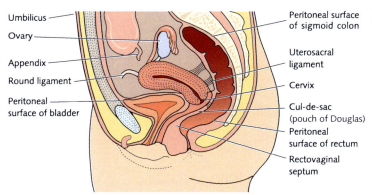

Fig. 1.3 External anatomy.

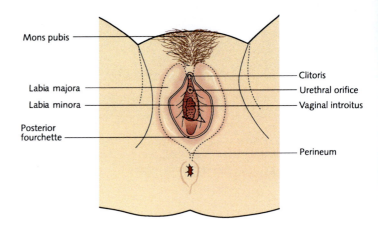

Mons pubis
Labia majora
Labia minora
Posterior fourchette
Clitoris
Urethral orifice
Vaginal introitus
Perineum

Fig. 1.4 Anatomy of pelvic floor muscles.

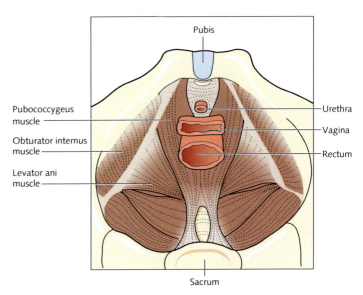

Pubis
Pubococcygeus muscle
Obturator internus muscle
Levator ani muscle
Urethra
Vagina
Rectum
Sacrum

Abdominal mass

Inspect for any abdominal masses. A gravid (pregnant) uterus can often be seen per abdomen from approximately 12 to 14 weeks' gestation. The shape and size of the abdomen should be noted. Are there any additional masses visualized, for example, an umbilical hernia.

Stigmata of pregnancy

Striae gravidarum (stretch marks) are caused by pregnancy hormones that stimulate the splitting of the dermis and can occur relatively early in pregnancy. New striae appear red and sometimes inflamed and can be sore and itchy; old striae from previous pregnancies are pale and silvery. They usually appear on the lower abdomen, upper thighs, buttocks and breasts.

Increased skin pigmentation can occur in pregnancy and results in the linea nigra – midline pigmentation from the xiphisternum to the symphysis pubis. Other areas that can undergo pigmentation in pregnancy include the nipples, the vulva, the umbilicus and recent abdominal scars.

Surgical scars

It is important to examine carefully for surgical scars as they can often be well-healed. Previous caesarean section scars are transverse suprapubic scars often hidden in the pubic hairline. Minimal access laparoscopy scars will usually have an umbilical scar site and additional abdominal sites. If scars are noted, it is important to confirm what surgical procedures have been performed (history taking).

Palpation

Before palpating the abdomen always enquire about areas of tenderness and palpate these areas last. On obstetric palpation there are a number of features which are being assessed:

- uterine size
- number of fetuses
- fetal lie, presentation, engagement and position

Uterine size

Uterine size is assessed by palpation and is a skill that is acquired and improved with increased experience. A rough guide to the uterine size and corresponding gestation can be made from assessment of the fundal height in relation to the following anatomical landmarks: the symphysis pubis (12 weeks), umbilicus (20 weeks) and xiphisternum (36 weeks; see Fig. 1.5). The fundus of the uterus is not palpable abdominally until 12 weeks' gestation. By 36 weeks the fundus should be approximately at the level of the xiphisternum, following which it drops down as the fetal head engages into the maternal pelvis.

When palpating the uterine fundus, always start at the xiphisternum and work towards the umbilicus using the medial border of the left hand or the fingertips. This technique should ensure that you always palpate the upper extent of a pelvic mass. Measuring the distance from the fundus to the symphysis pubis in centimetres [symphysis fundal height (SFH)] is a more objective method of assessing fundal height than using topography alone. After 24 weeks' gestation, the SFH measurement ± 3 cm should equal the gestation (e.g., at 34 weeks' gestation the SFH should be between 31 and 37 cm). This is a crude measurement technique and varies in precision between measurers, but is used to highlight patients measuring small for dates (e.g., growth-restricted babies) and large for dates (possible increased amniotic fluid levels).

Clinical assessment of liquor volume is not as accurate as objective assessment using ultrasound. However, subjective assessment can alert the examiner to the possibility of reduced or increased liquor volume and instigation of the necessary investigations. Reduced liquor volume might be suggested when the uterus is small for dates with easily palpable fetal parts producing an irregular firm outline to the uterus. Increased liquor volume causes a large-for-dates uterus that is smooth and rounded and in which the fetal parts are almost impossible to distinguish. If there are concerns regarding uterine size, an ultrasound scan should be ordered to assess fetus growth and amniotic fluid index.

Number of fetuses

The number of fetuses present can be calculated by assessing the number of fetal poles present. 'Fetal pole' is the term used to denote the head or the breech (buttocks). In a singleton pregnancy, two poles should be palpable unless the presenting part is deeply engaged in the pelvis. In multiple pregnancies, the number of poles present *minus one* should be palpable. For example, four poles are present in a twin pregnancy and only three should be palpable as one is usually tucked away out of reach. More commonly, the patient has already had an ultrasound scan detailing the number of fetuses.

Fetal lie, presentation, engagement and position

The fetal 'lie' is the relationship between the long axis of the fetus and the long axis of the uterus. This can be longitudinal, transverse or oblique (Fig. 1.6).

The fetal 'presentation' is the part of the fetus that presents to the maternal pelvis. If the head (also known as the 'vertex') is situated over the pelvis, this is termed a 'cephalic presentation'. In a breech presentation the buttocks occupy the lower segment, and in an oblique lie the shoulder generally presents (Fig. 1.7). Any presentation other than a vertex presentation is called a 'malpresentation'.

The fetal head is said to be engaged when the widest diameter of the head (the biparietal diameter) has passed through the pelvic brim. Abdominal palpation of the head

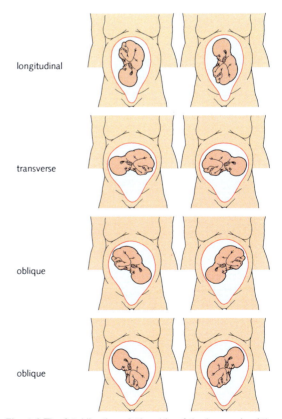

longitudinal

transverse

oblique

oblique

Fig. 1.6 The fetal lie; the relationship of the long axis of the fetus to the long axis of the uterus.

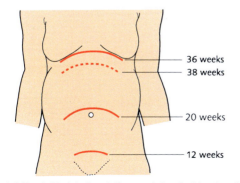

36 weeks
38 weeks

20 weeks

12 weeks

Fig. 1.5 Fundal height in relation to abdominal landmarks.

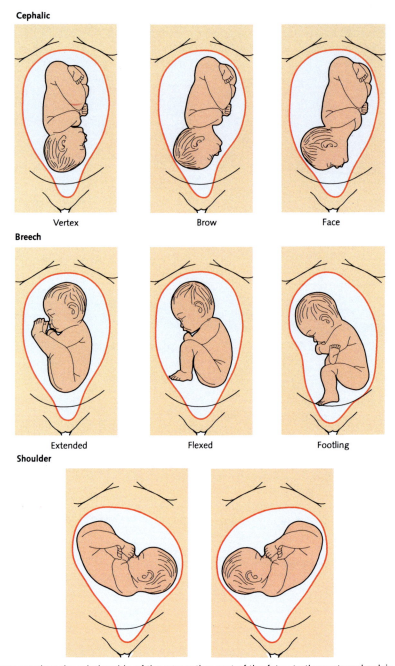

Cephalic

Vertex   Brow   Face

Breech

Extended   Flexed   Footling

Shoulder

Fig. 1.7 The fetal presentation; the relationship of the presenting part of the fetus to the maternal pelvis.

is assessed in fifths and is measured by palpating the angle between the head and the symphysis pubis (Fig. 1.8). When three or more fifths of the head are palpable abdominally the head is not engaged because the widest diameter of the head has not entered the pelvic brim. When two or fewer fifths of the head are palpable the head is clinically engaged. This should equate to the station found on vaginal examination.

The position of the presenting part is defined as the relationship of the denominator of the presenting part to the maternal pelvis. The denominator changes according to the presenting part: the occiput in a cephalic presentation, the mentum (chin) in a face presentation and the sacrum in a breech presentation. For example, if the fetal presentation is directly face downwards, the position is occiput anterior (direct occiput anterior). It is possible to assess position on abdominal palpation by determining the position of the fetal back (see Fig. 1.9), but this requires experience and practice (see Table 1.1). The position of the presenting part can be assessed more accurately by vaginal examination.

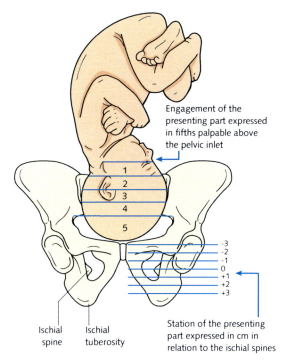

Engagement of the presenting part expressed in fifths palpable above the pelvic inlet

Ischial spine   Ischial tuberosity

Station of the presenting part expressed in cm in relation to the ischial spines

Fig. 1.8 Engagement of the fetal head.

Auscultation

In an obstetric patient the fetal heart should be auscultated using a Pinard or a Sonicaid. After 28 weeks it is appropriate for cardiotocography monitoring to be used to monitor both the fetal heart and contractions of the uterus.

ETHICS

It is crucial that before any intimate examination is performed informed consent is taken from the woman and a chaperone is advised. Routine presence of a chaperone is advised whether a male or female clinician.

Obstetric pelvic examination

Obstetric pelvic examination is not routinely performed at appointments, but indications for doing so include assessment in labour, assessment of membrane rupture and per vaginal bleeding, for example. The examination should include:

- external inspection of the vulva
- internal inspection of the vagina and cervix
- vaginal examination if indicated

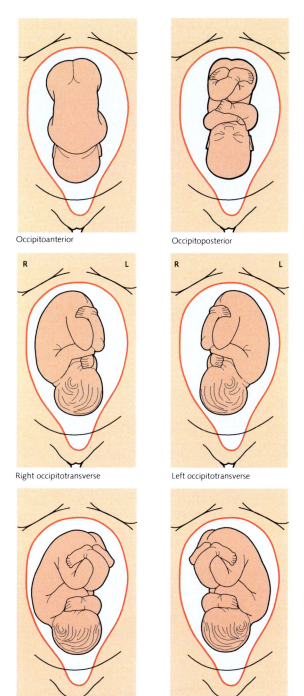

Occipitoanterior   Occipitoposterior

Right occipitotransverse   Left occipitotransverse

Right occipitoposterior   Left occipitoposterior

Fig. 1.9 The fetal position.

External examination

The blood flow through the vulva and vagina increases dramatically in pregnancy. The vulva might look swollen and oedematous secondary to engorgement. The presence of vulval varicosities should be noted. Look for presence of vaginal discharge, leaking amniotic fluid or any bleeding.

Table 1.1 Situations where fetal parts may be difficult to palpate

Types of reason	Description
Maternal reasons	Maternal obesity Muscular anterior abdominal wall
Uterine reasons	Anterior uterine wall fibroids Uterine contraction/Braxton Hicks contraction
Fetoplacental reasons	Anterior placenta Increased liquor volume

In certain ethnic groups, it may be appropriate to assess the vaginal introitus for signs of female genital mutilation.

Internal inspection of the vagina and cervix

Examination of the vagina and cervix with a sterile Cusco's speculum should be performed using an aseptic technique. Increased vaginal and cervical secretions are normal in pregnancy. Inspection of the cervix might reveal amniotic fluid draining through the cervical os. Digital examination in the presence of ruptured membranes is likely to increase the risk of ascending infection and is, therefore, usually avoided unless there are regular uterine contractions. Exclusion of cervical pathology is important in the presence of bleeding, such as a cervical polyp or ectropion.

Vaginal examination

This should be performed under aseptic conditions in the presence of intact membranes. Once the cervix has been identified, the following characteristics should be determined:

- dilatation
- length
- position of cervix
- consistency
- station of presenting part
- position of presenting part

Cervical dilatation is assessed in centimetres using the examining fingers. One finger-breadth is roughly 1–1.5 cm. Full dilatation of the cervix is equivalent to 10-cm dilatation. When not in established labour, the normal length of the

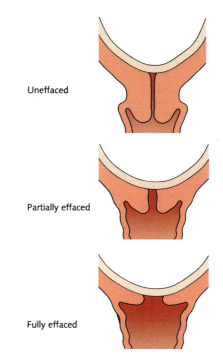

Uneffaced

Partially effaced

Fully effaced

Fig. 1.10 Effacement of the cervix.

cervix is about 3 cm. Shortening occurs as the cervix effaces, becoming part of the lower segment of the uterus, in the presence of regular uterine contractions (Fig. 1.10). Softening of the cervix occurs as pregnancy progresses, aiding cervical effacement and dilatation. The consistency of the cervix can be described as firm, mid-consistency or soft. The position describes where the cervix is situated in the anteroposterior plane of the pelvis. As the cervix becomes effaced and dilated, it tends to become more anterior in position.

The 'station' of the presenting part is determined by how much the presenting part has descended into the pelvis. The station is defined as the number of centimetres above or below a fixed point in the maternal pelvis, the ischial spines. This should equate to the engagement found on abdominal palpation (see Fig. 1.8).

Using the aforementioned characteristics, Bishop devised a scoring system (the Bishop score) to evaluate the 'ripeness' or favourability of the cervix (Table 1.2). This

Table 1.2 The Bishop score system

Cervical characteristic	Score			
	0	1	2	3
Dilatation (cm)	0	1–2	3–4	>4
Length (cm)	3	2	1	<1
Station (cm)	3	2	1 or 0	+1 or +2
Consistency	Firm	Medium	Soft	
Position	Posterior	Mid	Anterior	

system is used as an objective tool when inducing labour to assess the cervix. The higher the score, the more favourable the cervix and the more likely that induction of labour will be successful.

Defining the position of the presenting part

With a cephalic presentation, the anterior and posterior fontanelles and the sagittal sutures should be identified. The posterior fontanelle is Y shaped and is formed when the three sutures between the occipital and parietal bones meet. The anterior fontanelle is larger, diamond-shaped and formed by the four sutures between the meeting of the parietal and temporal bones (Fig. 1.11). The position of the presenting part can be defined as shown in Fig. 1.12. The presence of caput and moulding should also be assessed. Caput is the subcutaneous swelling on the fetal scalp that can be felt during labour and this increases if the labour is prolonged with failure of the cervix to dilate. 'Moulding' is the term used to describe the overlapping of the skull bones that occurs as labour progresses.

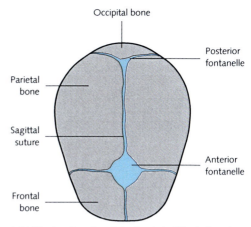
Fig. 1.11 The landmarks of the fetal skull including the anterior and posterior fontanelles.

GYNAECOLOGY EXAMINATION

Similar to obstetric examination, the general gynaecological examination follows the systemic review by:

- observation
- inspection
- palpation
- vaginal and bimanual examination

Observation and inspection

- Abdominal distention
- Abdominal mass
- Surgical scars

Observations and inspections follow the same technique as above for obstetric examination.

During inspection an abdominal mass may suggest a gravid uterus, but other causes should be considered including a pelvic mass, ascites or hernia.

Palpation

Before palpating the abdomen always enquire about areas of tenderness and palpate these areas last.

Using the palm of the hand, gently palpate the four quadrants of the abdomen for areas of tenderness, and for evaluating whether this is generalized or focussed. Assess whether the tenderness is deep or superficial and if you are eliciting any guarding or signs of peritonism.

Palpate for any abdominal mass and if found asses for:

- size
- shape
- position
- mobility
- consistency
- tenderness

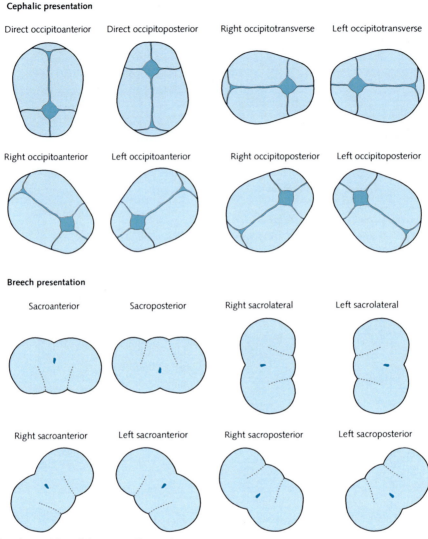

Cephalic presentation

Direct occipitoanterior   Direct occipitoposterior   Right occipitotransverse   Left occipitotransverse

Right occipitoanterior   Left occipitoanterior   Right occipitoposterior   Left occipitoposterior

Breech presentation

Sacroanterior   Sacroposterior   Right sacrolateral   Left sacrolateral

Right sacroanterior   Left sacroanterior   Right sacroposterior   Left sacroposterior

Fig. 1.12 Defining the position of the presenting part.

For example, fibroids can be palpated during an abdominopelvic examination, which classically appear as an enlarged, firm and irregular pelvic mass that is mobile and usually nontender.

You should ascertain whether the mass is arising from the pelvis. If you cannot palpate the lower aspect of the mass, it is probably arising from the pelvis. Percussion can help outline the borders of a mass in an obese patient. The size of a pelvic mass can be described similar to a pregnant abdomen (e.g., '20-week size' is equivalent to umbilical level).

Gynaecological pelvic examination

- External inspection of the vulva.
- Internal inspection of the vagina and cervix via a speculum.
- Bimanual examination of the pelvis.

The most common position for carrying out a pelvic examination is the dorsal position with the woman lying on her back with her knees flexed. Make sure that the patient is as comfortable as possible and only exposed appropriately. If the patient is a virgo intacta, external inspection only may be appropriate.

External examination of the vulva

Examine the anatomy of the vulva for inflammation, ulceration, swellings and lesions, atrophic changes and tissue discolouration. Parting the labia with the left hand, inspect the clitoris and urethral orifice (see Fig. 1.3). The presence of abnormal discharge on the vulva should be noted. A deficient or scarred perineum is a clue to previous trauma due to vaginal delivery. Vaginal or uterine prolapse through the introitus is assessed with and without the patient bearing down and stress incontinence might be demonstrated when the patient coughs.

Internal inspection of the vagina and cervix

To inspect the vagina and cervix, a speculum is used – either the Cusco's speculum (bivalve) or the Sims speculum (Fig. 1.13) with adequate gel for lubrication. Patients should be advised prior to assessment that speculum examination may be uncomfortable.

The Cusco's speculum is used with the patient in the dorsal position and consists of two blades hinged open at the vaginal introitus. When the blades are opened, the anterior and posterior walls of the vagina are separated allowing the vaginal fornices and cervix to be visualized.

The Sims speculum is used to inspect the anterior and posterior walls of the vagina and is an excellent tool for assessing uterovaginal prolapse. With the patient in the left lateral position the Sims blade is inserted into the vagina and used to retract either the anterior or the posterior walls. Uterovaginal prolapse can then be assessed with the patient bearing down. The vaginal tissue should be examined along with the cervix. Examine for any abnormalities of the vaginal tissue such as atrophy, inflammation or lesions. Ensure the cervix appears normal with no visible growths, ulcers or polyps.

Bimanual examination

A bimanual examination is performed to further elicit any pelvic masses or tenderness and asses the uterus.

It is usual to perform an internal examination using the lubricated index and middle fingers of the right hand. In nulliparous and postmenopausal women it might be necessary to use only the index finger. Palpation of the vaginal walls is important to exclude scarring, cysts and tumours that can easily be missed on inspection. The vaginal fornices should be examined for scarring, thickening and swellings that will suggest pelvic pathology. The size, shape, position,

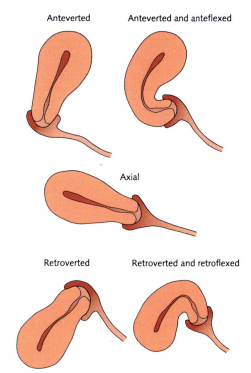

Anteverted   Anteverted and anteflexed

Axial

Retroverted   Retroverted and retroflexed

Fig. 1.14 Positions of the uterus.

consistency, angle and mobility of the cervix should be assessed. Moving the cervix from side to side might elicit cervical motion tenderness and elevating the cervix anteriorly, thereby stretching the uterosacral ligaments, might cause pain in the presence of endometriosis.

The fingers of the right hand are then used to elevate or steady the uterus while the left hand palpates abdominally. An anteverted uterus is usually palpable between the two hands. A retroverted uterus is usually felt as a swelling in the posterior fornix. The different combinations of version and flexion of the uterus are shown in Fig. 1.14. The size, position, consistency, outline and mobility of the uterus should all be noted. To examine the adnexa, the fingers of the right hand should be positioned in one of the lateral fornices and the adnexal region palpated between the two hands. Normal premenopausal ovaries are not always palpable depending on the size of the patient. Fallopian tubes and postmenopausal ovaries should not be palpable. If an adnexal mass is discovered, then its size, shape, consistency, mobility and whether it is fixed to the uterus or not should all be noted. The presence and degree of tenderness should be noted.

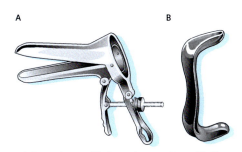

A   B

Fig. 1.13 Speculums: (A) Cusco's speculum; (B) Sims vaginal speculum.

● Chapter Summary

Knowledge of basic pelvic anatomy and examination techniques is essential in obstetrics and gynaecology to identify, diagnose and manage both normal and pathological presentations.

Taking a history is one of the first skills learnt in medical training. The history plays a vital role, often giving pointers to a diagnosis that is not always evident from examination and investigation of the patient alone. An obstetric and gynaecology history differs from the general medical clerking (Figs 2.1 and 2.2), so you will have to adapt your usual routine to incorporate the extra details required. Many women are embarrassed by having to discuss their personal problems, especially with someone who is often younger than they are, so it is important to overcome this by developing a confident, but sensitive manner. Always introduce and present yourself in an acceptable manner, be courteous and friendly without being overfamiliar and always pay attention. Remember to ask who has accompanied the patient – do not assume it is her partner – and consider whether she may want to answer personal questions in front of a family member.

It is therefore vital to ask the patient what she sees as her primary complaint and document this – preferably in her own words. If there are multiple symptoms, document each one in order of severity.

During the examination, investigations and treatment, never lose track of the presenting complaint, otherwise management plans may not always be appropriate. For example, it would not be helpful to suggest a Mirena coil for treatment of menorrhagia to a woman whose main concern is trying for a pregnancy. Conversely, the presenting complaint might be a cover for a different problem that the patient has difficulty discussing. For example, the patient may complain about vaginal discharge, although her main concern is pain during intercourse. Always ask if there is anything else bothering the patient that she wishes to discuss.

THE PATIENT'S DETAILS

It is surprising how often the patient's details are omitted from a history. They are vital for information governance reasons. Always record the following:

1. name, date of birth, age and address (sticky labels with this information are usually available)
2. marital status, ethnic group and occupation
3. the date, time and place of the consultation
4. source of referral (e.g., general practitioner referral, self-referral to accident and emergency or labour ward)

HINTS AND TIPS

It is useful to get into the habit of writing certain details in the top right-hand corner of the clerking sheet, so they are not omitted, for example:

- Age
- Parity
- Date of last menstrual period
- Date of last smear

PRESENTING COMPLAINT

The presenting complaint may be documented in the referral letter or the casualty card, but this does not always correlate with what the patient perceives as the main problem.

HISTORY OF PRESENTING COMPLAINT

Details of the history of the presenting complaint should be ascertained:

- **How long has the complaint been present?** For example, a woman might complain that she has always had heavy periods, but they have only been a problem for the last 2 years.
- **Was the onset of symptoms sudden or gradual?** For example, severe hirsutism of rapid onset is more likely to be due to an androgen-producing tumour.
- **Was the onset associated with a previous obstetric or gynaecological event?** For example, stress incontinence and childbirth.
- **Are there any relieving or exacerbating factors?** For example, symptoms of prolapse are often worse on standing and better on lying down.
- **Are there any associated symptoms?** For example, the painful periods of endometriosis are sometimes associated with deep dyspareunia (deep pelvic pain with intercourse).

If pain is the presenting complaint, then the following characteristics should be noted:

- **Site**: Is the pain pelvic or abdominal? For example, ovarian pain can be felt quite high in the abdomen.
- **Severity**: How severe is the pain and to what extent does it disrupt everyday life? For example, the cyclical pain of endometriosis might necessitate regular time off work.

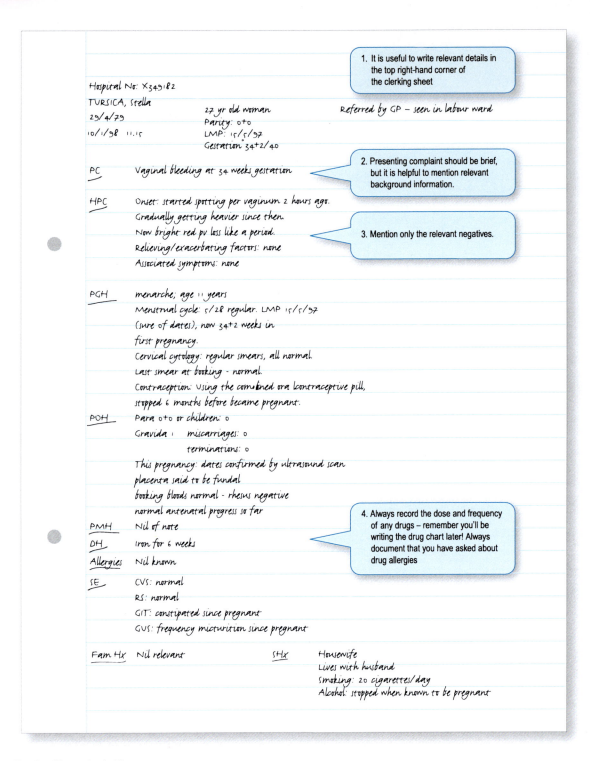

Fig. 2.1 Obstetric clerking.

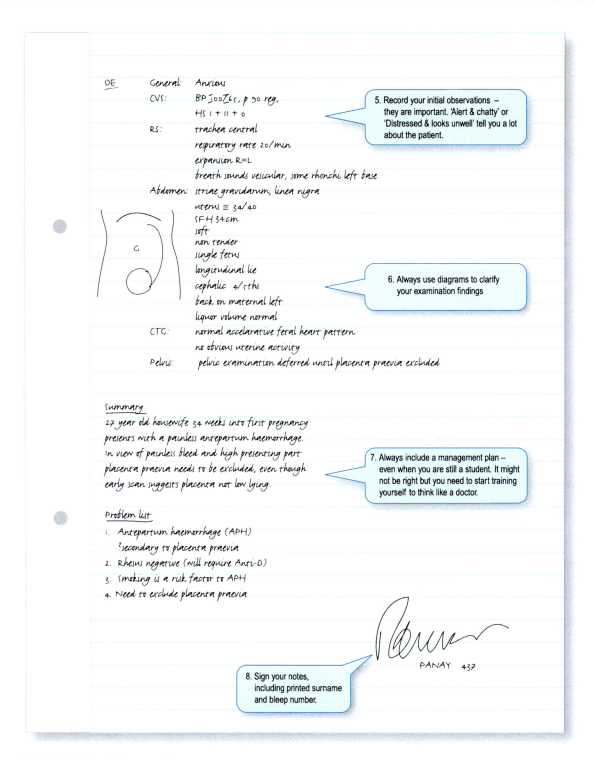

OE   General: Anxious
            CVS: BP 100/65, p 90 reg,
                        HS I + II + 0

> 5. Record your initial observations – they are important. 'Alert & chatty' or 'Distressed & looks unwell' tell you a lot about the patient.

            RS: trachea central
                        respiratory rate 20/min
                        expansion R=L
                        breath sounds vesicular, some rhonchi left base
            Abdomen: striae gravidarum, linea nigra
                        uterus ≡ 34/40
                        SFH 34cm
                        soft
                        non tender
                        single fetus
                        longitudinal lie
                        cephalic 4/5ths
                        back on maternal left
                        liquor volume normal

> 6. Always use diagrams to clarify your examination findings

            CTG: normal accelarative fetal heart pattern
                        no obvious uterine activity
            Pelvis: pelvic examination deferred until placenta praevia excluded

Summary

27 year old housewife 34 weeks into first pregnancy presents with a painless antepartum haemorrhage. In view of painless bleed and high presenting part placenta praevia needs to be excluded, even though early scan suggests placenta not low lying.

> 7. Always include a management plan – even when you are still a student. It might not be right but you need to start training yourself to think like a doctor.

Problem list

1. Antepartum haemorrhage (APH)
   ?secondary to placenta praevia
2. Rhesus negative (will require Anti-D)
3. Smoking is a risk factor to APH
4. Need to exclude placenta praevia

PANAY 437

> 8. Sign your notes, including printed surname and bleep number.

Fig. 2.1 Obstetric clerking, cont'd

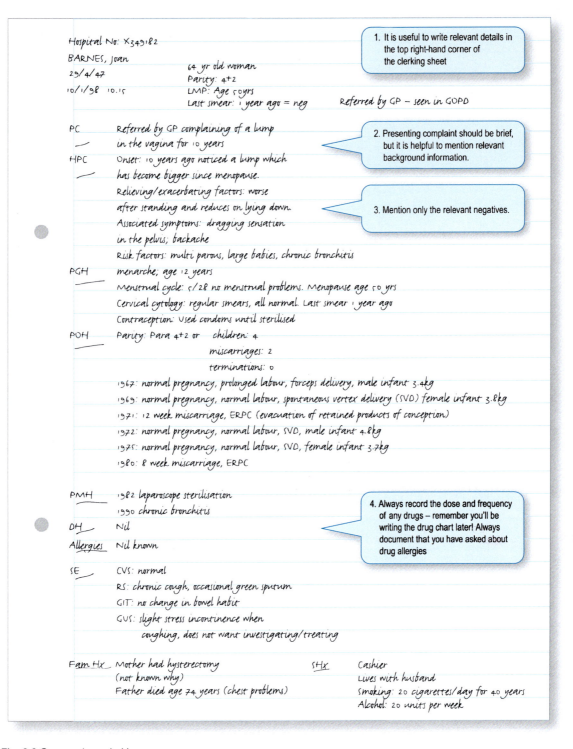

Hospital No: X349182

BARNES, Joan

29/4/47

10/1/98 10.15

64 yr old woman
Parity: 4+2
LMP: Age 50 yrs
Last smear: 1 year ago = neg   Referred by GP – seen in GOPD

1. It is useful to write relevant details in the top right-hand corner of the clerking sheet

PC   Referred by GP complaining of a lump
      in the vagina for 10 years

2. Presenting complaint should be brief, but it is helpful to mention relevant background information.

HPC   Onset: 10 years ago noticed a lump which
      has become bigger since menopause.
      Relieving/exacerbating factors: worse
      after standing and reduces on lying down.

3. Mention only the relevant negatives.

      Associated symptoms: dragging sensation
      in the pelvis; backache
      Risk factors: multi parous, large babies, chronic bronchitis

PGH   menarche; age 12 years
      Menstrual cycle: 5/28 no menstrual problems. Menopause age 50 yrs
      Cervical cytology: regular smears, all normal. Last smear 1 year ago
      Contraception: Used condoms until sterilised

POH   Parity: Para 4+2 or   children: 4
                            miscarriages: 2
                            terminations: 0
      1967: normal pregnancy, prolonged labour, forceps delivery, male infant 3.4kg
      1969: normal pregnancy, normal labour, spontaneous vertex delivery (SVD) female infant 3.8kg
      1971: 12 week miscarriage, ERPC (evacuation of retained products of conception)
      1972: normal pregnancy, normal labour, SVD, male infant 4.8kg
      1975: normal pregnancy, normal labour, SVD, female infant 3.7kg
      1980: 8 week miscarriage, ERPC

PMH   1982 laparoscope sterilisation
      1990 chronic bronchitis

4. Always record the dose and frequency of any drugs – remember you'll be writing the drug chart later! Always document that you have asked about drug allergies

DH   Nil

Allergies   Nil known

SE   CVS: normal
      RS: chronic cough, occasional green sputum
      GIT: no change in bowel habit
      GUS: slight stress incontinence when
           coughing, does not want investigating/treating

Fam Hx   Mother had hysterectomy   SHx   Cashier
         (not known why)   Lives with husband
         Father died age 74 years (chest problems)   Smoking: 20 cigarettes/day for 40 years
                                                Alcohol: 20 units per week

Fig. 2.2 Gynaecology clerking.

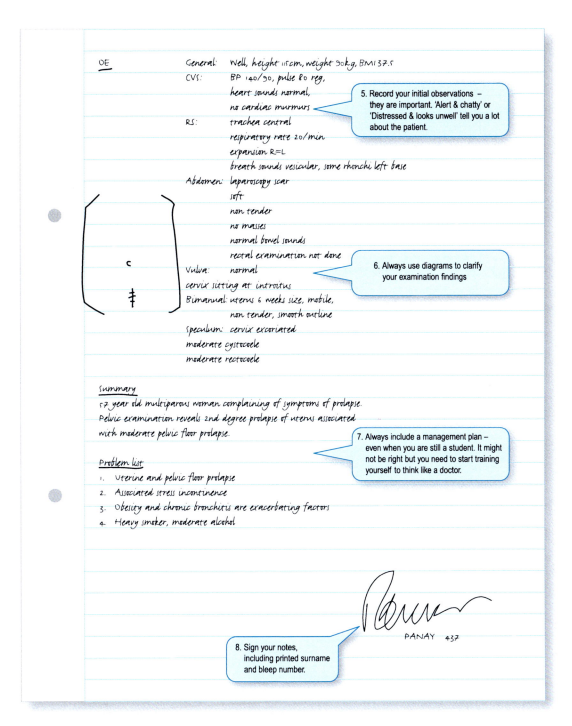

OE

General: Well, height 115cm, weight 90kg, BMI 37.5

CVS: BP 140/90, pulse 80 reg,
heart sounds normal,
no cardiac murmurs

> 5. Record your initial observations – they are important. 'Alert & chatty' or 'Distressed & looks unwell' tell you a lot about the patient.

RS: trachea central
respiratory rate 20/min
expansion R=L
breath sounds vesicular, some rhonchi left base

Abdomen: laparoscopy scar
soft
non tender
no masses
normal bowel sounds
rectal examination not done

> 6. Always use diagrams to clarify your examination findings

Vulva: normal
cervix sitting at introitus

Bimanual: uterus 6 weeks size, mobile,
non tender, smooth outline

Speculum: cervix excoriated
moderate cystocoele
moderate rectocoele

Summary

57 year old multiparous woman complaining of symptoms of prolapse. Pelvic examination reveals 2nd degree prolapse of uterus associated with moderate pelvic floor prolapse.

> 7. Always include a management plan – even when you are still a student. It might not be right but you need to start training yourself to think like a doctor.

Problem list

1. Uterine and pelvic floor prolapse
2. Associated stress incontinence
3. Obesity and chronic bronchitis are exacerbating factors
4. Heavy smoker, moderate alcohol

PANAY   437

> 8. Sign your notes, including printed surname and bleep number.

Fig. 2.2 Gynaecology clerking, cont'd

- **Onset**: Sudden or gradual? For example, the pain from a torted ovarian cyst is usually of very sudden onset.
- **Character**: Is the pain sharp, knife-like, dull, heavy, dragging, colicky, stretching or twisting? Many adjectives have been used to describe pain or discomfort of gynaecological origin. For example, women with uterine prolapse might describe a pulling or a dragging pain/sensation, dysmenorrhoea might be likened to labour pain.
- **Duration**: Is the pain constant or intermittent? What is the frequency if intermittent? The pain of a degenerating fibroid in pregnancy will be constant, whereas that of threatened premature labour will be intermittent and frequent.
- **Radiation**: Does the pain radiate? For example, endometriosis pain might radiate to the back or into the upper thighs.
- **Relieving/exacerbating features**: Does anything make the pain better or worse and this should include self-prescribed analgesia? For example, endometriosis symptoms are usually cyclical and associated with menstruation.
- **Associated symptoms:** For example, symptoms of peritonitis may be associated with nausea and vomiting, or advanced malignancy may be associated with weight loss.

HINTS AND TIPS

The acronym SOCRATES can be used for assessing pain:

Site
Onset
Character
Radiation
Associations
Time course
Exacerbating/relieving factors
Severity

GYNAECOLOGICAL HISTORY

Menstrual history

The following characteristics of menstruation and the menstrual cycle should be noted:

- Age at menarche.
- Last menstrual period = first day of last period.
- Menstrual cycle: usually denoted as 5/28, where the numerator is the length of the period in days and the denominator is the length of the cycle in days

from first day to first day. If period and cycle length are variable, the shortest and longest are noted (e.g., 3–10/14–56).
- Menstrual flow: whether light, normal or heavy. This is often very subjective, therefore if heavy, the presence of clots, flooding, night-time soiling and the number of sanitary pads used should be noted.
- Menstrual pain or dysmenorrhoea: is the pain mild, moderate or severe? Has it been present since menarche or is it of recent onset? Is the pain worse before (primary dysmenorrhoea) or during the period (secondary dysmenorrhoea)?
- Associated symptoms: for example, bowel or bladder dysfunction, nausea.
- Other bleeding: intermenstrual bleeding, postcoital bleeding, premenstrual or postmenstrual spotting.
- Age at menopause.

COMMUNICATION

A useful way to ask sensitive questions may be to consider a logical order: after menstrual cycle, ask about bleeding between periods, then bleeding after intercourse (postcoital bleeding) and then pain with intercourse (dyspareunia) either superficial (around the opening of the vagina) or deep.

Sexual activity and contraception

Has the patient ever been sexually active? Is the patient currently sexually active or in a relationship? Does the patient suffer from dyspareunia and if so is it superficial or deep? Is she or her partner using contraception and if so what? If she is on the pill or has a Mirena coil, was it prescribed for contraceptive purposes or menstrual disorder?

Cervical screening

Has the patient undergone regular cervical screening? When was the last smear taken and what was the result? Have there ever been abnormal smears? Has she had the vaccination for human papilloma virus?

Vaginal discharge

Is vaginal discharge present and if so, is it normal for the patient or abnormal? If abnormal, what is the colour and consistency, and is it irritant? Was the onset associated with a change in sexual partner? Is there a history of past sexually transmitted infections?

ETHICS

Particularly for women who come from countries in the Horn of Africa (e.g., Somalia, Eritrea, Ethiopia), either themselves or their families, a history should be elicited regarding female circumcision or female genital mutilation. This procedure usually occurs as a child in their country of origin, being illegal in the UK since 2003. It is defined as all procedures involving partial or total removal of the external female genitalia or other injury to the female genital organs, whether for cultural or other nontherapeutic reasons. As an adult, it can cause significant problems including dyspareunia, recurrent urinary tract infections, trauma and haemorrhage during childbirth, as well as psychological issues. Such a history must therefore be approached in a sensitive manner and then reported to the national register. If the patient is under the age of 18 years, her details must be referred to the police and to social services.

OBSTETRIC HISTORY

The parity and gravidity should be noted. Parity denotes the number of livebirths or stillbirths after 24 weeks gestation and gravidity the total number of pregnancies including the current one if pregnant (see Chapter 19). Use of the terms 'parity' and 'gravidity' can become very complicated, especially with a history of multiple pregnancies. After a previous multiple pregnancy the gravidity would count as 1 and if they were delivered after 24 weeks, then the parity would be 2. An alternative way of documenting previous pregnancies is to document the number of:

- C = children
- M = miscarriages
- T = terminations

Document the details of each pregnancy:

- The number of children with gestational age and birth weight. Note any complications of pregnancy, labour and the puerperium.
- The number of miscarriages, their gestation and complications if any.
- The number of terminations of pregnancy, their gestation, method, indication and complications if any.

MEDICAL HISTORY

This should include medical disorders such as hypertension or diabetes which may be relevant to suitability for surgery or because they are risk factors for complications in pregnancy. Surgical history should be documented as this may complicate any further planned operations. In the case of previous caesarean sections and pregnancies, there may be added risks in the current pregnancy such as placenta praevia (see Chapter 20). Psychiatric history is particularly important in obstetrics, for planning both antenatal and postnatal care, with the risk of postnatal depression (see Chapter 31).

DRUG HISTORY AND ALLERGIES

A careful drug history should be taken and should include hormonal contraception and hormone replacement therapy, which are often overlooked by the patient. Drugs are important for pregnancy (e.g., antiepileptics can be associated with fetal neural tube defects, or β-blockers with intrauterine growth restriction). Document any known or suspected allergies and the reaction that occurs.

SYSTEMS ENQUIRY

A brief systems enquiry should be made with particular reference to:

- general symptoms: weight gain or loss, loss of appetite
- gastrointestinal tract: change in bowel habit, especially with menstruation
- genitourinary system: urinary frequency, nocturia, dysuria, incontinence

FAMILY HISTORY

For gynaecology, enquire as to a family history of ovarian, uterine and breast disease. In obstetrics, diabetes, hypertension and pre-eclampsia may all have relevance to the current pregnancy. There may also be rare disorders that run in families; for example, autosomal recessive disorders are more common if a couple are related to each other.

SOCIAL HISTORY

Occupation, smoking habits and alcohol consumption should be noted. If gynaecological surgery is contemplated, what is the support network at home? Should social services be involved in planning the appropriate care for the new-born baby?

FURTHER READING

Royal College of Obstetricians and Gynaecologists (RCOG), May 2009. Female genital mutilation management: RCOG green top guideline no. 53. RCOG, London, UK.

COMMUNICATION

Clear documentation is very important in the patient notes as they form a legal document and can be called upon for medico-legal cases.

Chapter Summary

- Taking a thorough history is an important skill to learn.
- Keep the presenting complaint brief but include any relevant background information.
- In the gynaecology history remember to ask about cervical smears, sexual activity and contraception.
- In the obstetric history remember that gravidity refers to the total number of pregnancies and parity refers to the number of livebirths or stillbirths after 24 weeks' gestation.
- Present relevant negative points in the history.

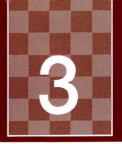

Common investigations

3

INTRODUCTION

A wide range of investigations are used for diagnosis and management in obstetrics and gynaecology. When considering investigations, always request the simplest first, working your way to the more invasive and complex investigations when necessary.

GYNAECOLOGY BEDSIDE TESTS

Urine

In patients presenting with abdominal pain, a urine dipstick is useful to identify a urinary tract infection or haematuria, and urine can be sent for microscopy and culture. A urinary pregnancy test should be performed in all women of child-bearing age with abdominal pain to identify pregnancy.

CLINICAL NOTES

Urine pregnancy tests use antibodies to detect human chorionic gonadotropin. It is a good detector of pregnancy as it rises rapidly and consistently in early pregnancy. Most current pregnancy test kits have a sensitivity of 10–25 mIU/mL and can reveal positive results as early as 3–4 days after implantation; by 7 days 98% will be positive.

Blood tests

Blood tests can provide a variety of information which, along with history and examination, can guide diagnosis and management. A full blood count can identify high inflammatory markers, suggestive of infection, and low haemoglobin due to an acute or chronic anaemia. Serum human chorionic gonadotropin levels over 25 mIU/mL can confirm pregnancy. When investigating menstrual complications hormone profiles can be performed, which can highlight conditions such as polycystic ovarian syndrome and anovulation. Tumour marker blood tests, such as Ca-125, can be performed if there is concern regarding malignancy but are not performed routinely as they can also be raised with benign gynaecological pathology.

Swabs

In patients with signs and symptoms of infection, for example, abnormal vaginal discharge or pyrexia, swabs should be taken for microbiology cultures. High vaginal swab should be performed to test for infections such as *Candida* infection, endocervical swabs to test for chlamydia and gonorrhoea. If the woman has had a recent operation, the wound is a potential source of infection and should be swabbed.

Smears

The National Screening in Cervical Cytology Programme recommends performing a smear in women between the ages of 25 and 49 years every 3 years, and every 5 years after that until the age of 64 years if smears are normal. The aim of the screening is to prevent cancer by detecting and treating abnormalities of the cervix (see Chapter 12). Using a Cusco's speculum the visible cervix is gentle swept through 360° five times with a cervical Cytobrush (Fig. 3.1). The sample is then placed into a medium and sent for liquid-based cytology. Smears must be taken prior to any other swabs or vaginal examination to avoid dislodging cells on the surface of the cervix.

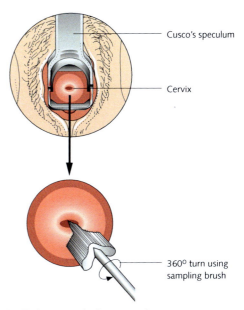

Cusco's speculum

Cervix

360° turn using sampling brush

Fig. 3.1 Taking a cervical smear using a Cytobrushcytobrush. The cervix must be visualized and a 360° sweep must be performed.[use ednfig]

GYNAECOLOGY PROCEDURES

Imaging

Imaging techniques are used widely in both obstetrics and gynaecology. Results of imaging tests should be interpreted carefully in the light of the history and clinical findings.

Ultrasound examination is the most common investigation in obstetrics and gynaecology and is a safe and reliable method of examining the pelvis. Ultrasound waves passing through the pelvis are reflected in varying degrees depending on the density of the tissues. For instance, bone is very echogenic and reflective, appearing white on the monitor, whereas fluid is less echogenic and appears dark on the monitor.

Transvaginal scanning provides the clearest images of the pelvis, but is invasive and is not appropriate in children, and may be declined in women who have not had sexual intercourse. It requires an empty bladder for clear examination of pelvic organs. Transabdominal scan is a noninvasive alternative but views can be limited, for example, in obese patients. The position and size of the uterus can be assessed, and the myometrium for pathology such as adenomyosis and fibroids. The midline echo corresponds to the endometrial cavity and can be assessed for endometrial thickness and hyperplasia, endometrial polyps and submucosal fibroids. Intrauterine contraceptive devices can also be visualized. The size and position of the ovaries can be assessed. Ovarian cysts, tumours and polycystic ovaries (see Chapter 15) can be identified, and follicular tracking is possible in women trying to conceive. Ovarian tumours can be identified by ultrasound and there are some characteristics of benign and malignant tumours that can be noted (Table 3.1), but differentiation between benign and malignant tumours cannot be made with certainty. The fallopian tubes are not normally visible by ultrasound. However, if they are blocked and distended with fluid (hydrosalpinx or tubo-ovarian abscess), they will appear as cystic structures.

Use of X-rays is generally minimized due to radiation exposure. Hysterosalpingography can be used to assess uterine cavity and patency of the fallopian tubes in investigations of subfertility (see Chapter 16). Radio-opaque dye is introduced via the cervix through the uterus and

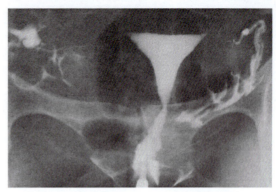

Fig. 3.2 Hysterosalpingography showing patent fallopian tubes with dye 'fill and spill'. In patients who have had previous surgery, a laparoscopy and dye test are recommended instead.

an X-ray is taken to look for passage of the dye. Blockage can be caused by internal or external tubal factors or tubal spasm (Fig. 3.2). This is not a suitable investigation if there is clinical evidence of current pelvic infection, and antibiotic prophylaxis is given routinely. An alternative is hysterosalpingo-contrast-ultrasonography performed using Doppler ultrasound to monitor the passage of fluid via the cervix through the uterus and tubes.

Magnetic resonance imaging and computed tomography scanning are used but not in routine investigations.

CLINICAL NOTES

In patients with a high chance of tubal blockage, such as those with a history of pelvic inflammatory disease or tubal surgery, an hysterosalpingography should not be performed. Ideally tubal potency can be assessed with a laparoscopy and dye test (see discussion in text) and then any pelvic pathology can be identified and treated at the same time.

Hysteroscopy

A hysteroscopy is an investigation using an endoscope (fine camera) inserted through the cervix to inspect the uterine cavity (Fig. 3.3). A distension medium such as normal saline or inert media such as glycine may be used to distend the uterine cavity. It is seen as the gold standard investigation of abnormal uterine bleeding and can identify endometrial polyps, fibroids and endometrial carcinoma. During operative hysteroscopy procedures such as polypectomy, endometrial biopsy and transcervical resection of fibroids can be performed. Hysteroscopy can be performed under general anaesthetic or as an outpatient procedure. Complications of the procedure include uterine perforation, and therefore potential damage to surrounding bowel, bladder and ureters.

Table 3.1 Ultrasound features to distinguish benign and malignant tumours. Borderline tumours cannot be identified with certainty using ultrasound alone

	Benign	Malignant
Size (cm)	<5	>5
Laterality	Unilateral	Bilateral
Cyst walls	Thin	Thick
Septa	Absent	Thick, incomplete
Solid areas	Absent	Present
Ascites	Absent	Present

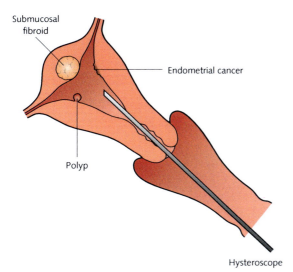

Fig. 3.3 A hysteroscope is used to visualize the endocervix and uterine cavity. This can identify polyps, fibroids or malignancy. Risks include uterine perforation, infection and bleeding.

Cystoscopy

A cystoscopy, similarly to a hysteroscopy, is an investigation using an endoscope (fine camera) inserted through the urethra into the bladder. It can identify bladder polyps or diverticulum, chronic inflammation and filling abnormalities. It can be performed under general anaesthetic or as an outpatient procedure.

Laparoscopy

Laparoscopy is the mainstay of investigating pelvic pain. It is used to diagnose pelvic disease such as endometriosis and adhesions, and to treat conditions such as ovarian cysts. It is the best method to image pelvic and other intraabdominal organs.

Laparoscopy is performed under general anaesthetic. Having emptied the bladder, and instrumented the uterus if manipulation is required, a Veress needle is inserted into the lower abdomen through an umbilical incision. After checking the Veress needle is correctly placed, carbon dioxide is pumped into the peritoneal cavity to produce a pneuma-peritoneum of 20 mmHg, to allow insertion of a laparoscopy port. The laparoscope can then be passed through the port into the pelvis and the organs can be visualized. Additional ports can be inserted using the camera to visualize entry, and laparoscopic instruments can be used to manipulate the organs (Fig. 3.4).

At the time of laparoscopy, a tubal dye test can be performed. Methylene blue dye is inserted via the cervical canal, and patent fallopian tubes will allow free spill of blue dye into the pelvis, which can be seen via the laparoscope.

Complications of laparoscopy include bowel, bladder, ureteric and vascular injury (<1%). If laparoscopy is not possible, there are complications, or a large specimen needs to be removed (such as dermoid cyst), the laparoscopic procedure may need to be extended and a laparotomy performed.

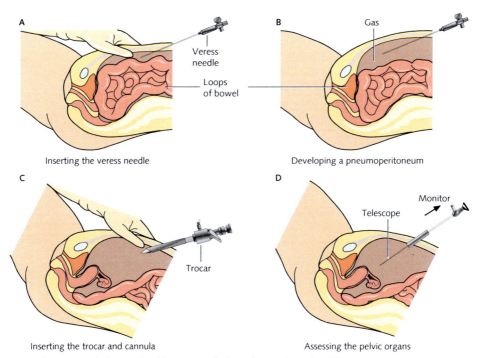

Fig. 3.4 Laparoscopic entry technique using Veress needle insertion and gas insufflation.

● Chapter Summary

- It is important to use investigations in conjunction with a thorough history and examination to aid diagnosis.
- Investigations should be planned to aid the diagnosis and avoid overinvestigation or inappropriately used invasive tests.
- Hysteroscopy, cystoscopy and laparoscopy can all be used as both diagnostic and operative procedures.

Abnormal uterine bleeding

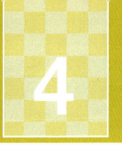

4

BACKGROUND

Abnormal uterine bleeding is a common problem experienced by women and a common presentation to primary and secondary care. For normal menstruation to occur, the following are necessary:

- hypothalamic function
- pituitary function
- ovarian function
- endometrial function
- patent cervix and vagina

Abnormal uterine bleeding can be caused by malfunction or disease at any of these levels.

Causes can be physiological or pathological and, as long as serious pathology is excluded, might not require treatment.

Since 2010, the International Federation of Gynaecology and Obstetrics introduced a classification system to identify possible causes of abnormal uterine bleeding for premenopausal women. The acronym PALM-COEIN stands for:

- *p*olyps
- *a*denomyosis
- *l*eiomyoma (fibroids)
- *m*alignancy and hyperplasia
- *c*oagulopathy
- *o*vulatory cause
- *e*ndometrial causes
- *i*atrogenic
- *n*ot classified

MENORRHAGIA

Definition

Menorrhagia [heavy menstrual bleeding (HMB)] is defined as excessive menstrual loss over several consecutive cycles, which interferes with physical, social and emotional quality of life. It can occur alone or in combination with other symptoms.

Mean menstrual blood loss is typically 30–40 mL per period, but clinical menorrhagia is defined as a total menstrual blood loss of >80 mL in each menstruation. As diagnosis is usually based on a woman's own subjective evaluation, only about half of women complaining of heavy periods actually have menorrhagia >80 mL.

Two-thirds of women with genuine menorrhagia will have iron-deficiency anaemia.

Associated conditions, such as fibroids, may be associated with menorrhagia (see Chapter 5), but it can exist in the absence of pathology, known as 'dysfunctional uterine bleeding (DUB)'.

Prevalence

HMB is common, affecting up to a quarter of the female population in Western Europe. It is estimated that 1.5 million women consult primary care each year with HMB in England and Wales, and menstrual disorders account for about 20% of all referrals to specialist gynaecology services.

Early menarche, late menopause, reduction in family size with concurrent reduction in periods of lactational amenorrhoea have all contributed to an almost tenfold increase in the number of periods that women experience during their reproductive life. This has meant that excessive menstrual bleeding has become one of the most common causes of concern for health in women.

Aetiology

The causation of HMB and mode of action are varied (Table 4.1):

- local pathology
- systemic conditions
- iatrogenic
- DUB

Table 4.1 Causes of menorrhagia

Classification	Specific cause of menorrhagia
Systemic disorders	Thyroid disease Clotting disorders
Local causes	Fibroids Endometrial polyps Endometrial carcinoma Endometriosis/adenomyosis Pelvic inflammatory disease Dysfunctional uterine bleeding
Iatrogenic causes	Intrauterine contraceptive devices Oral anticoagulants

Local pathology

Any pathology that enlarges the uterine cavity or is associated with increased endometrial tissue, will increase the surface area of the menstruating endometrium, and therefore can cause HMB. Examples include fibroids, endometrial polyps, endometriosis and adenomyosis. Fibroids may also produce prostaglandins, which have been implicated in the aetiology of menorrhagia (Chapter 5).

Premalignant and malignant endometrium may present with menorrhagia and must always be excluded.

Menstrual blood loss in the presence of pelvic pathology, such as pelvic inflammatory disease (see Chapter 9), is variable and often in the normal range. Menorrhagia is therefore associated with, but not necessarily caused by, these conditions.

Systemic conditions

Systemic disease is a rare cause of HMB and more common in adolescents. Coagulation disorders are found in up to one-third of young women admitted to hospital with profound menorrhagia and up to 90% of women with bleeding disorders have menorrhagia.

Hypothyroidism can cause menorrhagia, thought to be as a consequence of anovulatory dysfunctional bleeding, but is a rare cause of HMB. Untreated hypothyroidism and hyperthyroidism in most women will cause amenorrhoea.

Iatrogenic causes

The presence of an intrauterine contraceptive device may increase menstrual blood loss and is the most common iatrogenic cause of menorrhagia. Menorrhagia and iron-deficiency anaemia are up to five times more common in intrauterine contraceptive device users than with other forms of contraception.

Roughly one-half of women taking oral anticoagulants have objective evidence of menorrhagia.

Dysfunctional uterine bleeding

DUB is the most common cause of menorrhagia and is the term used when there are no apparent local or systemic causes for menorrhagia. It is therefore a diagnosis made by exclusion. Altered endometrial prostaglandin metabolism seems to have an important role in the aetiology of DUB. This is supported by the fact that prostaglandin inhibitors decrease menstrual blood loss in women with DUB.

DIAGNOSIS

Diagnosis of menorrhagia tends to be based on women's own subjective evaluation, as objective measurement is practically difficult to perform and pictorial blood loss assessment charts are not commonly used. However, a focused history highlighting the features below is strongly supportive of an HMB diagnosis:

- passing large clots
- need for double sanitary protection (towels and tampons)
- need for frequent changes of towels and tampons (every 2 hours or less)
- flooding through clothes or to bedding

History

A full medical and gynaecological history should be taken. The length and frequency of menstruation should be noted, together with any intermenstrual bleeding (IMB) and postcoital bleeding (PCB). Symptoms of iron-deficiency anaemia might be present, including lethargy and breathlessness.

HISTORY

What was the date of your last menstrual period? How long is your menstrual cycle? How many days are your periods? How many pads or tampons do you use per day? Do you suffer from overflow bleeding or flooding? Quantifying the extent of menorrhagia is important to understand the symptoms and what management may be appropriate. The date and result of the last cervical smear test should be checked, as well as a history of irregular or postcoital bleeding, which might be associated with malignancy.

Do you suffer with period pain? At what point during your cycle is the pain worst? Menstrual pain, or dysmenorrhoea, is often associated with menorrhagia and usually occurs when the flow is heaviest. Premenstrual pain can indicate endometriosis (see Chapter 6). Fever, pelvic pain, dyspareunia and vaginal discharge are common symptoms of pelvic inflammatory disease (see Chapter 9).

Are you currently using contraception? A contraceptive history is important. Normal periods experienced after stopping the combined oral contraceptive pill (COCP) may appear heavier than the withdrawal bleeds associated with the COCP. Symptoms of heavy or painful periods dating from the insertion of an intrauterine contraceptive device would suggest that it is the cause.

The history should include a thorough medical and surgical history. Symptoms of thyroid disease or clotting disorders can indicate a systemic cause of menorrhagia. Inquire about how menorrhagia affects activities of daily living, for example, going to school or taking time off work.

Examination

General examination aims to identify signs of systemic conditions such as iron-deficiency anaemia or thyroid disorders. This includes clubbing, swelling or soreness of the tongue; cracks in the sides of the mouth, or with thyroid disease dry skin and hair loss.

Is there abdominal distension? Determine the size, tenderness, mobility and nodularity of the mass. Fibroids can be palpated during an abdominopelvic examination, classically as an enlarged, firm and irregular pelvic mass. Abdominal examination might also reveal ascites, suggestive of malignancy.

Speculum examination may reveal vaginal discharge and cervical pathology, including cervicitis or frank malignancy. Occasionally, endometrial polyps or pedunculated fibroids will be seen prolapsing through the cervical os.

Vulval lesions should be evident on vaginal examination. A bimanual vaginal examination should be performed and the adnexa should be examined. It may reveal an enlarged uterus due to fibroids, pelvic tenderness and nodules associated with endometriosis or pelvic inflammatory disease and the presence of any adnexal masses. Postmenopausal ovaries should not be palpable on bimanual examination.

Investigations are aimed at excluding the systemic and local causes of menorrhagia (Fig. 4.1).

Blood tests

A full blood count to asses for anaemia should be performed in all cases. Thyroid function and clotting studies should only be performed if clinically suspected from history and examination. Testing for coagulation disorders such as von Willebrand disease should only be performed if women have had HMB since menarche or family/personal history suggesting a clotting disorder.

Pelvic ultrasound

A pelvic ultrasound will identify uterine enlargement caused by fibroids and any adnexal masses. Endometrial polyps or submucous fibroids may be seen or may be suspected if the endometrial thickness (ET) is excessive for the time of the menstrual cycle.

Specialist tests

A cervical smear should also be performed when this is due, or sooner if there is a history of IMB or PCB.

An endometrial biopsy should be performed on all women aged over 45 years and in women under 45 years if there are risk factors in the history such as persistent IMB or suspicious findings on ultrasound scan (see Chapter 12) to rule out endometrial hyperplasia or carcinoma. This can be performed either in the outpatient clinic or under general anaesthesia. A pipelle biopsy has high levels of patient acceptability, lower complication rates and does not require inpatient admission or general anaesthesia. However, it may miss benign and malignant endometrial pathology and must therefore be considered inadequate for the further investigation of menorrhagia that has persisted despite medical therapy.

Diagnostic hysteroscopy is the most effective way of excluding intrauterine pathology. This can be performed in the outpatient setting without analgesia and will identify endometrial polyps, submucous fibroids, endometritis and most endometrial carcinomas. It can be performed under a general anaesthetic to remove pathology such as polyps, and endometrial biopsy can be taken.

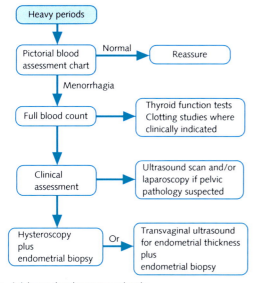

Fig. 4.1 Investigating menorrhagia.

Treatment of HMB aims to reduce menstrual blood loss, reduce iron-deficiency anaemia and improve the quality of life of the women. It is important to primarily use appropriate medical therapy for heavy periods without focal pathology and to avoid unnecessary surgical intervention.

Treatment of menorrhagia should be tailored to the patient's needs, fertility wishes and also to the findings of investigations. Practically, this includes:

- correcting iron-deficiency anaemia
- treating systemic disorders
- treating focal pathology
- control of menorrhagia by medical treatment
- surgical treatment if symptoms not managed medically

Treatment of menorrhagia secondary to fibroids is considered in Chapter 5.

Medical

The main forms of conservative or medical treatment for menorrhagia are:

- watchful waiting
- complementary and alternative treatments
- antifibrinolytics
- hormonal preparations

The efficacy of medical treatment varies from one individual to another. The reduction of mean menstrual blood loss for different medical therapies is shown in Table 4.2.

An important consideration with medical treatments is that they are not always suitable for long-term use, and some are associated with adverse side-effects.

Antifibrinolytics and haemostatics

Tranexamic acid is an antifibrinolytic agent that inhibits the activation of plasminogen to plasmin. It reduces the excessive fibrinolytic activity found in the endometrium of menorrhagic women. It is widely used for the treatment of heavy periods as it is effective for a substantial proportion of women. Its most important side-effect is the risk of thrombosis, although uncommon. In women with menorrhagia, who have no history or family history of thrombosis, it should be regarded as the first line of medical treatment.

Prostaglandin inhibitors

Several nonsteroidal antiinflammatory drugs (NSAIDs), including ibuprofen, aspirin, indomethacin and mefenamic acid, inhibit the cyclooxygenase enzyme system, which controls the production of cyclic endoperoxides from arachidonic acid. NSAIDs improve menstrual blood loss, dysmenorrhoea and menstrual headaches. NSAIDS are taken during menstruation, so side-effects such as indigestion and diarrhoea are usually better tolerated than with drugs that are taken throughout the menstrual cycle.

CLINICAL NOTES

Ongoing use of nonsteroidal antiinflammatory drugs or tranexamic acid is recommended for prolonged use if it is beneficial. However, they should be stopped if there is no symptomatic improvement in 3 menstrual cycles.

Hormonal therapy

Intrauterine systems

Intrauterine contraceptive systems with levonorgestrel dramatically reduce HMB as well as acting as contraception and are considered a first-line management. The Mirena intrauterine system releases 20 µg of levonorgestrel every 24 hours into the endometrium from a silicone barrel. As a result of minimal systemic absorption, side-effects are usually limited to irregular spotting in the initial year of use. Women should be advised of anticipated changes in the bleeding pattern, particularly in the first few cycles and maybe lasting longer than 6 months. They should therefore be advised to persevere for at least six cycles to see the benefits of the treatment.

Amenorrhoea occurs in up to 50% of long-term users because of endometrial atrophy. As a contraceptive, it is as effective as sterilization, although fertility returns almost immediately once it is removed. Since it was granted its license in the UK for the treatment of menorrhagia for up to 5 years per system, the use of the Mirena IUS for the treatment of heavy periods has increased dramatically.

CLINICAL NOTES

If an initial pharmaceutical treatment is ineffective, consider a second pharmaceutical treatment rather than immediate referral to surgery.

Table 4.2 Mean percent reduction in measured menstrual blood loss in women with menorrhagia treated with medical therapy

Drug	Mean % menstrual blood loss reduction
Nonsteroidal antiinflammatory drugs	
Ibuprofen	25
Mefenamic acid	47
Antifibrinolytics	
Tranexamic acid	54
Hormonal therapy	
Combined oral contraceptive pill	50
Danazol	60
Levonorgestrel intrauterine system	97
Luteal phase progestogen	15

Combined oral contraceptive pill

When taken in a cyclical fashion, the combined oral contraceptive pill (COCP) inhibits ovulation and produces regular shedding of a thin endometrium. This makes it an effective long-term medical treatment for some women with menorrhagia. Thrombogenic side-effects should be discussed with older women and smokers who are considering using COCP for therapeutic reasons.

Progestogens

Oral progestogens (typically norethisterone 15 mg daily from days 5 to 26 of the menstrual cycle) or injected long-acting progestogens can be used to treat menorrhagia. Side-effects can include weight gain, irregular bleeding, amenorrhoea and premenstrual-like syndrome.

CLINICAL NOTES

Additional medical therapies such as ulipristal acetate are available to women with heavy menstrual bleeding and fibroids of 3-cm plus size (see Chapter 5). Gonadotropin-releasing hormone agonists suppress pituitary–ovarian function and effectively produce a temporary, reversible menopausal state. They are used as a preoperative medication to reduce fibroid size and reduce surgical blood loss.

Guidelines for managing menorrhagia are shown in Fig. 4.2.

Surgical

The required surgical procedure used to treat menorrhagia depends on the underlying diagnosis:

- Hysteroscopy: Intrauterine pathology such as endometrial polyps and submucous fibroids should be removed hysteroscopically (see Chapter 3).
- Myomectomy or uterine artery embolization: For large symptomatic fibroids where the uterus is to be conserved (see Chapter 5).

- Endometrial ablation: Minimally invasive surgical management with rapid recovery.
- Hysterectomy: Management when other treatment options have failed, are contraindicated or are declined by women.

Endometrial ablation

Endometrial ablation is a day-case procedure that reduces menstrual blood loss by producing an 'iatrogenic' Asherman syndrome. Endometrium is destroyed using laser, resection, thermal or microwave ablation techniques and the ensuing intrauterine adhesions reduce endometrial regrowth from deep within crypts or glands. It is therefore not suitable for women wishing to conceive.

Although this does not guarantee amenorrhoea as hysterectomy does, advantages include speed of surgery, quicker recovery, rapid return to work and the use of local as opposed to general anaesthesia. Following endometrial ablation, menstrual blood loss has been shown to be reduced by up to 90%.

Complications of the procedure include:

- Uterine perforation – this commonly occurs where the uterine wall is thinnest, such as the cornual regions and the cervical canal. Perforation could then lead to damage to surrounding gastrointestinal and genitourinary tracts and major blood vessels, resulting in peritonitis or haemorrhage.
- Fluid overload – the use of nonelectrolytic solutions, such as 1.5% glycine, for electrosurgery and the pressures needed to distend the uterine walls predispose to the absorption of large quantities of fluid, which can result in hyponatraemia due to dilutional effects of the irrigating fluid. In extreme overload congestive cardiac failure, hypertension, neurological symptoms, haemolysis and coma can occur.
- Haemorrhage – this can occur if the myometrium is resected too deeply or if the uterus is perforated.
- Infection – the true incidence of pelvic infection following endometrial ablation is difficult to quantify.

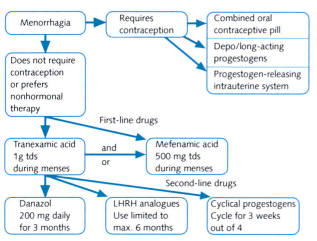

Fig. 4.2 Algorithm for investigating and managing menorrhagia. *LHRH,* Luteinizing hormone-releasing hormone; *tds,* three times a day.

Hysterectomy

Hysterectomy a surgical option in the event that other treatment options have failed, are contraindicated or are declined by the woman, there is a wish for amenorrhoea, the woman requests it and no longer wishes to retain her uterus and fertility.

Hysterectomy is a commonly performed procedure in the UK with up to one in five of all women having a hysterectomy before the age of 60 years, with HMB found to be the presenting complaint for approximately 40%. However, HMB incidence continues to fall due to better diagnostic abilities, better medical treatment and the development of focal and ablative hysteroscopic techniques.

Hysterectomy can be vaginal, laparoscopic or abdominal, depending on the uterine findings. Total abdominal hysterectomy is useful for women with large uteri, multiple large fibroids, adenomyosis, pelvic adhesions and endometriosis. Hysterectomy can be a 'subtotal' procedure, where the cervix is left behind and can include removing the ovaries, to reduce the risk of ovarian cancer (oophorectomy). Typically, if the ovaries are not removed, a bilateral salpingectomy is still performed, due to evidence that ovarian cancer may originate in the fallopian tubes. If the cervix is left behind, cervical smears must be continued.

Almost half the women undergoing abdominal hysterectomy and one-quarter of those undergoing vaginal hysterectomy experience a complication. Complications of the procedure include:

- fever
- urinary tract or bowel damage
- haemorrhage requiring transfusion
- long-term complications such as chronic pelvic pain
- mortality

Fever is the most common complication following abdominal hysterectomy, with one in three women experiencing this. In one-quarter of cases the source of infection is not identifiable; the most common identifiable infection is urinary tract infection, followed by wound or vaginal cuff infection. The use of prophylactic antibiotics is associated with a lower rate of infection.

Damage to the ureter or bowel occurs in approximately 1 in every 200 hysterectomies, with trauma to the bladder occurring in approximately 1 in 100. The ureter is likely to be damaged at the infundibulopelvic ligament, beneath the uterine artery and adjacent to the cervix. Predisposing factors to ureteric damage include congenital anomaly of the renal tracts and distortion of normal anatomy from pelvic inflammatory disease, endometriosis and malignancy. Risk factors predisposing to bowel damage are obesity, previous laparotomy, adhesions, intrinsic bowel problems (e.g., chronic inflammatory bowel disease) and irradiation.

Bowel dysfunction following hysterectomy is well documented, with constipation occurring in up to half the patients during the first 2 weeks of the abdominal approach. One in five patients will continue to experience constipation in the first 3 postoperative months.

When the uterus is removed, the pelvic floor and its nerve supply are disrupted. This can predispose to pelvic floor laxity with subsequent prolapse, as well as bladder and bowel dysfunction. Even when the ovaries are conserved, disruption of their blood supply can interfere with their function, and might even predispose to premature ovarian failure, a risk factor for cardiovascular disease and osteoporosis.

Mortality rate following hysterectomy for benign disease is very low, approximately 6 per 10,000 and is usually a consequence of cardiovascular disease and sepsis.

INTERMENSTRUAL BLEEDING AND POSTCOITAL BLEEDING

Definition

IMB is unscheduled bleeding that occurs between the menstrual periods not related to hormonal contraceptive breakthrough bleeding. It can sometimes be difficult to differentiate true IMB from irregularly frequent periods. PCB is defined as nonmenstrual bleeding, which is immediately precipitated by intercourse.

IMB and PCB are common symptoms and must be investigated as they can indicate serious underlying pathology. Although malignancy is an uncommon cause of bleeding in young women, it must be considered and ruled out in all patients.

Causes and prevalence

Evidence has shown that of women presenting to primary care with menstrual problems, one-third reported IMB or PCB in addition to heavy menstrual loss.

Causes of IMB and PCB are similar, and can be of vaginal, cervical or endometrial origin (Table 4.3):

- vaginal – atrophy, vaginitis, carcinoma (rare)
- cervical – polyp, ectropian, erosion/cervicitis, trauma, carcinoma
- endometrial – polyp, endometritis, submucous fibroids, hyperplasia, malignancy

History

History and examination are similar to those taken for menorrhagia (see above). It is important to ask additional questions regarding the presenting complaint of IMB or PCB as well as fully assessing a sexual health and smear history.

HISTORY

How long have you been experiencing bleeding for? When did the bleeding start? How heavy is the bleeding? Is there any pain associated with the bleeding? Has this happened before? The nature of the unscheduled bleeding may suggest its origin.

Examination

See menorrhagia examination above.

Table 4.3 Causes of intermenstrual and postcoital bleeding

Affected region/system	Specific cause
Cervical	Ectopy
	Polyps
	Malignancy
	Cervicitis
Intrauterine	Polyps
	Submucous fibroids
	Endometrial hyperplasia
	Endometrial malignancy
	Endometritis
Hormonal	Breakthrough bleeding

CLINICAL NOTES

Intermenstrual and postcoital bleeding can be a sign of cervical malignancy, so a history of cervical smears and sexually transmitted infections must be taken. Clinical inspection of the cervix and an up-to-date smear are essential (see Chapter 12).

Investigations

Urine test

A urine pregnancy test should be performed to exclude pregnancy as the cause. A midstream urine sample should be sent to exclude a urinary tract infection.

Vaginal swabs

Microbiology swabs and a screen for sexually transmitted infections, including high and low vaginal swabs, endocervical swabs and urethral swabs, should be performed. *Chlamydia* infection can be tested by an endocervical swab or a urine sample.

Pelvic ultrasound

Transvaginal ultrasound may identify pathology such as thickened endometrium, uterine fibroids or polyps.

Specialist tests

If abnormalities are noted on the cervix, or cervical smear is due, a cervical smear or biopsy may be taken.

If malignancy is suspected or IMB is persistent, hysteroscopy with endometrial sampling can be performed as an outpatient procedure or under a general anaesthesia.

Laparoscopy could be performed if intraabdominal pathology is suspected or to manage acute pelvic inflammatory disease (see Chapter 9).

Treatment

Treatment is dependent on the origins of the unscheduled bleeding. A summary of common treatments includes:

- Atrophic vaginitis – vaginal moisturizing cream or topical oestrogen (see Chapter 13).
- Infective vaginitis – treatment is according to results of the infective screen, for example, *Candida* and bacterial vaginosis (see Chapter 8).
- Cervical or endometrial polyps – excision of cervical polyps can be performed in outpatients, whereas endometrial polyps require hysteroscopic removal.
- Cervical ectropion or erosion – treatment can be with cryocautery.
- Cervicitis – treatment is according to results of the infective screen (see Chapter 8).

There are several causes of postcoital bleeding, intermenstrual bleeding and postmenopausal bleeding, but the easiest way to remember them is to consider the causes anatomically from the vulva ascending to the vagina, cervix, uterus and then ovaries.

Table 4.4 Causes of postmenopausal bleeding

Affected structure	Cause of postmenopausal bleeding
Ovary	Carcinoma of the ovary Oestrogen-secreting tumour
Uterine body	Myometrium: submucous fibroid Endometrium:: atrophic changes, polyp Hyperplasia: simple or atypical carcinoma
Cervix	Atrophic changes Malignancy: squamous carcinoma, adenocarcinoma
Vagina	Atrophic changes
Urethra	Urethral caruncle Haematuria
Vulva	Vulvitis Dystrophies Malignancy

POSTMENOPAUSAL BLEEDING

Definition

Postmenopausal bleeding (PMB) is vaginal bleeding occurring more than 12 months after the menopause other than the expected cyclic bleeding that occurs in women taking cyclic postmenopausal hormone therapy.

Prevalence

PMB is a common disorder occurring in approximately 4%–11% of postmenopausal women and accounts for approximately 5% of gynaecology referrals. The incidence of bleeding appears to correlate with time since menopause, with the likelihood of bleeding decreasing over time. Prompt investigation is required to exclude malignancy. Of all women in the UK with PMB, 9% will be found to have a malignancy.

Atrophic changes to the genital tract are the most common cause but must not be assumed to be the cause until other pathology, especially malignancy, have been excluded.

Aetiology

There are many causes of PMB (Table 4.4), but the most important causes to exclude are malignancy of the endometrium, cervix and ovary.

Atrophic changes to the lower genital tract due to oestrogen deficiency can cause bleeding and, in fact, are the most common cause of PMB. Atrophic changes can occur to the endometrium, cervix and vagina. Urethral caruncle (prolapse of the urethral mucosa) is also associated with oestrogen deficiency.

Submucous fibroids or uterine polyps can cause PMB, although these are likely to have existed from before the menopause. The endometrium should be inactive in the postmenopausal years and atrophic endometritis is a common consequence. Endometrial polyps might be benign, contain areas of atypical hyperplasia or be malignant.

Endometrial hyperplasia can arise de novo or be secondary to oestrogen stimulation. Exogenous unopposed oestrogens and endogenous oestrogens arising from peripheral conversion of precursors in adipose tissue, or from oestrogen-secreting ovarian tumours, can result in endometrial hyperplasia and adenocarcinoma. Adenocarcinoma of the endometrium is an important cause of PMB and must always be considered in the differential diagnosis.

Cervical carcinoma and squamous carcinoma of the vulva can present with PMB and, although the nonneoplastic epithelial disorders of the vulva (vulval dystrophies) do not themselves usually cause PMB, scratching because of pruritus vulvae may.

Disease of the ovary in postmenopausal women is uncommon but can present with PMB. An oestrogen-secreting tumour causes PMB by stimulating the endometrium in the absence of progesterone. This can cause hyperplasia and even carcinoma of the endometrium. Ovarian carcinoma usually causes PMB by direct invasion through the uterine wall.

RED FLAG

Always investigate postmenopausal bleeding promptly to exclude malignancy. Uterine malignancy is often detected early because it presents with abnormal uterine bleeding. Cervical malignancy can present with intermenstrual and postcoital bleeding, or smear abnormalities.

DIAGNOSIS

History

A full medical and gynaecological history should be taken as per menorrhagia and PMB/IMB as above. A focused history of the nature of the PMB is useful for considering differential diagnosis. Family history, drug history [including the use of hormone replacement therapy (HRT)] and smear history are particularly important. Medical comorbidities such as obesity and coagulation disorders should also be noted.

Examination

See menorrhagia examination above.

Investigations

Pelvic ultrasound

Transvaginal ultrasound should be performed on all women presenting with PMB. A normal postmenopausal ET is <5 mm. The ovaries can also be assessed using ultrasound, although postmenopausal ovaries are not always visualized on ultrasound scan.

Endometrial biopsy and hysteroscopy

A sampling of endometrial tissue should be made in the event of:

- ET >5 mm
- high risk for endometrial cancer, for example, Tamoxifen, HRT use, high body mass index, diabetes
- normal ET but persistent episodes of PMB
- previously normal biopsy but persistent episodes of PMB

Endometrial biopsy can be taken in the outpatient setting using a 'pipelle' endometrial sampler; however, it only samples 4% of the uterine cavity. Intrauterine pathology is best excluded by hysteroscopic examination of the uterine cavity. This can be done under local anaesthesia with pipelle endometrial biopsy, or under general anaesthesia with a more substantial endometrial biopsy.

Blood tests

If history and ultrasound findings suggest an oestrogen-secreting tumour, circulating oestradiol levels should be measured. If malignancy is suspected, tumour markers may be performed. This is usually only done in secondary care to work out the 'Risk of Malignancy Index', as multiple conditions, such as endometriosis, can cause falsely high results and considerable patient concern (see Chapter 12).

Vaginal swabs

Microbiology swabs and a screen for sexually transmitted infections, including high and low vaginal swabs, endocervical swabs and urethral swabs, should be performed. *Candida* infection is less common in the postmenopausal population, therefore should trigger ongoing investigations for potential immunocompromised state.

Specialist tests

If any focal lesions are noted during examination, this should prompt vulval, vaginal or cervical biopsies. If smear test is due or cervical abnormality is seen, this should prompt smear test or colposcopy referral. If gynaecological investigations have been completed and there is concern that the bleeding could originate in the rectum or bladder, a cystoscopy and sigmoidoscopy should be performed. Fig. 4.3 provides an algorithm for the diagnosis and investigation of PMB.

Treatment

Treatment depends on the underlying pathology. The most common cause of PMB is atrophic change and, therefore, oestrogen replacement is indicated not only to prevent a recurrence of PMB, but also to treat other symptoms associated with oestrogen deficiency (e.g., dyspareunia). Most women in this situation prefer to use topical oestrogen. The newer 17β-oestradiol-releasing creams, rings and vaginal tablets avoid the risk of endometrial hyperplasia by minimizing systemic absorption. If systemic HRT is requested, then oestrogen therapy must be combined with a progestogen in women who have a uterus.

Small urethral caruncles might recede with oestrogen cream, but larger areas of prolapsed urethral mucosa may require surgical excision.

The treatment of vulval, cervical and ovarian malignancy is discussed in detail in Chapter 12, and fibroids are discussed in Chapter 5.

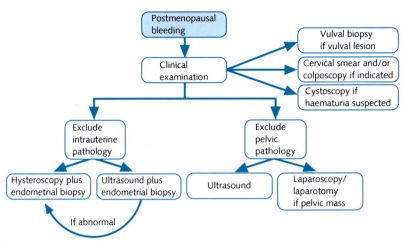

Fig. 4.3 Algorithm for postmenopausal bleeding.

Chapter Summary

- The topics covered in this chapter are common presentations to gynaecology outpatients.
- The key to treatment of menorrhagia, postcoital bleeding, intermenstrual bleeding and postmenopausal bleeding is identifying the underlying cause, as this will guide treatment.
- Investigations should be initiated promptly, particularly with postmenopausal bleeding, as a differential diagnosis we must consider is malignancy.
- It is crucial that as healthcare providers we emphasize the importance of screening programmes such as the cervical screening programme to reduce incidence of malignancy diagnoses.

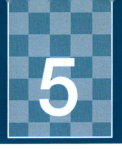

BACKGROUND

Definition

Uterine fibroids (otherwise known as 'leiomyomas') are benign tumours of the myometrium. Histologically they are composed of whorling bundles of smooth muscle cells that resemble the architecture of normal myometrium. They are categorized by position within the myometrium (Fig. 5.1).

Prevalence

They are the most common benign tumours found in women and occur in over 50% of women over the age of 40 years. Incidence is increased in women in certain ethnic populations, particularly African and Afro-Caribbean. Fibroids are affected by exposure to oestrogen; therefore, they can be stimulated to grow with increasing age, in hyperoestrogenic state of pregnancy and decrease in size in postmenopausal women. At hysterectomy, 70% of all uteruses are found to have microscopic fibroids.

Malignant changes are rare (1:1000) but it is possible for fibroids to develop into sarcoma.

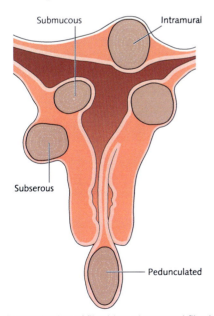

Fig. 5.1 Categorization of fibroids: submucosal fibroids impact on the endometrial cavity, intramural fibroids lie within the uterus wall, subserosal fibroids lie on the outer surface of the womb. Pedunculated fibroids are attached to the uterus through a stalk.

Submucous — Intramural — Subserous — Pedunculated

CLINICAL NOTES

RISK FACTORS AND PROTECTIVE FACTORS FOR FIBROIDS

Increased incidence with:	Decreased incidence with:
African–Caribbean women	Cigarette smoking
Increasing age	Use of combined oral contraceptive pill
Nulligravidity	Full-term pregnancy
Obesity	

Symptoms

Approximately 50% of patients have fibroids diagnosed incidentally, for example, at the time of obstetric ultrasound scan, and are asymptomatic. In asymptomatic cases no routine intervention is required.

CLINICAL NOTES

SYMPTOMS ASSOCIATED WITH UTERINE FIBROIDS
- Asymptomatic
- Menstrual abnormalities
- Abdominopelvic mass
- Subfertility
- Pressure symptoms
- Urinary symptoms secondary to pressure
- Pregnancy complications
- Pain

The most common presenting symptom of fibroids is menstrual abnormalities, particularly menorrhagia, which occurs in approximatively one-third of women with fibroids. The increased menstrual loss is secondary to the increased endometrial surface area, distorted by submucosal fibroids or an enlarged uterine cavity with increased endometrial blood supply. This can secondarily cause iron-deficiency anaemia and patients often present with symptomatic anaemia.

Symptoms also include pelvic pressure from large fibroids growing within the abdominal cavity, which can cause abdominal swelling or distension. Pressure on the bladder can cause urinary frequency, urgency and nocturia. Extensive fibroids can press on the ureters and can affect renal function. Pain can result from degeneration (breakdown) of fibroids, torsion of pedunculate fibroid and presence of pelvic varicosities.

Women can present with reproductive dysfunction, including subfertility, early and late miscarriage and premature birth; however, many women with fibroids have uncomplicated pregnancies. Theories include that subfertility is secondary to anatomical distortion and alteration in uterine environment. There is evidence that suggests pre-in vitro fertilization surgical treatment of fibroids improves in vitro fertilization success.

CLINICAL NOTES

A complication of fibroids is degeneration, where the fibroid breaks down, causing abdominal pain. In pregnancy, a type of haemorrhagic infarction can occur known as 'red degeneration'.

DIAGNOSIS

History

A full medical, gynaecological and obstetric history should be taken in addition to these focussed questions. The extent and type of symptoms may help guide the appropriate management for the woman.

HISTORY

What was the date of your last menstrual period? How long is your menstrual cycle? How many days are your periods? How many pads or tampons do you use per day? Do you suffer from overflow bleeding or flooding? Quantifying the extent of menorrhagia is important to understand the symptoms and what management may be appropriate.

Do you have any dysuria or increasing urinary frequency? Do you have any difficulty opening your bowels? Have you noticed an abdominal mass? How quickly did this develop? These pressure symptoms may suggest large fibroids within the abdominal cavity. Very rapid development of an

---

abdominal mass may increase suspicion of a quick growing mass such as sarcoma.

Do you have any children? Have you been pregnant before? Are you using any contraception? A complete obstetric history is essential to take. The management of fibroids will depend on whether fertility preservation is desired.

How does this effect your quality of life? Symptoms of prolapse can be very troubling to women and can affect their day-to-day life. It is important to consider this when deciding most appropriate management.

Examination

Fibroids can be palpated during an abdominopelvic examination, which classically presents as an enlarged, firm and irregular pelvic mass.

Is there abdominal distension? Determine the size, tenderness, mobility and nodularity of the mass. A large fibroid uterus can extend out of the pelvis and be palpated abdominally. The size of a fibroid uterus can be described similar to a pregnant abdomen (e.g., "20-week size' is equivalent to umbilical level).

A bimanual vaginal examination should be performed and the adnexa should be examined. A fibroid may be mobile or move along with the uterus.

INVESTIGATIONS

Blood tests

Full blood count to assess current haemoglobin (Hb) levels and assess for anaemia. In patients with large fibroids that may be pressing on the ureters, check renal function (urea and electrolytes).

Transvaginal ultrasound

Transvaginal ultrasound is the diagnostic tool of choice for diagnosis of fibroids. It should enable location and size of individual fibroids. The images can be limited by multiple fibroids, very large fibroid uterus or adiposity. It is also not always possible to distinguish between fibroids and ovarian or broad ligament masses.

Specialist tests

If imaging is not sufficient with transvaginal ultrasound, diagnosis is unclear or surgical intervention is being considered, magnetic resonance imaging is the next imaging of choice. Hysteroscopy is the best method of imaging submucosal fibroids.

CLINICAL NOTES

COMPLICATIONS OF FIBROIDS

Gynaecological complications

- Degeneration – may include red degeneration or calcification
- Torsion – of pedunculated fibroids
- Malignancy – the risk of leiomyosarcoma is 0.1%–0.5%

Pregnancy-related complications

- Infertility
- Obstructed labour
- Risk of postpartum haemorrhage

TREATMENT

Medical

Medical therapy is predominantly useful as an adjunct to surgery and as an aid to correcting anaemia prior to surgery. Fibroids commonly regrow to their original size within 3 months of ceasing medical therapy without subsequent surgical intervention.

Gonadotropin-releasing hormone (GnRH) analogues produce a hypogonadotropic hypogonadal state leading to a temporary, reversible, chemical menopause. This can result in up to a 40% reduction in fibroid volume in 6 months and a considerable improvement in bleeding pattern. At surgery this may allow a smaller, transverse surgical incision, reduced blood loss and a reduced risk of hysterectomy as a complication of myomectomy. The long-term use of GnRH analogues is limited due to their side-effects, which include menopausal symptoms, and bone density reduction (osteoporosis). Low-dose hormone replacement therapy as 'add back' can be used to alleviate adverse effects and reduce bone loss density.

Other medical options include selective progesterone receptor modulators such as ulipristal acetate, which are thought to stimulate apoptosis and inhibit cell proliferation in fibroids. Trials have shown amenorrhoea and median fibroid volume reduction of 45%.

Surgical

Surgical intervention depends on the location of fibroids and extent of symptoms.

Smaller submucous fibroids can be removed using an operative hysteroscope in a procedure called a 'transcervical resection of fibroids'.

Myomectomy is the removal of fibroids with preservation of the uterus and can be performed either open at laparotomy, or laparoscopically (Fig. 5.2). This is more suitable for larger fibroids whether they are pedunculated, subserosal or intramural. It is a procedure with a high complication rate, most commonly haemorrhage, which can require blood transfusion, and potentially hysterectomy. Adhesion formation is common, and fibroid regrowth is likely to occur in 40% of patients, with reoperation required in up to one-fifth of cases.

For ultimate removal of fibroids the surgical procedure of choice is hysterectomy, in women who have completed their families, although not all women wish to have their uterus removed. Surgical treatment by hysterectomy has less morbidity than myomectomy.

Other techniques

Uterine artery embolization is a minimally invasive alternative to surgery that involves the radiological embolization of fibroids. A catheter is inserted into the femoral artery, and then small silicone microbeads are injected into the arteries supplying the fibroids, causing thrombosis and fibroid infarction. This procedure is performed by interventional radiologists, and the patients are assessed first to determine suitability. Complications include postoperative pain, infection, and failure of treatment. It is not advised for women wishing to preserve fertility, as reproductive outcomes are significantly lower than following surgical intervention.

Magnetic resonance-guided high-intensity focused ultrasound is a procedure involving thermal coagulation of targeted fibroids. Research is ongoing into radiofrequency ablation and gene therapy.

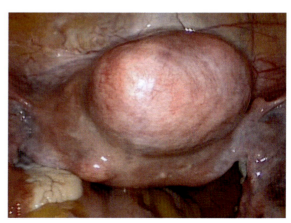

Fig. 5.2 Fibroids at laparoscopy.

Chapter Summary

- Fibroids are very common, and range in presentation from asymptomatic to severe menstrual abnormalities, pain and pressure symptoms.
- During management patient symptoms and severity should be considered.
- Patients should be counselled regarding benefits and adverse effects of treatment options in addition to potential effect on fertility.

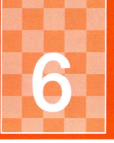

Endometriosis 6

BACKGROUND

Definition

Endometriosis is the presence of endometrial-like tissue (uterine lining) outside of the uterine cavity, which induces a chronic, inflammatory reaction. Endometrial cells occurring in the myometrium (uterine muscle) are known as 'adenomyosis'. The most common sites for endometriosis are the ovaries, the uterosacral ligaments and the pouch of Douglas. Although endometriosis has been reported in nearly every organ, extrapelvic endometriosis is rare (Fig. 6.1).

Prevalence

The true incidence of endometriosis is difficult to ascertain as not all patients are symptomatic. It is thought to occur in about 10% of the female population in reproductive years but has been diagnosed in up to 25% of women at diagnostic laparoscopy. It is one of the most common gynaecological conditions and therefore seen regularly in gynaecology outpatients.

Symptoms

- Cyclical pain prior to period.
- Painful periods (dysmenorrhoea).
- Chronic pelvic pain.
- Pain during intercourse (dyspareunia).
- Pain opening bowels (dyschezia).

The main symptom of endometriosis is cyclical pain typically prior to menstruation. This occurs because the deposits of endometriosis respond to the hormonal cycle, and the subsequent bleeding from the deposits cause local irritation and inflammatory responses. Other classic symptoms of endometriosis include dysmenorrhoea and chronic pelvic pain. Deep endometriosis of the rectovaginal septum is associated with symptoms such as dyschezia and deep dyspareunia.

If endometriosis develops within an ovary, it can form a cyst called an 'endometrioma', otherwise known as a 'chocolate cyst' due to its characteristic liquid brown contents (Fig. 6.2). Similar to other causes of an ovarian cyst, they can cause symptoms by torsion or rupture and release of the irritant chocolate material, causing peritonism.

The site of ectopic deposits of endometriosis dictate the location of the pain and symptoms. Endometriosis of the lung, bladder, bowel or umbilicus will produce cyclical bleeding from these sites associated with menstruation (Fig. 6.3).

DIAGNOSIS

History

Symptoms that are suggestive of endometriosis should be elicited with a focused history. This will help differentiate from other conditions such as irritable bowel syndrome and pelvic inflammatory disease.

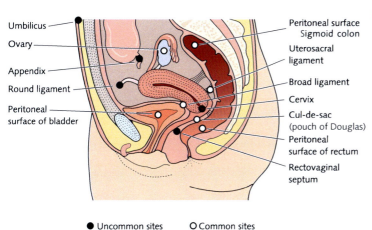

Fig. 6.1 Common sites of endometriosis.

Umbilicus
Ovary
Appendix
Round ligament
Peritoneal surface of bladder

Peritoneal surface Sigmoid colon
Uterosacral ligament
Broad ligament
Cervix
Cul-de-sac (pouch of Douglas)
Peritoneal surface of rectum
Rectovaginal septum

● Uncommon sites   ○ Common sites

Endometriosis

Fig. 6.2 Symptoms of endometriosis.

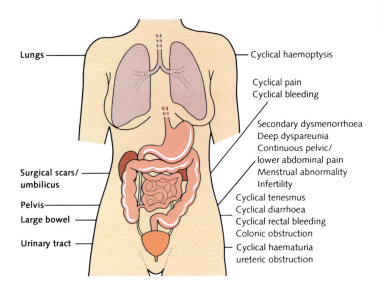

Lungs — Cyclical haemoptysis

Cyclical pain
Cyclical bleeding

Secondary dysmenorrhoea
Deep dyspareunia
Continuous pelvic/lower abdominal pain
Menstrual abnormality
Infertility

Surgical scars/umbilicus

Cyclical tenesmus
Cyclical diarrhoea
Cyclical rectal bleeding
Colonic obstruction

Pelvis

Large bowel

Urinary tract — Cyclical haematuria
ureteric obstruction

HISTORY

What was the date of your last menstrual period? How long is your menstrual cycle? Do you suffer with period pain? At what point during your cycle is the pain worst? Do you have to take analgesia for the pain? Do you have any pain opening your bowels or passing urine? Do you have deep pain during intercourse? Do you have any other bleeding during your period, for example, rectal bleeding? A detailed history of the menses should identify the typical symptoms of endometriosis.

Do you have any children? Have you been pregnant before? Are you using any contraception? A complete obstetric history is essential to take and may highlight subfertility issues.

How does this effect your quality of life? Endometriosis and chronic pelvic pain can have serious effect on women's quality of life and this may affect management options offered.

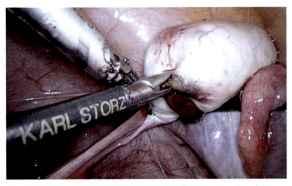

Fig. 6.3 Altered blood (chocolate fluid) seen seeping from a ruptured ovarian endometrioma.

Examination

Is there abdominal distension? Abdominal inspection may reveal a slightly distended abdomen and palpation may be tender, particularly around the time of menses.

A bimanual vaginal examination should be performed and the adnexa should be examined.

Pelvic examination may reveal a tender, retroverted, retroflexed, fixed uterus with thickening of the cardinal or uterosacral ligaments. Endometriotic nodules might be palpable in the posterior vaginal fornix and ovarian endometrioma might be evident on bimanual palpation. The pelvic anatomy might be normal with mild disease and a useful sign is to elicit pain on moving the cervix interiorly (cervical excitation). This stretches the uterosacral ligaments, which is painful in the presence of endometriosis. In the presence of adenomyosis, the uterus is typically smoothly enlarged (globular) and tender. Deeply infiltrating rectovaginal nodules may be most reliably detected by vaginal examination during menstruation.

INVESTIGATIONS

Transvaginal ultrasound

Ovarian endometrioma can be seen by ultrasound but differentiation from other ovarian pathology may be difficult without histological confirmation. The typical ultrasound appearance of an endometrioma is described as 'ground glass'.

Specialist tests

Diagnosis and severity of pelvic disease can only effectively be assessed by laparoscopy. The classic 'powder-burn' lesions of endometriosis might be seen, but these areas of haemosiderin pigmentation might represent 'burnt-out' endometriosis. Nonpigmented lesions can appear as opaque white areas of peritoneum, red lesions or glandular lesions. If there is doubt about the macroscopic appearance, then a biopsy should be taken. At the time of laparoscopy, the endometriosis can be classified and graded (Table 6.1).

More complex imaging such as magnetic resonance imaging may be performed if extensive disease is suspected prior to surgery.

COMPLICATIONS

Subfertility

Endometriosis is associated with infertility, and as many as one-third of infertile women are diagnosed with endometriosis. Adhesions, tubal and ovarian damage and distortion of pelvic structures can contribute. However, there is also association of mild endometriosis without structural damage with infertility. It is thought that this may be due to release of substances such as prostaglandins, which can affect ovulation or tubal motility. There is evidence that treating even mild endometriosis can improve fertility.

Malignant change within endometriotic lesions is rare and most commonly occurs in ovarian endometriosis.

CLINICAL NOTES

POSSIBLE THEORIES FOR AETIOLOGY OF ENDOMETRIOSIS
- Retrograde menstruation
- Lymphatic and venous embolization
- Coelomic metaplasia
- Genetic and immunological factors
- Composite theories

Retrograde menstruation/implantation theory

This is the theory that during menstruation, endometrial tissue spills into the pelvic cavity through the fallopian tubes. This ectopic endometrium then implants and becomes functional, responding to the hormones of the ovarian cycle. This theory is supported by the association

Table 6.1 American Fertility Society classification of endometriosis[a]

Anatomical site	Score	1	2	3	4	5
Peritoneum	Endometriotic lesion size	<1 cm	1–3 cm	>3 cm		
	Adhesions	Flimsy	Dense with partial pouch of Douglas occlusion	Dense with complete pouch of Douglas occlusion		
Ovary (points for each side involved)	Endometriotic lesion size		<1 cm		1–3 cm	>3 cm
	Adhesions		Filmy		Dense with partial ovarian coverage	Dense, completely enclosing ovary
Fallopian tubes (points for each side involved)	Endometriotic lesion size		<1 cm		>1 cm	Tubal occlusion
	Adhesions		Filmy		Dense and distorting tubes	Dense and completely enclosing tubes
		Stage I (mild) <5 Stage II (mod) 6–15			Stage III (severe) 16–30 Stage IV (extensive) > 31	

[a] Scores are: Stage 1 (mild) <5, stage II (mod) 6–15, stage III (severe) 16–30, stage IV (extensive) >31.

between endometriosis and prolonged periods, and by the fact that the most common sites for endometriosis are the ovaries and the uterosacral ligaments – areas in which retrograde menses spill. The implantation theory would also account for the rare cases of endometriosis found during surgical incision, for example, following open myomectomy or caesarean section. However, this theory does not account for the existence of endometriosis at the distant sites in the body (e.g., lungs). There is growing laparoscopic evidence to suggest that most women experience retrograde menstruation, in which case the incidence of endometriosis would be expected to be higher.

Lymphatic and venous embolization

This theory hypothesizes that endometrial tissue is transported through the body by the lymphatic or venous channels and would explain the rare cases of distant sites for endometriosis. However, distant endometriotic deposits would be expected to be more common if the lymphatic and venous embolization theories were the only mechanism for the development of endometriosis.

Coelomic metaplasia

This theory relies on the principle that tissues of certain embryonic origin maintain their ability to undergo metaplasia and differentiate into other tissue types. This is certainly true of peritoneum of coelomic origin, which can undergo metaplasia and differentiate into functional endometrium. However, this does not explain the distribution of endometriosis within the peritoneal cavity itself (most common in the lower part of the peritoneal cavity) or the presence of endometriosis in sites of the body that are not of coelomic origin.

Genetic and immunological factors

The role of a genetic influence is supported by the strong family history seen in endometriosis sufferers, but its exact role has not yet been characterized. It is possible that women with a genetic predisposition to endometriosis have an abnormal response to the presence of ectopic endometrium, which results in endometriosis developing. There is some evidence that an altered or defective cell-mediated response is implicated.

Composite theories

None of the above theories alone account for all cases of endometriosis, however, together all the theories could play a role.

TREATMENT

Treatment depends on the severity of the disease and should be tailored to the woman's individual needs. The aim of treatment is to alleviate symptoms, stop progression of disease and development of complications and improve fertility.

Endometriosis is a chronic condition with up to 40% of women developing recurring symptoms within 1 year of stopping treatment. Initial treatment should, therefore, be followed by maintenance therapy to reduce the chance of recurrence. Maintenance therapy is usually medical and aims to suppress or reduce the frequency of periods.

Medical

Endometriotic lesions regress during pregnancy and after the menopause. Medical treatment is, therefore, aimed at mimicking these physiological processes. Hormonal treatment for endometriosis can reduce pain and has no permanent negative effect on subsequent fertility but most will concurrently act as contraception (Table 6.2).

Analgesia

Simple analgesia such as paracetamol and nonsteroidal antiinflammatory drugs should be advised either alone or in combination with other medical treatments. In cases of chronic pelvic pain, neuromodulators are occasionally started in a pain clinic.

Table 6.2 Summary of medical treatment of endometriosis

Drug	Mode of action	Side-effects
Progestogens	Pseudopregnancy	Break-through bleeding, weight gain, oedema, acne, abdominal bloating, increased appetite, decreased libido
Danazol	Pseudomenopause	Increase weight, break-through bleeding, muscle cramps, decreased breast size, hot flushes, emotional lability, oily skin, acne, hirsutism, headache, increased libido, hoarseness or deepening of the voice
Gestrinone	Pseudomenopause	Similar to danazol
Luteinizing hormone-releasing hormone analogues	Pseudomenopause	Hot flushes, break-through bleeding, vaginal dryness, headaches, decreased libido, bone density loss

Combined oral contraceptive pill

The combined oral contraceptive pill (COCP) suppresses ovulation and the normal cyclical ovarian production of oestrogen and progesterone. Mild symptoms of endometriosis may be controlled using the COCP, but it is more often used as maintenance therapy following initial treatment. Tricycling the COCP can be used to reduce frequency of withdrawal bleeds.

Progestogens

Continuous progestogen therapy effectively induces a 'pseudopregnancy' state, causing endometriotic deposits to decidualize and then regress. Progestogens can be taken orally or as depot preparations, and treatment should be for 6 months.

Mirena coil

The Mirena coil releases small amounts of progesterone into the uterus and can be used for up to 5 years. Its advantages include the fact that it simultaneously acts as contraception and minimizes systemic side-effects. Studies have shown that it can reduce endometriosis-related pain and it is therefore a popular first-line treatment option.

Gonadotropin-releasing hormone analogues

These are synthetically modified versions of a naturally occurring hormone known as 'gonadotrophin-releasing hormone', which help to control the menstrual cycle. An example is the goserelin implant. Continued administration desensitizes pituitary gonadotrophs, leading to a temporary, reversible state of hypogonadotropic hypogonadism – in other words, a temporary chemical menopause. Gonadotropin-releasing hormone analogues are as effective as danazol in reducing the symptoms and severity of endometriosis and are usually used for 3–6 months. Their menopausal side-effects are often better tolerated than the androgenic side-effects of danazol and can be reduced using 'add-back' continuous combined hormone replacement therapy.

Danazol

Danazol is a testosterone derivative that produces a hypo-oestrogenic and hypoprogestogenic state, and it is this pseudomenopausal state that induces endometrial regression and atrophy.

The mechanism of action of danazol is complex; it acts at pituitary, ovarian and target tissue levels. It should be taken for 6–9 months and the dose should be titrated to the patient's response and presence of side-effects. It is now not commonly used, because of its side-effect profile.

Surgical

Surgical options should be considered if medical options are not controlling symptoms, or with regard to fertility investigations.

Laparoscopy is the gold-standard operative treatment, enabling division of adhesions, destruction of endometriotic lesions using diathermy or laser and removing endometriomas, which do not respond well to medical therapy. Complications include damage to other pelvic structures including bowel, bladder and ureters. Women must also be informed about potential recurrence of endometriosis, and no change to symptoms of pelvic pain. If at laparoscopy the endometriosis is extensive, involving bladder or bowel, a more invasive surgery may be planned, often with a surgical team in event of bowel surgery. As an adjunct to surgery for deep endometriosis involving the bowel, bladder or ureter, consider 3 months of gonadotrophin-releasing hormone agonists before surgery.

If the patient has fertility concerns, a tubal dye test can be performed at the same time. Pregnancy rates following conservative surgery are directly related to the severity of the disease and can improve within the 6 months postoperatively.

In patients who have completed their family and have exhausted more conservative measures, more extensive surgery can be considered. Hysterectomy with bilateral salpingo-oophorectomy is the procedure of choice together with excision of all endometriosis. This will effectively manage adenomyosis (if present) as well and will prevent the normal cyclical variation of oestrogen and progesterone that endometriosis responds to. As many of these women are relatively young, hormone replacement therapy is recommended. Oestrogen replacement may cause a recurrence of endometriosis in a small percentage of women and should, therefore, be kept to a minimum. Continuous combined oestrogen and progesterone replacement might further reduce the rate of recurrence because of the effects of progestogens on endometriosis.

ETHICS

Endometriosis is a chronic condition and can have a considerable effect on women's quality of life due to pelvic pain. There is a large amount of support and information available from organizations such as Endometriosis UK and clinicians should inform women about these services.

Chapter Summary

- Endometriosis is a chronic gynaecological condition characterized by cyclical pelvic pain caused by ectopic endometrial tissue.
- It is a common presentation seen in both primary and secondary care.
- Management of the condition, both medical and surgical, is aimed at symptomatic control and preventing further spread of the disease and should be individualized to each woman's needs.

Pelvic pain and dyspareunia

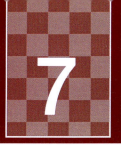

7

BACKGROUND

Pelvic pain is a common gynaecological presentation in accident and emergency, primary and secondary care. Chronic pain is thought to affect up to one in six adult women. Acute pelvic pain is sudden onset, often secondary to a new pathology, for example, an ovarian cyst torsion, whereas chronic pelvic pain is defined as intermittent or constant pelvic pain that lasts 6 months or more not occurring exclusively with menstruation, intercourse or pregnancy. It is a symptom therefore investigations must be made to identify a possible underlying diagnosis.

Symptoms

The type of pain experienced should be elicited through the history and examination. In terms of acute pain, it may be constant or intermittent, mild or severe, in a certain location in the pelvis with or without radiation and exacerbated by certain factors.

Chronic pain may be apparent as cyclical pain prior to a period, painful periods (dysmenorrhoea), pain passing urine or opening bowels (dyschezia) and pain during intercourse (dyspareunia). Dyspareunia can be classified as superficial or deep, depending on whether it is experienced superficially at the area of the vulva and introitus or deep within the pelvis (Table 7.1).

Table 7.1 Differential diagnosis of dyspareunia

Superficial	Deep
Congenital	**Congenital**
Vaginal atresia	Incomplete vaginal atresia
Vaginal septum	Vaginal septum
Infection	**Infection**
Vulvovaginitis (see Chapter 13)	Pelvic inflammatory disease (see Chapter 9)
Postsurgery	**Postsurgery**
Relating to childbirth	Relating to childbirth
Pelvic floor repair	Pelvic floor repair
Vulval disease	**Pelvic disease**
Bartholin cyst	Endometriosis
Vulval dystrophies	Fibroids
Carcinoma of vulva	Ovarian cyst/tumours
Psychosexual	**Psychosexual**
Vaginismus	Vaginismus
Atrophic changes	
Postmenopausal	

Differential diagnosis

If a woman presents with acute pelvic pain, urgent conditions should be considered initially. These include ectopic pregnancy, ruptured ovarian cyst, ovarian torsion and pelvic inflammatory disease (PID), of which ovarian cyst accidents and PID are the most common presentations. Nongynaecological causes must also be considered; for example, gastrointestinal conditions such as appendicitis, and urinary conditions such as urinary tract infection.

Chronic pelvic pain may be secondary to underlying endometriosis, adenomyosis or pelvic adhesions. Again, nongynaecological causes must also be considered, such as nerve entrapment or irritable bowel syndrome (Table 7.2).

Table 7.2 Differential diagnosis of pelvic pain

Acute	Chronic
Pelvic inflammatory disease (see Chapter 9)	Adenomyosis (see Chapter 6)
Tubo-ovarian abscess	Endometriosis
Posttermination of pregnancy	Adhesions
Postinsertion of intrauterine contraceptive device	Gynaecological operation
Posthysteroscopy	Pelvic inflammatory disease
	Appendicitis
Early pregnancy complications (see Chapter 18)	
Miscarriage	
Ectopic pregnancy	
Gynaecological malignancy (see Chapter 12)	Gynaecological malignancy
Ovarian cyst (see Chapter 11)	Gastrointestinal pathology
Rupture	Diverticulitis
Haemorrhage	Irritable bowel syndrome
Torsion	
Fibroid necrosis (see Chapter 5)	
Ovulation pain (mittelschmerz)	
Abscess	
Bartholin cyst	
Labial	
Urinary tract infection	
Renal calculi	
Appendicitis	

DIAGNOSIS

History

A detailed history of the pain is essential to distinguish between acute onset and chronic pain, and to differentiate between the diverse differential diagnosis. Important features in the history are:

- categorizing pain
- association with menstrual cycle
- associated symptoms
- gynaecological history
- medical and surgical history
- social history

HISTORY

How long have you suffered with this pain? Is it continuous or intermittent? Is it sharp or dull? Where is the pain and does it radiate anywhere? Does anything make the pain worse or better? Do you have to take analgesia for the pain? The nature of the pain will identify whether it is acute or chronic onset and may narrow down possible differentials. For example, ovarian torsion typically presents with unilateral acute pain, associated with nausea and vomiting, radiating to the upper thighs. It is important to make this diagnosis promptly because an operation to relieve the torsion might save the ovary from irreversible ischaemia.

It is important to assess the association of the pain with the menstrual cycle. Do you suffer with period pain? At what point during your cycle is the pain worst? Do you have to take analgesia for the pain? Do you have any pain opening your bowels or passing urine? Do you have deep pain during intercourse? Do you have any other bleeding during your period, for example, rectal bleeding? Chronic cyclical pains may be suggestive of endometriosis, typically starting up to 2 weeks before the period and usually being relieved when the bleeding starts. Mittelschmerz is an acute pain associated with ovulation. To make this diagnosis, it is, therefore, essential to know the timing of the pain in relation to the patient's menstrual cycle.

Associated symptoms along with the pain should be explored. Have you noticed any increase in or change to vaginal discharge? Have you had any nausea or vomiting? Have you had any high temperatures? Pelvic inflammatory disease

(PID) may or may not be associated with vaginal discharge. The pain is typically felt across the whole of the lower abdomen and there might be a history of fever. Appendicitis can be associated with nausea and vomiting. Diverticulitis is more likely to be associated with constipation and to affect the older population.

A general gynaecology history should be taken, including last menstrual period, to exclude current pregnancy and the possibility of a miscarriage or ectopic pregnancy. The date and result of the last cervical smear test should be checked, as well as a history of irregular or postcoital bleeding, which might be associated with malignancy. A history of sexually transmitted disease, previous PID or pelvic surgery could result in adhesion formation. Current use of contraception must be checked, both to exclude pregnancy and to determine the risk of PID. A recent change of partner increases the risk, particularly if no barrier contraception has been used. A sexual history must be taken in a sensitive manner with particular attention to a new partner, possible relationship issues or a history of abuse.

The history should include a thorough medical and surgical history, and a drug history will help elicit the amount of analgesia required to control the pain symptoms. Inquire about how chronic pelvic pain affects activities of daily living, for example, going to school or taking time off work.

Examination

See Chapter 1 for full gynaecological examination technique.

- Abdominal palpation
- Vulval/vaginal/cervical inspection
- Bimanual pelvic examination

Before palpating the abdomen always enquire about areas of tenderness and palpate these areas last.

Using the palm of the hand, gently palpate the four quadrants of the abdomen for areas of tenderness, and whether this is generalized or focussed. Assess whether the tenderness is deep or superficial and if you are eliciting any guarding or signs of peritonism. Palpate for any abdominal mass arising from the pelvis, for example, an enlarged fibroid uterus may be present. This could give symptoms of acute pelvic pain, if there is fibroid necrosis, or of deep dyspareunia. Some abdominal masses may not be palpable abdominally, such as an ovarian cyst, but may be palpable on bimanual examination.

Table 7.3 Vulval and vaginal inspection

Cause(s)	Symptoms and signs
Postmenopausal changes (see Chapter 17)	Vulval and vaginal skin appears thin and atrophic. This can cause superficial dyspareunia.
Vulval dystrophies (see Chapter 13)	There might be patches of inflammation, leucoplakia and ulceration, which cause superficial dyspareunia.
Episiotomy/ lacerations	Injury secondary to childbirth commonly causes superficial dyspareunia.
Abscesses	A Bartholin abscess is an abscess of the gland situated towards the posterior fourchette; labial abscesses are commonly situated on the labia majora. Both types cause acute pain and need incision and drainage.

Table 7.4 Investigations of pelvic pain and dyspareunia

Investigation	Procedure
Blood tests Pregnancy test	Full blood count/group and save/C-reactive protein
Infection screen	Midstream urine sample Vulval/high vaginal swabs Endocervical/urethral swabs
Radiological investigations	Pelvic ultrasound scan Abdominal X-ray
Biopsy for vulval disease	
Laparoscopy to exclude: endometriosis ovarian cyst ectopic pregnancy adhesions pelvic inflammatory disease	

Table 7.3 shows the diagnoses responsible for both pelvic pain and superficial dyspareunia that might affect the vulva and vagina. A speculum examination should be performed to look for discharge and cervical pathology.

A bimanual vaginal examination should be performed and the adnexa should be examined.

Generalized tenderness, including uterine, is more common with PID. This condition is also associated with cervical excitation (cervical motion tenderness), which indicates peritonism. The tenderness may be unilateral with an ovarian cyst or an ectopic pregnancy. A common site for endometriosis is the pouch of Douglas, and tender nodules can be palpated in the posterior fornix. If an adnexal mass is palpated, this could indicate a tubo-ovarian abscess, ovarian cyst or endometrioma, or ectopic pregnancy. The uterus is enlarged in pregnancy and a fixed, tender, retroverted uterus could be a result of endometriosis or PID. The uterus typically feels tender and bulky with adenomyosis.

INVESTIGATIONS

Target investigations for a specific differential as highlighted by the history if possible. A summary list of the investigations used in patients who present with pelvic pain and dyspareunia is shown in Table 7.4.

Observations

Regular observations are required, particularly in acute presentations to assess pulse, blood pressure, temperature, respiratory rate and oxygen saturation. Pyrexia and tachycardia are associated with PID. Rupture of an ovarian cyst

can cause intraperitoneal bleeding and, subsequently, hypotension with tachycardia. A ruptured ectopic pregnancy would also present with these signs. It should be noted that hypotension is a late sign in an otherwise healthy patient and its absence does not exclude these diagnoses.

Urine test

A urine pregnancy test is mandatory in a patient of reproductive age with acute abdominal pain. It must be performed regardless of the date of the last menstrual period or if the symptoms suggest a gastrointestinal cause. It may highlight or exclude pregnancy, ectopic pregnancy or miscarriage as the cause. A midstream urine sample should be sent to exclude a urinary tract infection.

Vaginal swabs

Swabs for sexually transmitted infection should be sent whether the pain history is chronic or acute. Most importantly these should include a test for *Chlamydia* infection, either an endocervical swab or a urine sample.

Blood tests

A full blood count to check haemoglobin and group-and-save sample are necessary if there is an early pregnancy complication with vaginal or suspected intraperitoneal bleeding. A white blood cell count and a C-reactive protein level will aid diagnosis of infection.

Pelvic ultrasound

A pelvic ultrasound scan is important in acute and chronic pain, as well as in case of deep dyspareunia. Pathology can include ovarian cysts, uterine fibroids or ectopic pregnancy.

Specialist tests

If the appearances of the vulva are abnormal, a biopsy may be indicated. This can be performed under local anaesthesia, depending on the size of the lesion. Depending on the suspected pathology a diagnostic or operative laparoscopy may be appropriate.

TREATMENT

Management of acute or chronic pelvic pain depends on the underlying diagnoses, which are explored in other chapters.

See Figs 7.1 and 7.2 for the algorithms to aid diagnosis of pelvic pain and dyspareunia.

ETHICS

As with all chronic pain it is important to consider psychological and social factors as well as physical causes of pain. Women must be supported and offered advice, for example, introduction to support groups, or referral to a pain clinic.

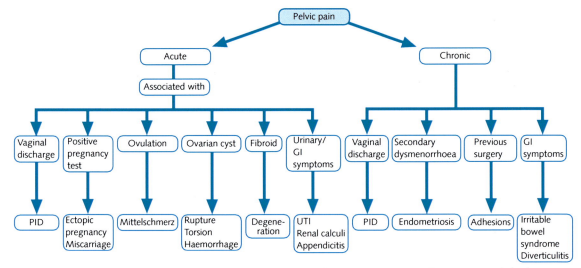

Fig. 7.1 Algorithm for pelvic pain. *GI,* Gastrointestinal; *PID,* pelvic inflammatory disease; *UTI,* urinary tract infection.

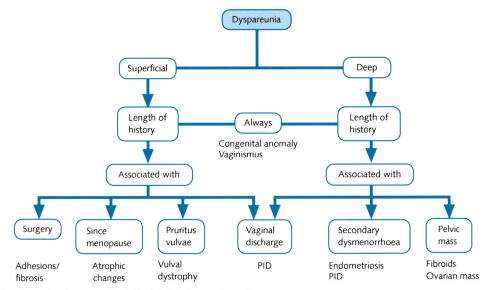

Fig. 7.2 Algorithm for dyspareunia. *PID,* Pelvic inflammatory disease.

Chapter Summary

- Ability to identify and diagnose both acute and chronic gynaecological conditions is crucial to enable timely and appropriate management.
- In presentations of acute abdominal pain, conditions that are considered a gynaecological emergency such as an ectopic and ovarian torsion should be considered and excluded first.
- Accurate diagnosis and effective management from the first presentation may help to reduce permanent ill effects of an acute presentation, or extensive investigations and operations in chronic conditions.
- There is a wide range of differential diagnosis for pelvic pain and dyspareunia that should be explored. It is, however, important to consider diagnosis that are nongynaecological.

Vaginal discharge and sexually transmitted infections

BACKGROUND

Vaginal discharge is a normal physiological process, which varies with the changing oestrogen levels associated with the luteal phase of the menstrual cycle and pregnancy. Other common physiological causes of vaginal discharge are:

- vaginal transudate
- cervical mucus
- residual menstrual fluid
- vestibular gland secretions

However, some vaginal discharge can be pathological, and these causes must be excluded before it is concluded as physiological. The differential diagnoses of pathological vaginal discharge are presented in Table 8.1. The most common pathological causes are infections, both sexually transmitted and nonsexually transmitted. The most significant pathologies are malignancies, such as cervical carcinoma, which must be considered and ruled out in the investigations.

> ### COMMUNICATION
>
> Do not forget to reassure the patient that vaginal discharge might simply be physiological, related to the menstrual cycle or to pregnancy. However, pathological causes need to be excluded.

Table 8.1 Differential diagnosis of pathological vaginal discharge

Diagnosis	Cause of discharge

Infective	Sexually transmitted infection
	   Chlamydia trachomatis
	   Trichomonas vaginalis
	   Neisseria gonorrhoeae
	Infection not sexually transmitted
	   Candida albicans
	   Bacterial vaginosis

Inflammatory	Allergy to soap/contraceptives, etc. Atrophic changes Postoperative granulation tissue
Malignancy	Vulval carcinoma Cervical carcinoma Uterine carcinoma
Foreign body	Retained tampon/condom Ring pessaries
Fistula	From bowel, bladder or urethra to vagina

DIAGNOSIS

History

In the history it is important to establish the nature of the discharge, along with associated symptoms such as abdominal pain or weight loss.

Description of the discharge can help identify the origin and you should ask:

- timing of onset
- colour
- odour
- presence of blood
- irritation

> #### HISTORY
>
> Have you noticed any increase or change to vaginal discharge? What colour is it? Is there an offensive smell? Some causes of vaginal discharge have a typical appearance, such as *Candida*, which appears as a thick, itchy and white discharge without an offensive smell, whereas with bacterial vaginosis there is typically a grey, fishy-smelling discharge.
>
> Associated symptoms should be explored. Do you have any abdominal pain? Have you had any nausea or vomiting? Have you had any high temperatures? Have you had any urinary symptoms? Have you recently noticed unintended weight loss or reduced appetite? Lower abdominal pain, backache and dyspareunia suggest infection in a younger woman, such as pelvic inflammatory disease (see Chapter 9), but could highlight malignancy in older age groups. Urinary symptoms, such as dysuria and frequency, might be present with a sexually transmitted infection.
>
> It is important to take a full gynaecological history, first whether the woman is premenopausal or postmenopausal. Do you have any gynaecological history, or did you have a previous surgery? Are you up to date with smear tests and have these been normal? The date of the menopause and the last cervical smear test are relevant, particularly if malignancy is suspected. A ring

pessary might previously have been sited to relieve genital prolapse, which could be causing excess discharge. Previous history of gynaecological surgery could be linked with development of a ureterovaginal or vesicovaginal fistula.

Are you currently or have you ever been sexually active? Have you previously been diagnosed with a sexually transmitted infection and if so was it treated? What contraception do you use and do you regularly use barrier contraception? A full sexual history should be explored to assess the patients individual risk of sexually transmitted infection. A history of sexual partners should also be explored, such as a new partner, or multiple recent partners. Recent change of partner increases the risk, particularly if no barrier contraception has been used.

Take a full medical and medication history, as conditions such as diabetes or recent antibiotic use can predispose to *Candida* infection.

To complete your history, enquire about vaginal hygiene or changes to washing powders or soaps, which can cause allergic reactions or irritation.

Pelvic examination may reveal adnexal tenderness, cervical motion tenderness or uterine tenderness, suggesting PID. An adnexal mass would be suspicious for a pelvic tumour.

CLINICAL NOTES

Thrush is a very common inflammatory dermatitis of the vagina and vulva caused by mucosal invasion of commensal yeast, most commonly *Candida albicans* (80%–92%). Symptoms include vulval and vaginal soreness and itch, and a vaginal discharge that is typically thick, white and nonoffensive. There might be signs of erythema, fissuring and oedema.

Diagnosis is made by a vaginal swab from the anterior fornix and wet film examination.

Treatment is with topical antifungal cream or pessary and has a cure rate of over 80%. Oral antifungals may be required for severe cases.

Thrush is associated with antibiotic use, pregnancy and immunocompromised conditions such as diabetes. Women with recurrent episodes should be advised to avoid tight fitting synthetic clothing and irritants such as perfumed products.

Examination

- General examination.
- Abdominal palpation.
- Vulval/vaginal/cervical inspection.
- Bimanual pelvic examination.

Does the patient appear well? General examination should be aimed at identifying signs of systemic infection, such as tachycardia, pyrexia, local lymphadenopathy or malignancy, such as cachexia or generalized lymphadenopathy.

Is there abdominal tenderness? Abdominal palpation should assess for pelvic tenderness, which may be present if the patient has pelvic inflammatory disease (PID), or an abdominal mass if malignancy is suspected. If a pelvic mass is felt, it should be assessed for size, tenderness, mobility and nodularity.

Can you identify any vulval, vaginal or cervical pathology? Inspect these areas carefully both externally and internally using a Cusco's speculum. Examine for:

- vaginal or cervical discharge
- vulval, vaginal or cervical inflammation
- vulval, vaginal or cervical ulceration
- vulval, vaginal or cervical lesions or polyps
- retained foreign bodies
- local tumours

A bimanual vaginal examination should be performed and the adnexa should be examined.

INVESTIGATIONS

Observations

Systemic illness suggests an infectious cause; pyrexia >38% and tachycardia are associated with PID (see Chapter 9).

Urine test

A urine pregnancy test should be performed to exclude pregnancy as the cause. A midstream urine sample should be sent to exclude a urinary tract infection.

Vaginal swabs

Microbiology swabs and a screen for sexually transmitted infections (STIs), including high and low vaginal swabs, endocervical swabs and urethral swabs should be performed. *Chlamydia* infection can be tested by an endocervical swab or a urine sample (Table 8.2).

Blood tests

Raised inflammatory markers (white blood cell count, C-reactive protein level and erythrocyte sedimentation rate) may highlight an infectious cause. Blood cultures should be performed in the event of pyrexia. Occasionally, if malignancy is suspected, tumour markers may be evaluated.

Table 8.2 Investigations for vaginal discharge

Investigation	Cause of discharge
Microbiological swabs	Vulval/high vaginal swab *Candida albicans* *Trichomonas vaginalis*
	Endocervical/urethral swab *Chlamydia trachomatis* *Neisseria gonorrhoeae*
Midstream urine specimen	Infection
Cervical cytology	Cervical disease
Endometrial sampling/ hysteroscopy	Uterine disease
Pelvic ultrasound scan	Pelvic mass
Laparoscopy	Pelvic inflammatory disease Pelvic malignancy

Pelvic ultrasound

Transvaginal ultrasound may identify pathology such as thickened endometrium.

Specialist tests

If abnormalities are noted on the cervix, or cervical smear is due, a cervical smear or biopsy may be taken.

If malignancy is suspected, hysteroscopy with endometrial sampling can be performed as an outpatient procedure or under general anaesthetic.

Laparoscopy could be performed if intraabdominal pathology is suspected or to manage acute PID (see Chapter 9).

CLINICAL NOTES

Bacterial vaginosis (BV) is the most common cause of abnormal discharge in women of childbearing age. In BV the pH of vaginal fluid is elevated above 4.5 and up to 6.0, which causes Lactobacilli, a physiological bacterium in the vagina, to have concentrations up to a 1000-fold greater than normal. Symptoms include a thin, white-grey, offensive 'fishy smelling' vaginal discharge. It is not associated with soreness, itching or irritation. Risk factors for developing the condition include vaginal douching, recent change of sexual partner, smoking and concurrent presence of a sexually transmitted infection.

Diagnosis is made with the presence of the typical discharge, clue cells on microscopy of wet mount and pH of vaginal fluid >4.5.

Treatment is with oral metronidazole, and conservative advice to avoid vaginal douching, shower gel and use of antiseptic agents or shampoo in the bath.

TREATMENT

Treatment of vaginal discharge depends on its origin, and whether this is physiological or pathological.

Treatment of conditions such as PID (Chapter 9), gynaecological malignancies (Chapter 12) and vulval disease (Chapter 13) are detailed in individual chapters.

Women with heavy physiological discharge should be educated that this is a normal process, and advised about female hygiene, as it can be exacerbated by practises such as excessive vaginal washing or douching (Fig. 8.1).

SEXUALLY TRANSMITTED INFECTIONS

Background

STIs are spread through sexual contact, including vaginal, anal and oral sex, although some can also spread via blood, or transmitted from mother to child during pregnancy and childbirth. More than 30 different bacteria, viruses and parasites are responsible for these conditions. Drug resistance, especially for gonorrhoea, is a major threat to the management of STIs worldwide.

Prevalence

The World Health Organization estimates that more than 1 million STIs are acquired every day. Young people are more likely to be diagnosed with an STI than older age groups, and there is also significant geographic variation in distribution.

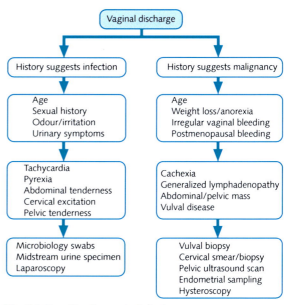

Fig. 8.1 Algorithm for vaginal discharge.

Table 8.3 Summary of common sexually transmitted infections

Organism	Symptoms	Diagnosis	Treatment
Chlamydia	• Asymptomatic (80%) • Postcoital or intermenstrual bleeding • Lower abdominal pain • Purulent vaginal discharge • Dysuria	Endocervical swab Urethral swab Vulvovaginal swab First catch urine less sensitive NAAT	Doxycycline 100 mg bd 7 days or azithromycin 1 g PO stat. Treatment regime may differ in pregnancy
Gonorrhoea	• Asymptomatic (50%) • Increased or altered vaginal discharge • Lower abdominal pain • Dysuria	Endocervical swab Urethral swab NAAT	Ceftriaxone 500 mg IM stat plus azithromycin 1 g oral. Treatment regime may differ in pregnancy
Anaerobes including *Gardnerella* and *Mycoplasma*	Asymptomatic (50%) Offensive fishy-smelling discharge	High vaginal swab for microscopy and culture + pH test > 4.5 + fishy odour with 10% KOH solution	Metronidazole 400 mg bd 7 days

bd, Twice a day; IM, intramuscular; NAAT, nucleic acid amplification test; PO, orally; stat, immediately.

Chlamydia is the most common bacterial STI diagnosed in England (up to 46% of all STIs) and genital warts are the most common viral STI. The following sections present a summary of the most common STIs associated with vaginal discharge (Table 8.3).

GONORRHOEA

Gonorrhoea is infection with the gram-negative diplococcus *Neisseria gonorrhoeae*. It can infect mucous membranes of the urethra and endocervix, and can also affect the rectum, pharynx and conjunctiva. Transmission is by direct inoculation of infected secretions from one mucous membrane to another. Commonly no abnormal findings are present on examination, but symptoms include:

- increased or altered mucopurulent discharge/vaginal discharge
- lower abdominal tenderness
- dysuria
- endocervical bleeding

Vaginal or endocervical swab specimens are equally sensitive for detecting *N. gonorrhoeae* by nucleic acid amplification test (NAAT). Treatment is usually with azithromycin and cephalosporins.

CHLAMYDIA

Chlamydia infection is caused by the obligate intracellular bacterium *Chlamydia trachomatis*. It has a high frequency of transmission and has highest prevalence in young adults. It is transmitted through penetrative sexual intercourse, although the organism can be detected in the conjunctiva and nasopharynx without concomitant genital infection. *Chlamydia* infection is associated with significant morbidity, such as PID (see Chapter 9). *Chlamydia* is asymptomatic in the majority of patients, but symptoms may include:

- increased vaginal discharge
- postcoital and intermenstrual bleeding due to mucopurulent cervicitis
- dysuria
- lower abdominal tenderness
- deep dyspareunia

A vulvo-vaginal swab is the specimen of choice in women, as endocervical and urethral swabs can be less sensitive. First-catch urine samples can also identify *Chlamydia* infection. Treatment is usually with doxycycline or azithromycin.

CLINICAL NOTES

There are a number of sexually transmitted infections (STIs) that are not associated with vaginal discharge.

Genital warts are the most common viral STI and are caused by the human papilloma virus. They are small fleshy growths typically around the vulva or anus and are spread by skin-to-skin contact. Treatments include creams and cryotherapy.

Genital herpes is a common infection caused by the herpes simplex virus, which is the same virus that causes cold sores. Small, painful blisters or sores appear around the vulva, which cause itching, pain and dysuria. Outbreaks can be managed with antiviral medications, but the virus remains in the body in a dormant state. In many cases the virus can become active again and cause further outbreaks of genital herpes.

Syphilis is a bacterial infection of *Treponema pallidum* that in the early stages causes a painless, but highly infectious, genital sore that can last up to 6 weeks. If not identified and treated promptly with antibiotics, patients can develop systemic symptoms such as flu-like illness and rashes. In the late stages of the condition it can cause serious conditions such as dementia symptoms, blindness and cardiac problems.

Human immunodeficiency virus (HIV) targets the immune system by destroying and impairing the function of immune cells, causing immunodeficiency. It is transmitted via a variety of body fluids such as blood, breast milk, semen and vaginal secretions. It is identified by blood tests to detect the presence or absence of antibodies to HIV-1/2 and/or HIV p24 antigen. Symptoms of HIV depend on stage of infection and individuals, but initially tend to be influenza-like illness. If the disease progresses, the state of immunodeficiency can cause severe illness including cancers such as lymphomas. Treatment is by suppression with combinations of antiretroviral therapy. This is not a cure for HIV, but suppresses viral replication.

TRICHOMONAS VAGINALIS

Trichomonas vaginalis is a flagellated protozoon that is found in the vagina, urethra and paraurethral glands. It is transmitted via direct inoculation intravaginally or intraurethrally. Up to 50% are asymptomatic, but the most common symptoms are:

- vaginal discharge, typically 'frothy yellow' with offensive odour
- vulval itching, inflammation or ulceration
- cervicitis, identified by the examination finding of a 'strawberry cervix'

A posterior fornix swab is the specimen of choice in women, and the organism is detected by NAAT. Treatment is usually with metronidazole.

COMPLICATIONS

Morbidity from STIs can be considerable, caused by the sequelae of PID (see Chapter 9). This includes:

- infertility
- ectopic pregnancy
- chronic pelvic pain
- recurrent episodes PID
- perihepatitis
- sexually acquired reactive arthritis in less than 1%

COMMUNICATION

Contact tracing (or partner notification) is the process of contacting and providing healthcare to sexual contacts who may have been at risk of infection from a confirmed case, including providing treatment. The British Association for Sexual Health and HIV advise that the length of time for tracing must include typically 6 months. This process not only protects individuals, but also important for public health to prevent onward infection and reinfection. This is most easily coordinated by a sexual health clinic, and must be done sensitively and confidentially.

● Chapter Summary

- Vaginal discharge can be a troubling symptom for patients, but does not always mean an underlying pathology.
- The most common pathological cause are infections, both sexually transmitted and non-sexually transmitted.
- Diagnosis is elicited from the history and examination, alongside sexually transmitted infection (STI) screening.
- STIs have a profound impact on sexual and reproductive health worldwide, and have significant associated morbidity.
- Sexual health education regarding STIs and the use of barrier contraception is essential to reduce this impact.

Pelvic inflammatory disease

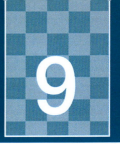

9

Definition

Pelvic inflammatory disease (PID) is defined as the clinical syndrome associated with ascending spread of microorganisms from the endocervix to the endometrium, fallopian tubes and related structures. It can cause endometritis, salpingitis, parametritis, oophoritis, tubo-ovarian abscess or pelvic peritonitis. Severe disease can cause the development of adhesions between the liver and the peritoneum, with perihepatitis, known as 'Fitz–Hugh–Curtis syndrome'.

It usually begins with an acute infection; this might resolve completely or develop a chronic course with repeated acute or subacute episodes.

Prevalence

The true incidence of PID is difficult to determine because of the difficulty in making a clinical diagnosis, and because it may be unrecognized if asymptomatic or presenting atypically. Studies have shown that PID is diagnosed in up to 2% of general practitioner visits for women of reproductive age.

PID is almost always a sexually transmitted disease, therefore its incidence is strongly correlated with the prevalence of sexually transmitted infections, and has increased in most countries (see Chapter 8). In the United States, the highest annual incidence is among sexually active women in their teenage years; 75% of cases occur in women under the age of 25. Table 9.1 outlines risk factors for the development of PID.

Table 9.1 Risk factors for the development of pelvic inflammatory disease

Risk factor	Description
Age	75% of patients are below 25 years
Marital status	Single
Sexual history	Young at first intercourse High frequency of sexual intercourse Multiple sexual partners
Medical history	History of sexually transmitted disease in patient or partner History of pelvic inflammatory disease in patient Recent instrumentation of uterus (e.g., termination of pregnancy)
Contraception	Use of intrauterine contraceptive device, especially insertion within 3 weeks

Aetiology

The most common causative agents for PID are *Neisseria gonorrhoeae* and *Chlamydia trachomatis*, which account for approximately a quarter of cases in the UK, with *Chlamydia* being the most common. They are thought to act as primary pathogens, causing damage to the protective mechanisms of the endocervix and allowing endogenous bacteria from the vagina and cervix into the upper genital tract as secondary invaders (see Chapter 8).

Aerobic and anaerobic organisms in normal vaginal flora, such as *Gardnerella vaginalis*, have also been implicated. *Mycoplasma genitalium* has also been associated with upper genital tract infection in women (see Chapter 8).

PID can also develop secondary to other disease processes, such as appendicitis. Rarely, it is part of more generalized disease such as tuberculosis. Very rarely, PID follows instrumentation of the uterus.

Symptoms

The diagnosis of PID is sometimes difficult to make, because it does not rely on one particular sign or symptom. However, the following symptoms are suggestive of PID:

- bilateral lower abdominal pain
- abnormal vaginal or cervical discharge that may be purulent
- deep dyspareunia
- abnormal vaginal bleeding

On examination you may note adnexal or cervical motion tenderness on bimanual vaginal examination and the patient may be systemically unwell with a fever.

The differential diagnoses include gynaecological conditions such as ovarian cyst accident, endometriosis and early pregnancy complications including ectopic pregnancy, in addition to nongynaecological conditions such as appendicitis, urinary tract infection or constipation (see Chapter 7: Pelvic pain and dyspareunia).

DIAGNOSIS

History

A diagnosis of PID is made on clinical grounds, therefore a focused history is important. The history should elicit any signs or symptoms of PID, and try to exclude possible differentials. A menstrual history and the use of contraception, in particular barrier methods, should be assessed.

Sensitivity is essential when taking a sexual history.

Do you have any pain? A full assessment of any pelvic pain may highlight bilateral lower abdominal pain sometimes found in association with pelvic inflammatory disease (PID).

Associated symptoms along with the pain should be explored. Have you had any nausea or vomiting? Have you had any high temperatures? Have you noticed any increase or change to vaginal discharge? What colour is it? Is there an offensive smell? PID may or may not be associated with vaginal discharge.

Are you currently or have you ever been sexually active? Have you previously been diagnosed with a sexually transmitted infection and if so was it treated? What contraception do you use and do you regularly use barrier contraception? A full sexual history should be explored to assess the patient's individual risk of developing PID. A history of sexual partners should also be explored, such as a new partner or multiple recent partners. Recent change of partner increases the risk, particularly if no barrier contraception has been used.

Examination

Is there abdominal tenderness? Abdominal palpation may identify pelvic and lower abdominal tenderness, which is most commonly bilateral. Right upper quadrant pain may be present due to Fitz–Hugh–Curtis syndrome, but this is uncommon.

Vaginal examination with a speculum may show abnormal cervical or vaginal mucopurulent discharge. This is often slight and may be transient.

A bimanual vaginal examination should be performed and the adnexa should be examined.

Pelvic examination may reveal adnexal tenderness (with or without a palpable mass), cervical motion tenderness or uterine tenderness.

INVESTIGATIONS

Observations

Observations are required, particularly in acute presentations, to assess pulse, blood pressure, temperature, respiratory rate and oxygen saturation. Pyrexia >38 °C and tachycardia are associated with PID.

Urine test

A urine pregnancy test is mandatory in a patient of reproductive age with abdominal pain and should be performed regardless of last menstrual period. It may highlight or exclude pregnancy, ectopic pregnancy or miscarriage as the cause. A midstream urine sample should be sent to exclude a urinary tract infection.

Vaginal swabs

A full screen for sexually transmitted infections, including high and low vaginal swabs, endocervical swabs and urethral swabs should be performed. *Chlamydia* infection can be tested by an endocervical swab or a urine sample. The swabs are examined using nucleic acid amplification tests which have high detection rates. It is important to remember that negative swab results do not rule out a diagnosis of PID.

Blood tests

The aim of blood tests is to establish and monitor signs of infection. White blood cell count, C-reactive protein level and erythrocyte sedimentation rate can be evaluated. However, these may be normal in mild or moderate PID. Blood cultures should be performed in the event of pyrexia. All patients should be offered screening for human immunodeficiency virus (HIV).

Pelvic ultrasound

Transvaginal ultrasound may identify pathology such as tubo-ovarian abscess or alternative diagnoses such as an ovarian cyst.

Specialist tests

Laparoscopy is considered to be the gold standard to diagnose acute PID. However, in practice, it is only considered if the patient fails to respond to antibiotic therapy, or if there is doubt about the differential diagnoses. In acute disease, the pelvis will appear generally inflamed, with pus seen around the fallopian tubes, which may be distended. In chronic disease, there may be generalized pelvic adhesions or evidence of old tubal disease or hydrosalpinges. Fitz–Hugh–Curtis syndrome indicates previous chlamydia infection, when the typical bow-string perihepatic adhesions are seen.

TREATMENT

There should be a low threshold for empirical treatment for PID, even in the absence of definitive diagnostic criteria, as delaying treatment increases the risk of long-term sequelae, such as ectopic pregnancy, infertility and pelvic pain. Treatment should therefore be started prior to obtaining the results of microbiology specimens.

The principle of treatment is:

- broad-spectrum antibiotic treatment
- surgery
- contact tracing

Antibiotic choice is based on therapy to cover gonorrhoea and chlamydia, and other aerobic and anaerobic bacteria commonly isolated from the upper genital tract in women with PID. There are various advised regimes that are usually influenced by local antimicrobial sensitivity patterns and guidelines. An example regime is ceftriaxone 2 g IV once daily, plus doxycycline 100 mg oral twice daily, plus metronidazole 400 mg oral twice daily.

Outpatient therapy with oral treatment has been shown be as effective as inpatient treatment for patients with clinically mild to moderate disease. In-patient treatment with intravenous antibiotics is indicated for more severe clinical disease, for example, pyrexia, tubo-ovarian abscess and signs of pelvic peritonitis. Admission should also be considered if there is lack of response to oral therapy or pregnancy. Intravenous therapy should be continued until 24 hours after clinical improvement and then switched to oral. If outpatient therapy is being used, review at 72 hours is recommended to ensure improvement in clinical symptoms and signs, or to highlight if further investigations or treatments are required.

If the patient fails to respond to antibiotic therapy, laparoscopy helps to resolve the disease by draining pelvic abscesses and dividing adhesions. Ultrasound-guided aspiration of pelvic fluid collections is less invasive and may be equally effective.

If a patient resumes sexual intercourse with a partner who is infected but untreated, there is obviously a high chance of re-infection. It is, therefore, important to trace all current partners so that they can all be given treatment, either empirically or as a result of microbiology results. Tracing of contacts within a 6-month period of onset of symptoms is recommended but this period may be influenced by the sexual history. This should be done in a sensitive manner and confidentiality is essential at all times. Contact tracing can be done more effectively by referring the patient to a genitourinary medicine clinic. The patient should avoid intercourse until all current partners have completed a course of treatment.

COMPLICATIONS

- Infertility
- Ectopic pregnancy
- Chronic pelvic pain
- Recurrent episodes of PID

The long-term morbidity associated with acute PID is considerable (Table 9.2), and therefore the need for prompt appropriate treatment is important. Early diagnosis and treatment are essential to reduce the risk of long-term complications.

Moderately severe disease is associated with inflammation and oedema in the fallopian tubes, with deposits of fibrin and subsequent adhesion formation between the pelvic and abdominal organs. Tubal morphology and

Table 9.2 Complications of pelvic inflammatory disease

Type of complication	Description
Short term	Pelvic abscess formation Septicaemia Septic shock
Long term	Infertility Ectopic pregnancy Chronic pelvic pain Dyspareunia Menstrual disturbances Psychological effects

ETHICS

Transmission of sexually transmitted diseases (STDs), and therefore pelvic inflammatory disease, is prevented using barrier methods of contraception. Therefore, it is hugely important to educate sexually active adults about the importance of contraception and the need to screen for STDs. This can be done both at routine appointments and opportunistically for those at risk, for example, a termination of pregnancy clinic.

function are affected, resulting in subfertility and an increased risk of ectopic pregnancy. As PID can be asymptomatic, patients may present many years after the acute infection with subfertility.

Adhesions in the pelvis may lead to chronic pain, either as a sole feature or in relation to menstruation or sexual intercourse.

● Chapter Summary

- Pelvic inflammatory disease (PID) is an infective condition of the genital tract associated most commonly with sexually transmitted infections.
- PID may be symptomatic or asymptomatic and there are no individual symptoms that are diagnostic of PID, but a general clinical picture.
- Primary prevention of the disease is of great importance as it is associated with high complication rates including tubal infertility, ectopic pregnancy and chronic pelvic pain.
- Early diagnosis and timely treatment reduces long-term risks.

Contraception and termination of pregnancy

INDICATIONS

Contraception is an important aspect of women's health acting as both birth control and protection from sexually transmitted infections (STIs). Up to 65% of women of reproductive age worldwide use some form of contraception.

Contraception options vary in their method of action, mode of delivery, reversibility, pregnancy prevention, STI protection and contraindications. It is therefore crucial to individualize contraception to each woman, educating them with accurate information and allowing them to make informed decisions about their choices. To be effective, contraception must be used correctly and consistently, which is directly related to the user.

When discussing contraception needs with women it is important to discuss the superior effectiveness of long-acting reversible contraception (LARC).

All forms of contraception have a failure rate, based on both 'user error' and integral failure rates (Table 10.1). 'Typical use' rates are therefore lower than 'perfect use' as it includes common incorrect use such as forgotten pills and incorrectly placed condoms.

Table 10.1 Methods of contraception and their relative effectiveness

Method	Perfect use	Typical use (%)
Sterilization female	Lifetime failure rate 1 in 200–500	—
Sterilization male	Lifetime failure rate 1 in 2000	—
Combined oral contraceptive pill	>99%	91
Progesterone-only pill	>99%	91
Depot injection	>99%	94
Contraceptive implant	>99%	>99
Intrauterine contraceptive device (IUCD)	>99%	>99
Mirena intrauterine system (has the lowest failure rate in IUCD)	>99%	>99
Condom: male	98%	82
Diaphragm	95%	79
Natural fertility methods	up to 99%	76

NATURAL METHODS

Fertile and infertile times of the menstrual cycle can be identified by changes in 'fertility indicators'. These include body temperature, cervical mucus and menstrual cycle length. Basal body temperature rises 0.2°C–0.4°C when progesterone is released from the corpus luteum. Women using the 'rhythm method' will only have intercourse within their infertile times.

'Coitus interruptus' or 'withdrawal method' is a contraceptive technique using withdrawal during intercourse prior to ejaculation.

Advantages

Natural methods can help to either avoid or plan a pregnancy. There are no unwanted physical side-effects as there is no hormone involvement and therefore safe with any co-existing medical conditions. It is also acceptable to all faiths and cultures.

Disadvantages

This method relies on regular menstrual cycles, record-keeping and commitment and can take three to six cycles to learn effectively. Events such as illness, stress or travel may alter the fertility indicators.

At fertile times partners must avoid sex or use barrier contraception, and natural methods do not protect against STI. The failure rate with coitus interruptus is high due to variable control of ejaculation and the presence of some sperm within pre-ejaculatory fluid.

Contraindications

There are no medical contraindications.

BARRIER CONTRACEPTION

Barrier contraception includes the male condom, female condom, female diaphragm and cervical cap. It was previously advised to use a spermicide (e.g., nonoxynol-9) to increase effectiveness of barrier contraception. However, more recent evidence, supported by the World Health Organization (WHO), shows that nonoxynol-9 offers no protection from STI, and may increase risk of human immunodeficiency virus (HIV) transmission.

Advantages

When used correctly barrier protection is effective and without side-effects. They are easily available and only need to be used at the time of intercourse. Crucially, condoms help to protect both partners against the transmission of STI and HIV.

Disadvantages

Barrier contraception must be applied prior to penetration and can reduce degree of sensation. The diaphragm and cap must be fitted and checked regularly by a trained professional. Condoms can slip or split if not used correctly or if of wrong size or shape and there can be difficulties in correct placement of a female condom. User error greatly increases barrier method failure rates.

Contraindications

Occasionally, people can also have sensitivities or allergy to latex condoms, although polyurethane and polyisoprene condoms are widely available.

HORMONAL CONTRACEPTION

Combined oral contraceptive pill

Since their introduction in 1961, various combinations of oestrogen and progestogens have been used to prevent pregnancy. These are most widely available as a contraceptive pill or alternatively as a skin patch or vaginal ring.

Combined oral contraceptives have several modes of action. They thicken the cervical mucus which prevents sperm from reaching the uterus, and thin the endometrial lining to discourage implantation. It inhibits ovulation by altering hormone levels – inhibiting follicular-stimulating hormone and preventing follicular ripening, and preventing the luteinizing hormone surge.

Advantages

The method is reliable if taken correctly, convenient and not intercourse related. It commonly reduces dysmenorrhoea, menorrhagia and premenstrual symptoms. It can reduce occurrence of functional ovarian cysts and incidence of ovarian, endometrium and colon cancer. Some combined oral contraceptive pill (COCP) preparations improve acne and menopausal symptoms. Vaginal rings can stay in place for up to 3 weeks.

Disadvantages

The pill can have some serious side-effects, but these are uncommon. The main risks are cardiovascular complications and thromboembolic disease. This includes hypertension, venous thrombosis [venous thromboembolism (VTE)], arterial thrombosis, heart attack or stroke. The risk of developing these complications increases with age, obesity, smoking, diabetes and hypertension.

Research suggests that there is a small increase in the risk of developing cervical intraepithelial neoplasia or cervical cancer following prolonged use. There is mixed evidence regarding increased risk of breast cancer while taking COCP.

More minor side-effects include weight gain, breakthrough bleeding, headaches, nausea, breast tenderness and mood changes.

The effectiveness of COCP is limited by some antibiotics, hepatic enzyme-inducing drugs, vomiting and diarrhoea. COCP does not have any protection against STI.

Contraindications

CLINICAL NOTES

Health professionals must ask women about their medication use including prescription, over-the-counter, herbal, recreational drugs and dietary supplements. Concurrent medications may increase or decrease serum levels of contraceptive hormones; similarly, hormonal contraception may increase or decrease serum levels of other medications. This can potentially cause adverse effects.

Guidance regarding drug interactions and contraception is available on the Faculty of Sexual and Reproductive Healthcare website and in the British National Formulary.

CLINICAL NOTES

The UK Medical Eligibility criteria for contraceptive use guidelines in full can be easily online via https://www.fsrh.org/ukmec.

UK medical eligibility criteria for contraceptive use (UKMEC) is a document produced by the Faculty of Sexual and Reproductive Healthcare that offers evidence-based guidance to providers of contraception regarding who can use contraceptive methods safely, particularly contraindications linked to particular medical conditions. It categorizes contraceptive options with various medical conditions from 'no restriction' to 'unacceptable health risk' (Table 10.2). Example of an absolute contraindications to COCP include

Table 10.2 Definition of UK Medical Eligibility criteria for contraceptive use (UKMEC) categories

UKMEC category	Definition
1	A condition for which there is no restriction for the use of the method.
2	A condition where the advantages of using the method generally outweigh the theoretical or proven risks.
3	A condition where the theoretical or proven risks usually outweigh the advantages of using the method. The provision of a method requires expert clinical judgement and/or referral to a specialist contraceptive provider, because use of the method is not usually recommended unless other more appropriate methods are not available or not acceptable.
4	A condition that represents an unacceptable health risk if the method is used.

Table 10.3 Contraindications to the combined oral contraceptive pill

Degree of contraindication	Description
Absolute	Heavy smoker Vascular disease/ischaemic heart disease/stroke History of/current venous thromboembolism Thrombogenic mutations Atrial fibrillation Migraine with aura Current breast cancer Liver disease Systemic lupus erythematosus with antibodies Pregnancy Oestrogen-dependant tumour
Relative	Family history of thrombosis Diabetes with nephropathic complications Hypertension Body mass index >35 kg/m²

atrial fibrillation and previous personal history of VTE (see Table 10.3). The COCP should be discontinued 4 weeks before major surgery due to the increased risk of VTE.

Progesterone-only contraception

Progesterone-only contraception has a similar mode of action to combined contraceptives with changes to cervical mucus and endometrium, but ovulation is only suppressed in 50%–60% of cycles. There are multiple different progesterone contraceptive options available, such as the progesterone-only pill (POP), depo-injections and implants.

Advantages
Progesterone-only methods are good contraceptive choices for women with contraindications for COCP, such as age over 35 and smokers. It also can help with premenstrual symptoms and painful periods. The contraceptive injection has varied lengths of efficacy, from 8–13 weeks, depending on the preparation used.

Disadvantages
Changes to the menstrual cycle, such as irregularity, increased frequency and breakthrough bleeding tend to settle within 6 months. Side-effects can also include spotty skin, breast tenderness, weight change and headaches. It is very important to take the POP at the same time every day; late pills, vomiting and severe diarrhoea can make it less effective. If you do become pregnant using the POP, there is a risk of it being an ectopic pregnancy.

Contraindications
As per UKMEC, there are few contraindications to progesterone-only methods. One absolute contraindication is a current diagnosis of breast cancer.

INTRAUTERINE AND IMPLANTED CONTRACEPTION

Intrauterine and implanted contraception are also known as 'LARC'. They are highly effective methods of preventing pregnancy, easy to use and patient friendly.

Contraindications to an intrauterine contraceptive device include:

- pregnancy
- undiagnosed uterine bleeding
- active or past history of pelvic inflammatory disease
- previous ectopic pregnancy or tubal surgery

Contraceptive implant

The contraceptive implant is a small, flexible rod put under the skin of the upper arm which releases progestogen. It is a highly effective contraception that can be left in place for 3 years, or removed earlier. It requires a small procedure under local anaesthesia for implantation and removal.

Mirena coil intrauterine system

The intrauterine system (IUS) is a small T-shaped plastic device that releases progesterone locally into the uterus for up to 5 years. Periods usually become shorter, lighter and can even stop, although this may take up to 6 months. Insertion of the IUS can cause discomfort particularly if the patient is nulliparous and often a local anaesthetic is injected into the cervix. Two fine threads are left hanging through the cervical os which can be examined to ensure the coil is still in place. Complications include expulsion or uterine perforation of the IUS, and if a pregnancy occurs, it is more likely to be ectopic. A 'Jaydess' is a newly available slightly smaller IUS that is felt to be easier to fit in nulliparous women.

Intrauterine device

The intrauterine device (IUD) is a small T-shaped plastic and copper device that works by both spermicidal action and thickening cervical mucus, and can remain in place for up to 10 years. Periods can become heavier or more painful with one in place. Insertion is by the same method as the IUS and the complication issues are the same (Fig. 10.1).

STERILIZATION

Sterilization is considered a permanent method of preventing pregnancy using surgical methods. As it is considered irreversible, it is important that the patient is adequately counselled, that their family is complete and that they have considered other forms of contraception.

Male sterilization

Male sterilization is known as a 'vasectomy'. It is ligation of the vas deferens bilaterally via incisions in the scrotum performed under a local anaesthetic. At 3 and 4 months postoperatively sperm samples must be tested to confirm azoospermia and barrier contraception should be used until

this is confirmed. There is a failure rate of this procedure of approximately 1:2000 after azoospermia is confirmed. A complication of the procedure is chronic testicular pain.

Female sterilization

Female sterilization is performed by cutting, sealing or blocking the fallopian tubes, therefore preventing fertilization. It can be performed laparoscopically or by laparotomy, for example, at the time of caesarean section. There is a failure rate of 1:200–500 with this method. There are no short- or long-term serious side-effects other than expected surgical complications.

COMMUNICATION

It must be emphasized to all women that nonbarrier contraception does not protect from sexually transmitted infections and should still be used, particularly with new or occasional partners. They should be advised to attend regular sexual health checks.

POSTNATAL CONTRACEPTION

Postnatal contraception is an important part of post-pregnancy counselling, to prevent unplanned pregnancies following childbirth. An interval of less than 12 months can increase preterm birth, low-birthweight and small-for-gestational age babies. This is relevant for both breastfeeding and nonbreastfeeding women as soon as possible, as ovulation can resume soon afterwards.

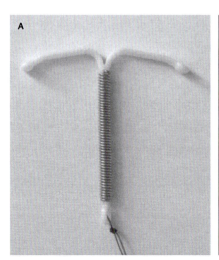
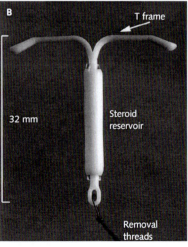

Fig. 10.1 Types of intrauterine contraceptive device: (A) Copper; (B) Mirena intrauterine system.

Most methods of contraception including POP and progesterone implants can be initiated safely immediately, with the exception of COCP. Women can initiate the COCP from 21 days after childbirth if they are not breastfeeding and have no additional VTE or hormonal contraception risk factors. If breastfeeding or any additional VTE risk factors are present, COCP can only be started from 6 weeks postnatally. IUDs can be inserted immediately after birth, even at the time of caesarean section, up to 48 hours after delivery. If 48 hours have passed, insertion should be after 28 days.

POST ABORTION/MISCARRIAGE

Abortion services should offer methods of contraception, particularly LARC to women prior to their discharge. In the event of miscarriage or ectopic pregnancy we should allow women to discuss their conception plans and offer contraception if requested.

Any method of contraception can be initiated after an uncomplicated abortion or miscarriage, as long as there is no presence of sepsis.

BREASTFEEDING

Breastfeeding can be an effective form of contraception if less than 6 months postpartum, amenorrhoeic and fully breastfeeding. However, if breastfeeding decreases, menstruation returns or if it is over 6 months postpartum, risk of pregnancy increases. Progesterone-based contraception methods have no adverse effects on lactation, infant growth or development. COCP should wait until 6 weeks postpartum if breastfeeding; due to minimal evidence of effect of COCP in breastmilk on child development.

EMERGENCY CONTRACEPTION

Emergency contraception is aimed to prevent unplanned pregnancy in the event of contraceptive failure or unprotected sexual intercourse (UPSI). Patients must be counselled about the risks of failure, and therefore pregnancy even after taking emergency contraception. Pregnancy must be excluded prior to providing the medication.

There are three methods currently available over-the-counter in the UK; levonorgestrel (Levonelle), ulipristal acetate (EllaOne) and the copper IUD (Cu-IUD).

Levonorgestrel is a synthetic progestogen taken in a single 1.5-mg tablet that must be used within 72 hours (3 days) of the episode of UPSI. If taken before the preovulation oestrogen surge, ovulation can be inhibited for 5–7 days and fertilization prevented. Side-effects include dizziness, nausea, headaches, breast tenderness or abdominal pain.

Vomiting occurs in approximately 1% of patients, and the treatment should be repeated if vomiting occurs within 2 hours of ingestion.

Ulipristal acetate is a selective progesterone receptor modulator taken in a single-dose 30-mg tablet that must be used within 120 hours (5 days) of UPSI. It inhibits ovulation and alters endometrial lining to prevent implantation. It has a similar side-effect profile to levonorgestrel.

Cu-IUD can be inserted up to 120 hours (5 days) following UPSI or more, if not more than 5 days after the earliest predicted date of ovulation. The copper has a toxic effect on the sperm and ovum, which prevents fertilization. It has the advantage of providing ongoing contraception.

It is important to offer a regular method of contraception and risk assessment for STIs following use of emergency contraception.

TERMINATION OF PREGNANCY

The Abortion Act 1967, amended by the Human Fertilisation and Embryology Act 1990, instructs abortion care in England, Scotland and Wales. Two registered medical practitioners must agree that an abortion is justified within the terms of the Act, agreeing on one of five circumstances. Over 98% of abortions are undertaken due to risk to mental or physical health of the woman or her children.

Medical

Medical abortions can be performed at any gestation using regimes of mifepristone, an antiprogesterone, and misoprostol, a prostaglandin analogue. In early pregnancy (<63 days) mifepristone (200 mg) is taken orally followed by misoprostol (800 mcg) after 24–48 hours orally or vaginally. At later gestations the misoprostol can be readministered every 3 hours up to four further doses. Fetocide should be performed before medical abortion after 21 weeks and 6 days of gestation to ensure there is no risk of a live birth. Complete abortion occurs in 95% of patients. If there is clinical evidence that the abortion is incomplete, then surgical evacuation may be required.

Surgical

Vacuum aspiration is an appropriate method of surgical abortion up to 14 weeks of gestation and is the most commonly used method up to 12 weeks. During vacuum aspiration, the uterus is emptied using a suction cannula. After 14 weeks surgical abortion by dilatation and evacuation can be performed; this may require uterine contents to be removed with forceps. Cervical preparation should be considered in all cases, particularly in nulliparous women, with either prostaglandin priming (misoprostol) or osmotic dilators at later gestation.

Complications

Abortion is a safe procedure with major complications being uncommon. Complications are more common with surgical methods. These include pain, infection, bleeding and trauma to the cervix and uterus including perforation. Prior to an abortion it is advised to screen for STIs and give prophylactic antibiotics. Retained products of conception following the procedure may result in heavier bleeding, and a second evacuation may be required. It is crucial to determine rhesus status, as if rhesus negative, anti-D is required.

ETHICS

It is crucial to appreciate the physical symptoms and psychological sequelae experienced after an abortion. It is important to provide women with information regarding counselling, support and contraceptive advice.

● Chapter Summary

- There is a huge variety of options available for women to manage their contraception and sexually transmitted infection protection, additionally having beneficial effects to their periods.
- Clinicians should educate women about these options, so they are able to make the most appropriate choice for them.
- It is important to identify risk factors and contraindications for various methods and encourage the use of long-acting reversible contraception method when appropriate.

Benign gynaecological tumours

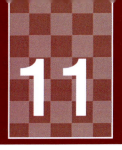

BACKGROUND

Prevalence

Among benign ovarian tumours, ovarian cysts are common, and in the majority of both premenopausal and postmenopausal women these cysts are asymptomatic and resolve spontaneously. The true prevalence is unclear due to the lack of consistent reporting and a high likelihood of spontaneous resolution. Almost all ovarian masses and cysts are benign in premenopausal women with an incidence of malignancy of 1:1000. In postmenopausal women over the age of 50 years the incidence of malignancy increases to 3:1000.

Excluding the physiological group, a germ-cell tumour is most common in premenopausal women, and in postmenopausal women epithelial tumours are the most common.

Risk factors for ovarian tumours include infertility treatment and use of ovulation-induction agents, tamoxifen therapy, hypothyroidism and smoking.

Uterine leiomyomas (fibroids) are covered in detail in Chapter 5 and cysts associated with endometriosis (endometriomas) in Chapter 6; premalignant conditions are also covered in Chapter 12. About 10% of suspected ovarian masses are ultimately found to be nonovarian in origin.

Symptoms

Benign ovarian tumours can be asymptomatic and therefore detected incidentally, for example, at the time of a routine antenatal scan. However, ovarian cyst pathology is one of the most common causes for gynaecological hospital admissions.

The presenting symptom is most commonly pain, which can be secondary to ovarian torsion, cyst rupture or haemorrhage within the cyst. In cyst rupture or ovarian torsion the pain can be severe and the patient may present with an acute abdomen. If the cyst is very large, the patient may present with abdominal swelling or pressure effects on the bowel or bladder. Rarely if the cyst or mass is secretory, they may present with hormonal effects.

RED FLAG

In any woman presenting with abdominal pain it is crucial to rule out an ectopic pregnancy by performing a urinary pregnancy test. It is also important to consider differential diagnoses that require urgent management, such as appendicitis (see Table 11.1).

DIAGNOSIS

History

The diagnosis of an ovarian cyst or tumour is helped by a thorough history alongside the examination. However, it is important to not miss an alternative diagnosis as individual symptoms could be related to different pathology (Table 11.1).

A full medical and gynaecological history should be taken. Important features include:

- characteristics of any pain
- menstrual and gynaecological history
- associated symptoms

HISTORY

Do you have pain? Describe the pain, is it acute or chronic? How severe is the pain? Is it constant or colicky? A full assessment of the pain is required. The nature of the pain may help narrow down the diagnosis and assess for risk of ovarian torsion. In torsion the pain is usually sudden onset and severe.

What was the date of your last menstrual period? Do you have regular periods? What are your periods like? It may be possible to attribute midcyclical pain to ovulation (mittelschmerz), but postovulation pain to a haemorrhagic corpus luteal cyst, for example.

Do you have any prior gynaecological history? Have you previously had ovarian cysts? Cysts such as physiological cysts and endometriomas can reoccur, so a prior history of cysts may increase the index of suspicion.

Are you experiencing any dyspareunia or vaginal discomfort? Have you noted any abdominal swelling or urinary symptoms? These symptoms are more common with a larger pelvic mass, or cysts in the pouch of Douglas.

Are you up-to-date with smear tests? Do you have any family or personal history of ovarian or breast cancer? Have you been systemically unwell or noted unintentional weight loss? It is important to assess risk factors for malignancy.

Have you had any nausea or vomiting? Do you have any gastrointestinal or urinary upset? These symptoms could indicate an alternative diagnosis, but can also be associated with a cyst accident. Infective symptoms could also suggest a diagnosis of pelvic inflammatory disease.

Table 11.1 Differential diagnoses for ovarian tumours

Symptom	Differential diagnosis
Pain	Ectopic pregnancy Spontaneous miscarriage Pelvic inflammatory disease Appendicitis Diverticulitis
Abdominal swelling	Pregnancy Fibroid uterus Full bladder
Pressure effects	Constipation Urine frequency Vaginal prolapse
Hormonal effects	Menstrual irregularity Postmenopausal bleeding Precocious puberty

Examination

General observations are important in the assessment. Does the patient look well or unwell? Is she pale and shocked? Is her pain under control? This first snapshot assessment will highlight a patient who may be acutely unwell with an acute abdomen.

Is there abdominal distension? This may be visible due to the cyst, or secondary to ascites if the cyst is malignant. Determine the size, tenderness, mobility and nodularity of the cyst. A large ovarian tumour can extend out of the pelvis and be palpated abdominally. Ascites should be excluded by testing for shifting dullness.

Is there pain? Examining the abdomen you may illicit tenderness if a cyst is present; typically the focus of pain is in the iliac fossa. Assess for guarding or peritonism.

A bimanual vaginal examination should be performed and the adnexa should be examined. If the patient has a cyst or tumour, it commonly causes fullness and tenderness on the affected side. If a mass is felt, determine the size, tenderness, mobility and nodularity.

If bimanual examination is normal, this suggests a nongynaecological cause for symptoms. Assessing the size of the uterus may exclude fibroids.

Investigations

Observations

Reviewing the observations is crucial to assess whether the patient is haemodynamically stable. A patient unwell with an ovarian torsion or ruptured haemorrhage cyst may have raised pulse and low blood pressure. Significant pain may also result in elevated pulse and blood pressure.

Urinary pregnancy test or serum β-human chorionic gonadotropin

To exclude pregnancy.

Blood tests

Full blood count to assess current haemoglobin levels (Hb) and assess for new anaemia, which may be indicative of a ruptured haemorrhagic cyst. White blood cell count and C-reactive protein would likely be within the normal range.

Transvaginal ultrasound

Transvaginal ultrasound is the diagnostic tool of choice for diagnosis of an ovarian pathology. Because of typical ultrasound appearances of ovarian cysts, both the presence and the type of cyst can often be identified. Transabdominal scan can be performed if it is not appropriate for a vaginal scan.

High vaginal/endocervical swabs

These are important if there is suspicion of pelvic inflammatory disease or a tubo-ovarian abscess (see Chapter 9).

Specialist tests

If malignancy is suspected, further imaging such as computed tomography scanning may be required. Tumour marker blood tests such as Ca-125 may be performed if concerned about malignancy, but should not be performed routinely as they can be raised with benign gynaecological pathology such as fibroids, and can cause undue anxiety. Ca-125 levels are required to calculate the risk of malignancy index (RMI; see discussion later in this chapter). Serum α-fetoprotein and human chorionic gonadotropin (HCG) levels can be assessed if germ-cell tumours are suspected.

TYPES OF TUMOUR

Ovarian tumours can be physiological (functional) or pathological (either benign or malignant). Their classifications depend on the ovarian tissue from which they arise (Table 11.2).

Table 11.2 Classification of benign ovarian tumours

Type of tumour	Name
Physiological	Follicular cysts Luteal cysts
Benign epithelial tumours	Serous cystadenoma Mucinous cystadenoma Endometrioid cystadenoma Brenner
Benign germ-cell tumours	Mature cystic teratoma (dermoid cyst) Mature solid teratoma
Benign sex cord stromal tumours	Theca cell tumours Fibroma Sertoli–Leydig cell tumour
Other benign ovarian tumours	Endometriotic cyst

Physiological cysts

These are often asymptomatic and tend to occur in younger women. As suggested by their name they are cysts that occur as the result of a normal physiological process.

Follicular cysts

These are simple cysts that occur as a result of nonrupture of the dominant follicle during the normal ovarian cycle, or failure of atresia of the nondominant follicle. Smaller cysts commonly resolve spontaneously. Intervention is required if the patient is symptomatic or follow-up scans show increase in size.

Luteal cysts

These are cysts that originate from the corpus luteum following ovulation. They are typically haemorrhagic and can rupture and cause intraperitoneal bleeding. Because of their origin, they typically rupture on days 20–26 of the menstrual cycle, and are more common on the right side.

Theca lutein cysts

These are the least common physiological cysts that result from excessive physiological stimulation, such as high levels of β-HCG, for example, during pregnancy. They are often bilateral cysts, which can be very large, and the majority resolve spontaneously.

Benign epithelial

The majority of ovarian cysts arise from the ovarian epithelium. They develop from the coelomic epithelium over the gonadal ridge of the embryo and are, therefore, derived from any of the pelvic organs or the renal tract.

Serous cystadenoma

This is the most common benign epithelial tumour. They contain thin serous fluid, usually within a unilocular cavity, and histologically appear to have tubal origin. They are bilateral in approximately 10% of cases.

Mucinous cystadenoma

These tumours are typically unilateral and multilocular with thick mucoid fluid. They are typically larger than serous cystadenomas. The mucus-secreting cells are likely to indicate an endocervical derivation.

Brenner tumours

The majority of these tumours are benign, but it is possible for them to be malignant. They arise from uroepithelial cell lines and contain transitional epithelium. They are solid, sharply circumscribed and pale yellow–tan in colour with 10%–15% being bilateral.

Endometrioid tumours

These tumours are derived from endometrial cells, but the majority are malignant.

Benign germ cell

These tumours are the most common in premenopausal women. The tumours arise from totipotential germ cells, and therefore can contain elements of all three layers of embryonic tissue. This includes ectodermal derivatives such as teeth and hair, endodermal tissue such as intestine and mesodermal tissue such as bone.

Mature cystic teratoma

This tumour is commonly known as a 'dermoid cyst'. It has a median age of presentation of 30 years and approximately 10% are bilateral. Most are asymptomatic, but they can undergo torsion (10%), or, rarely, rupture.

Mature solid teratoma

This is a predominantly solid tumour commonly with neural elements. It is much less common than the dermoid cyst (mature cystic teratoma). They must be histologically distinguished from an immature solid teratoma, which is malignant.

Benign sex cord stromal

These tumours are uncommon, accounting for approximately 4% of benign ovarian tumours. Because of their origin, many secrete hormones and therefore present with hormonally mediated symptoms.

Theca cell tumours

These cysts are nearly always benign solid tumours. Many secrete oestrogen, and therefore have systemic effects such as postmenopausal bleeding. They commonly present over the age of 50. Theca-granulosa types are malignant tumours.

Fibroma

These tumours are rare, mostly derived from stromal cells with intersecting bundles of spindle cells producing collagen. They can be associated with ascites, and Meigs syndrome is seen in 1% of cases, which is the triad of ascites, pleural effusion and a benign ovarian tumour.

Other

Leiomyoma

Known as 'fibroids', these are very common as benign smooth muscle tumours (see Chapter 5).

Endometrioma

Women with endometriosis may develop cysts, known as 'endometriomas' (chocolate cyst), which can enlarge and become large cysts that typically do not resolve spontaneously. The have a typical 'ground glass' ultrasound appearance as a result of haemorrhagic debris (see Chapter 6).

Non-ovarian

Non-ovarian causes of a pelvic mass can include a paratubal cyst, hydrosalpinges or a tubo-ovarian abscess.

MANAGEMENT

Management of benign ovarian cysts should be tailored to the specific patient. Contributing factors to consider include the severity of presenting symptoms, the patient's age and fertility needs, and any risk of malignancy.

Conservative

Ovarian cysts can generally be managed conservatively if they are asymptomatic, depending on the woman's age and size of the cyst. In younger women (under 40 years of age) the risk of malignancy is reduced, and with cyst size <5 cm the cyst is small and torsion risk is low. The cyst should be monitored with serial transvaginal ultrasound; they would usually resolve over two to three menstrual cycles. A thin-walled, simple cyst is likely to resolve spontaneously, but if it persists or increases in size, then cystectomy might be indicated (Fig. 11.1). Simple cysts 5–7 cm can be managed with yearly ultrasound follow-up, but should be considered for either further imaging or surgical intervention.

The combined oral contraceptive pill is thought to be effective in preventing formation of functional tumours, but its effectiveness in shrinking or resolving cystic tumours has not yet been proven.

Conservative management is preferred in premenopausal women who wish to retain fertility, as along with

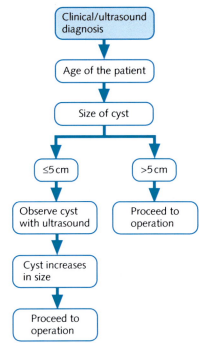

Fig. 11.1 Management of an asymptomatic benign ovarian tumour in a premenopausal woman.

common surgical risks, cystectomy has additional risks of more extensive surgery requiring laparotomy and possible oophorectomy (removal of the ovary) to remove the cyst or for haemostasis.

CLINICAL NOTES

The risk of malignancy of any ovarian cyst can be suggested by calculating the 'Risk of Malignancy Index' (RMI). Higher RMI has a greater risk of ovarian cancer.

$$RMI = Ultrasound\ score\,(U) \times Menopause\ score\,(M) \times Ca\text{-}125\ level\,(IU/mL)$$

Ultrasound scan findings (U) are scored a point for each of the following characteristics: multilocular, solid areas or bilateral cysts, metastasis, ascites.

$$No\ 'U'\ characteristics = 0$$
$$1\ 'U'\ characteristic = 1$$
$$2\ or\ more\ 'U' = 3$$

Menopausal score (M) is based on menopausal status: M = 1 premenopausal, M = 3 postmenopausal

<25 = low risk (<3%)
25–250 = moderate risk (20%)
>250 = high risk (30%)

Surgical

Surgical management of ovarian cysts should be considered depending on several factors. If the cyst is large (>5 cm) or if there is any concern regarding malignancy, a cystectomy should be advised. Surgery is also advised if there is failure of conservative measures and the cyst is not resolving or increasing in size. This is ideally planned as an elective procedure. Up to 10% of women will have some form of surgery during their lifetime for the presence of an ovarian cyst or tumour.

Vaginal or laparoscopic aspiration of ovarian cysts is less effective and is associated with a high rate of recurrence.

If a woman presents with severe acute pain and there is concern regarding ovarian torsion or cyst rupture, an emergency laparoscopy or laparotomy may be required. This is particularly crucial in women of childbearing age as prolonged ovarian torsion can cause decreased perfusion, and therefore unrecoverable necrosis of the ovary requiring oophorectomy.

To reduce surgical risk, improve recovery time and decrease blood loss and hospital stay, cystectomy is ideally performed laparoscopically. However, this is dependent on the operator, patient body mass index, previous surgery and risk of malignancy. A laparotomy may need to be performed if there is suspected malignancy, a large cyst not appropriate for laparoscopy, or for operative need (e.g., conversion from laparoscopy intraoperatively). Again, the patient should be counselled and consented for oophorectomy.

> ● **Chapter Summary**
>
> - Ovarian cysts are a common acute gynaecological presentation to hospital.
> - Any woman presenting with lower abdominal pain must be investigated for possible differential diagnosis such as ectopic pregnancy and appendicitis.
> - A true ovarian torsion should be treated as an emergency as the ovary twisting can cause decreased perfusion, and therefore unrecoverable necrosis of the ovary requiring oophorectomy.
> - Transvaginal ultrasound is the optimum investigation to highlight an ovarian cyst and identify its probable aetiology.
> - Management should be tailored to the particular patient considering their age, cyst size and risk of malignancy as calculated using the Risk of Malignancy Index.

Gynaecological malignancies 12

BACKGROUND

Gynaecological malignancies include cancers affecting the ovary, uterus, cervix, vagina, vulva and fallopian tubes. Because of the diverse group of tumours with differing pathological features, there are differing clinical presentations and treatment strategies.

Ovarian and uterine cancers are among the most common cancers in women in the UK.

HISTORY

The aim of the history is to elicit any concerning history or symptoms that may support a diagnosis of malignancy. Key factors include:

- red flag symptoms
- general malaise – weight loss, loss of appetite
- family or personal history of cancer

HISTORY

Have your periods stopped? If so, for how long? What was the date of your last menstrual period? How long is your menstrual cycle? How many days are your periods? Have you noted any unscheduled bleeding between periods/after sex/in the postmenopausal period? Establishing bleeding patterns is crucial to establish any abnormal bleeding. It is important to establish the timeline of any abnormal bleeding and associations. It is also crucial to establish any associations, for example, with abdominal pain, vaginal discharge.

Do you have pain? Describe the pain, is it acute or chronic? Have you noted any abdominal bloating or fullness? A full assessment of any pain is required. The nature of the pain may help narrow down the diagnosis and assess for risk of ovarian pathology. Are you experiencing any dyspareunia or vaginal discomfort? Have you noted any abdominal swelling or urinary symptoms? These symptoms are more common with a larger pelvic mass, or cysts in the pouch of Douglas.

Do you have any prior gynaecological history? Have you previously had ovarian cysts? Are you up-to-date with smear tests? Do you have any family or personal history of ovarian or breast cancer? Have you been systemically unwell or noted unintentional weight loss? It is important to assess these red flag risk factors for malignancy.

Do you have any medical conditions? A medical history such as immunosuppression may increase your suspicion of malignancy. Have you had any nausea or vomiting? Do you have any gastrointestinal or urinary upset? These symptoms could indicate an alternative diagnosis, but can also be associated with an underlying malignancy.

EXAMINATION

- General examination.
- Abdominal palpation.
- Vulval/vaginal/cervical inspection.
- Bimanual pelvic examination.

General examination aims to identify signs of systemic illness such as cachexia, pallor and clubbing.

Is there abdominal distension? Is the uterus enlarged? Determine the size, tenderness, mobility and nodularity of any pelvic mass, including the uterus itself. Abdominal examination might also reveal ascites, suggestive of malignancy.

Vulval and vaginal inspection may identify lesions or masses.

Speculum examination may reveal cervical pathology, such as frank malignancy.

A bimanual vaginal examination should be performed and the adnexa should be examined. It may reveal the presence of any adnexal masses. Postmenopausal ovaries should not normally be palpable on bimanual examination.

OVARIAN CANCER

Background

In the UK ovarian cancer is the fifth most common cancer in women (behind breast, bowel, lung and uterus) with around 7000 new cases being diagnosed each year. This equates to a

Table 12.1 Staging of ovarian carcinoma

Stage	Description	Treatment	Survival rates at 5 years (%)
I	Limited to the ovaries	Surgery	80
A	One ovary, capsule intact, no ascites		
B	Both ovaries, capsules intact, no ascites		
C	Breached capsule(s) or ascites present		
II	Presence of peritoneal deposits in pelvis	Surgery then chemotherapy	60
A	On uterus or tubes		
B	On other pelvic organs		
C	With ascites		
III	Peritoneal deposits outside pelvis	Surgery then chemotherapy	25
A	Microscopic deposits		
B	Macroscopic < 2 cm diameter		
C	Macroscopic > 2 cm diameter		
IV	Distant metastases	Surgery for palliation only	5–10

BOX 12.1 RISK FACTORS FOR OVARIAN CARCINOMA

Increased risk	Reduced risk
Hormone replacement therapy	Pregnancies
Few or no pregnancies	Treatment with the combined pill
Treatment with ovulation-induction drugs	Black/Asian
White (Caucasian)	Blood group O
Blood group A	
Higher socioeconomic status	
Late age of first conception	
Family history	

13), or Lynch II syndrome (an autosomal dominant inherited disorder that predisposes to breast, endometrial, colon and ovarian cancer). There is new evidence that strongly suggests that some ovarian carcinoma originates from the fallopian tubes. Risk factors for ovarian cancer are associated with an increased exposure to oestrogen, and therefore include:

- increasing age
- nulliparity
- early menarche
- late menopause
- smoking
- obesity

Pregnancy, breastfeeding and exercise are thought to be protective factors (Box 12.1).

Symptoms

Ovarian cancer is often labelled the 'silent killer' as it may not have symptoms. There should be a high index of suspicion of even vague symptoms especially in at-risk groups (women over 50 years of age or with a family history). Patients presenting with these symptoms need careful assessment to rule out ovarian cancer:

- abdominal pain
- bloating, distension or ascites
- abdominal mass
- postmenopausal bleeding
- loss of appetite, early satiety or unexplained weight loss

Investigations

Pelvic ultrasound

The most common first-line investigation for women suspected to have ovarian cancer is a pelvic ultrasound. Ideally

general practitioner being likely to diagnose approximately one person with ovarian cancer every 3–5 years. It has a peak incidence between the ages of 60 and 64 years and it is the leading cause of death in women with a gynaecological cancer. The staging, treatment and survival rates are shown in Table 12.1.

There are different types of ovarian cancers depending upon which cell they arise from. Most commonly tumours are from the epithelial cells, but others can arise from germ cells, ovarian stroma, ovarian mesenchymal cells or metastatic disease from other sites.

Aetiology

The aetiology of ovarian cancer is not completely understood, although various risk factors have been identified. Women with a familial predisposition to ovarian cancer probably account for around 10% of cases, and most of these will have either the BRCA1 or BRCA2 mutations (chromosomes 17 and this should be performed transvaginally, but can be performed transabdominally and can identify both ovarian and uterine pathology. Suspicious features that may be identified on scan include:

- multilocular cysts
- solid areas of cysts
- bilateral lesions
- ascites

Blood tests

Tumour markers are also used in the investigation of ovarian cancer, especially Ca-125, which is often raised in patients with epithelial cell tumours. Normal serum Ca-125 is <35 IU/mL. Younger patients (i.e., <40 years old) suspected of having ovarian cancer should have serum α-fetoprotein, β-human chorionic gonadotrophin and Ca-125 levels measured to identify other tumour types.

Specialist tests

Patients suspected of having ovarian cancer should have a computed tomography (CT) scan of their pelvis, abdomen and chest to establish the extent (or stage) of the disease.

CLINICAL NOTES

As ovarian cysts are very common (especially in premenopausal women), it is important to distinguish between benign and malignant cysts. To identify women with a high risk of ovarian cancer, the risk of malignancy index (RMI) has been devised.

The RMI uses ultrasound features as well as the patient's menopausal status and Ca-125 level to give a risk score (see Chapter 11).

$$RMI = Ultrasound\ score\,(U) \times Menopause\ score\,(M) \times Ca\text{-}125\ level\,(IU/mL)$$

Those with a score of >250 should be referred to a specialist multidisciplinary team.

Treatment

Surgery is the main modality of treatment in ovarian cancer and can be both diagnostic and curative (in early stage disease). It is performed by a gynaecological oncologist in a tertiary centre and involves a midline laparotomy, peritoneal washings, a total abdominal hysterectomy with bilateral salpingo-oophorectomy, omentectomy and biopsy of any suspicious areas. In addition, those patients who are suspected of having a mucinous tumour also undergo an

appendicectomy. In patients with advanced disease the objective is to remove all visible tumour tissue. This allows accurate staging which will then dictate further management.

Chemotherapy may be needed following surgery based on the staging and type of tumour. In patients with low-risk stage I disease (grade 1 or 2, stage 1a or 1b) chemotherapy is not recommended. Patients with high-risk stage I disease (Grade 3 or stage 1c) or greater are recommended to have chemotherapy.

The choice of chemotherapy depends upon the individual patient. Most commonly a combination of a platinum-based agent and paclitaxel is used for six cycles.

Common side-effects of chemotherapy agents include nephrotoxicity, nausea, alopecia, mucositis, hypersensitivity reactions and neurotoxicity.

CLINICAL NOTES

The rationale for screening for ovarian cancer is to reduce the late presentation that currently results in poor survival. Unfortunately, screening for this condition is difficult, partly because there is no premalignant stage, but also because there is no single test to diagnose ovarian cancer. Currently, research is being carried out into screening to see which approach is more effective.

Prognosis

In the UK ovarian cancer survival is improving and has almost doubled in the last 40 years. Prognosis is better in younger women and decreases with increasing age. Approximately three-quarters of women survive the disease for 1 year or more, almost half for 5 years or more, and more than a third survive for over 10 years.

ENDOMETRIAL CANCER

Background

In the UK endometrial cancer is the most common gynaecological cancer, with around 8000 new cases being diagnosed each year. This equates to a general practitioner being likely to diagnose approximately one person with endometrial cancer every 3–5 years. Endometrial cancer predominantly occurs in postmenopausal women over the age of 50 years. These women may present with postmenopausal bleeding and it is essential they are appropriately investigated. A small number of cases occur in younger women (aged <40 years) who may have a genetic predisposition. The probability of endometrial cancer in women presenting with postmenopausal bleeding is 5%–10%.

Aetiology

Obesity is the main potentially avoidable risk factor for endometrial cancer, linked to an estimated 34% of cases in the UK. Body mass index of >29 kg/m^2 are said to have a threefold increase in risk. Other risk factors include:

- polycystic ovary syndrome
- nulliparity
- unopposed oestrogen use
- tamoxifen use
- genetic syndromes (hereditary nonpolyposis colorectal cancer)

Endometrial cancer is an adenocarcinoma, the most common type being endometrioid. Other subtypes are serous, clear cell, mixed and small cell. Spread initially involves local myometrial invasion and then transperitoneal. Lymphatic spread occurs to the paraaortic nodes. Staging is shown in Table 12.2.

Endometrial hyperplasia

Endometrial hyperplasia is a premalignant condition that if left untreated can progress to cancer. It is divided into hyperplasia without atypia and atypical hyperplasia. Diagnosis of endometrial hyperplasia requires histological examination (biopsy) of the endometrial tissue. The risk of endometrial hyperplasia without atypia progressing to endometrial cancer is less than 5% over 20 years and that the majority

of cases will regress spontaneously during follow-up. Progesterone treatment (such as Mirena coil) can encourage regression, and women are under surveillance at 6-month intervals. The presence of atypia has a high likelihood of progression to cancer, and in many cases might indicate that a carcinoma is already present in another part of the uterus. Women with atypical hyperplasia should undergo a total hysterectomy because of the risk of underlying malignancy or progression to cancer.

> **RED FLAG**
>
> Women with atypical hyperplasia of the endometrium have up to 40% chance of progression to endometrial cancer (if left untreated), so the option of definitive surgery (i.e., hysterectomy) should be discussed.

Symptoms

The most common presenting symptom of endometrial cancer is unexpected vaginal bleeding – most commonly postmenopausal bleeding. Others include:

- intermenstrual bleeding
- watery or blood stained vaginal discharge
- unscheduled bleeding on hormone replacement therapy
- suspicious pre/perimenopausal bleeding (e.g., new-onset heavy bleeding)

In late stages it could present with back pain, anorexia and lethargy.

Investigations

Pelvic ultrasound

This should be performed to measure the endometrial thickness and also for endometrial sampling. Endometrial cancer causes thickening of the endometrium and in the postmenopausal state should be less than 5 mm.

Endometrial biopsy

The endometrium can be sampled in an outpatient setting using a pipelle biopsy. It involves the passage of a thin plastic tube through the cervix into the uterine cavity and uses aspiration to obtain an endometrial biopsy. This technique, however, only samples 4% of the endometrial surface area and may miss the cancer if present. More commonly patients are advised to undergo a hysteroscopy and endometrial biopsy (gold standard). This allows direct visualization of the endometrial cavity and a more representative sample to be taken. The procedure can be done under a local or general anaesthetic.

Table 12.2 Staging of endometrial cancer

Stage	Structures involved	Survival rates at 5 years (%)
I	Body of uterus	85
A	Endometrium only	
B	Extension into inner half of myometrium	
C	Extension into outer half of myometrium	
II	Extension from the body of uterus to cervix	60
A	Endocervical glands only	
B	Cervical stroma	
III	Outside uterus, within pelvis	40
A	Spread to adnexae, or positive peritoneal cytology	
B	Metastases in vagina	
C	Pelvic or paraaortic lymphadenopathy	
IV	Distant spread	10
A	Involvement of bladder or bowel mucosa	
B	Distant metastases	

Specialist tests

Once a tissue diagnosis is obtained, a magnetic resonance imaging (MRI) scan is performed to assess the extent of myometrial invasion and thus differentiate between stages Ia, Ib and those above (see Table 12.2). Stages Ia and Ib can be treated locally; higher stages should be treated in a regional cancer centre. The decision as to where to treat should be discussed in a multidisciplinary team meeting.

Treatment

Surgery is the mainstay of treatment for patients with endometrial cancer. In stage I disease complete surgical staging is recommended. This includes a laparotomy (or laparoscopy) with peritoneal washing being taken for cytology, inspection of the pelvis and abdomen and a total abdominal (or laparoscopic) hysterectomy plus bilateral salpingo-oophorectomy. Stage II or high-risk disease is treated by a midline laparotomy and stage III disease is again surgically managed with the aim of debulking disease prior to radiotherapy. In stage IV disease a combination of surgery, radiotherapy and palliation may be required depending upon individual circumstances.

Prognosis

The overall 5-year survival rates for all stages of endometrial carcinoma are around 83%–86%. Those with disease confined to the uterus, however, have a much better prognosis with a 5-year survival rate of 95%–97%.

UTERINE SARCOMA (NONENDOMETRIOID CANCER)

Background

Gynaecological sarcomas are rare, accounting for only 2% of all gynaecological malignancies, typically with an aggressive nature and poor prognosis. They are categorized as:

- mesenchymal tumours (such as leiomyosarcoma)
- endometrial stromal tumours (low grade or high grade)
- miscellaneous (such as rhabdomyosarcoma)

Leiomyosarcoma

Leiomyosarcoma is a type of soft-tissue sarcoma that could be described as a 'malignant fibroid', although only 5%–10% of them arise within an existing fibroid; they are macroscopically very similar, benign tumours of smooth muscle cells. They account for 1% of all uterine cancers and 35%–40% of all uterine sarcomas, and therefore are the most common gynaecological sarcomas.

An index of suspicion is raised in women who present with fast growing masses, which on imaging appear to be consistent with a fibroid. However, it is most commonly reported as an incidental finding in hysterectomy specimens posthysterectomy. Leiomyosarcoma has a poor prognosis with recurrence rate of up to 70% and overall 5-year survival rate for all stages of 39%.

Stromal sarcoma

Tumours of stromal cells can be divided into the following categories:

- endometrial stromal nodule – low grade
- endometrial stromal sarcoma – low grade: cells have delicate vasculature resembling normal proliferative-phase endometrial stroma
- undifferentiated endometrial sarcoma – high grade: aggressive neoplasm with extensive cell atypia and necrosis

Diagnosis of low-grade stromal tumours is made difficult by a lack of clear tumour circumscription and similarity to proliferative phase endometrium. One-third to half of the low-grade tumours present with spread outside the uterus.

Investigations

Specialist tests

These pathologies can be identified by biopsy, but predominantly are identified postsurgery.

Treatment

Patients with sarcoma should be treated by specialist multidisciplinary teams. Standard treatment for uterine sarcomas is a total hysterectomy and bilateral salpingectomy with oophorectomy for endometrial stromal sarcoma.

Advanced or metastatic uterine leiomyosarcoma and undifferentiated endometrial sarcoma are treated systemically with the same chemotherapy drugs as soft-tissue sarcomas at other sites, such as gemcitabine. Advanced/metastatic endometrial stromal sarcoma can be treated with antioestrogen therapy, with an aromatase inhibitor or progestogen.

Prognosis

Five-year survival rates are poor (approximately 50%) with very high recurrence rates despite surgical management.

CERVICAL CANCER

Background

Cervical cancer is the second most common cancer in women (under the age of 35 years), and in the UK approximately 2700 new cases of cervical cancer are diagnosed each year, around three-quarters identified at cervical screening. In terms of incidence there appear to be two peaks in ages with the first occurring between 30 and 34 years and the second between 80 and 84 years. Five-year survival rate is approximately 65%. Risk factors for developing cervical cancer include:

- human papilloma virus (HPV)
- smoking
- first intercourse/pregnancy at young age
- smoking
- oral contraceptive pill
- human immunodeficiency virus (HIV)

Symptoms

Cervical cancer may be completely asymptomatic and only identified by cervical cytology. Patients who present with postcoital bleeding, intermenstrual bleeding, persistent vaginal discharge (may be blood stained) or postmenopausal bleeding should all be examined to identify any abnormality on the cervix, and any features of concern should prompt referral for colposcopic examination.

Human papilloma virus

HPV is a virus belonging to the Papovaviridae family, which has over 100 different subtypes causing, for example, warts. In the 1980s HPV was linked with cervical cancer and since then research has identified certain types responsible. HPV can be transmitted by sexual contact and, therefore, any female who is sexually active is at risk. HPV types 16, 18, 6 and 11 are all known to cause cervical cancer with 16 and 18 known as 'high-risk subtypes'.

HPV infection is the main potentially avoidable risk factor for cervical cancer, linked to an estimated 100% of cervical cancer cases in the UK. Based on this research in the UK a vaccination programme is in place to vaccinate young girls before their first sexual contact and prevent cervical cancer. Girls are invited to have the vaccination between the ages of 13 and 14 years, which involves a course of three injections. It should be noted, however, that vaccination does not currently replace screening.

Screening

The UK has an established screening programme that invites women to have cervical smears performed on a 3-year basis between the ages of 25 and 49 years and on a 5-year basis from the ages of 50–64 years. If results show borderline or low-grade abnormal cell changes (dyskaryosis), laboratories will perform a high-risk HPV test. Patients with abnormal smears and HPV-positive results will be offered a colposcopy and may need more frequent smears depending upon findings and treatment. When high-risk HPV is not detected, women are returned to routine screening.

Premalignant changes (cervical intraepithelial neoplasia)

The natural progression of the disease means that squamous cell cervical cancers (accounting for >90% of cervical cancers) exist in a premalignant form, which can be detected by cervical cytology. Cervical intraepithelial neoplasia (CIN) grading describes the premalignant condition and is made up of three stages, which are thought to represent a continuum from low grade (CIN I) to high grade (CIN II to CIN III; Fig. 12.1). CIN grade is identified histologically at the time of biopsy.

Patients with an abnormal smear result may then be referred for a colposcopy. At colposcopy the cervix is inspected

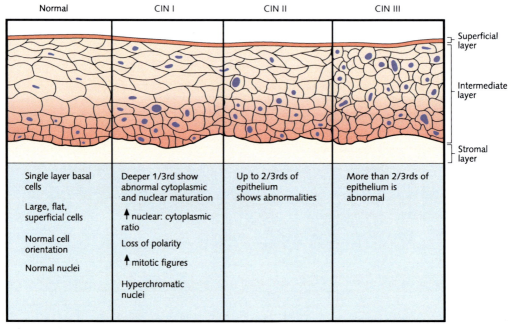

Normal	CIN I	CIN II	CIN III
Single layer basal cells	Deeper 1/3rd show abnormal cytoplasmic and nuclear maturation	Up to 2/3rds of epithelium shows abnormalities	More than 2/3rds of epithelium is abnormal
Large, flat, superficial cells	↑ nuclear: cytoplasmic ratio		
Normal cell orientation	Loss of polarity		
Normal nuclei	↑ mitotic figures		
	Hyperchromatic nuclei		

Fig. 12.1 Grades of cervical intraepithelial neoplasia.

for suspicious features (see clinical notes). Abnormal areas can be biopsied, meaning that the patient will be invited back at a later date for treatment if appropriate, or treatment can be performed at this point.

Treatment consists of either excising or destroying the transformation zone. Excision techniques include large loop excision of transformation zone (LLETZ), needle excision of transformation zone and cone biopsy; these allow the tissue removed to be sent for histology and examined to confirm the diagnosis and to check the margins, ensuring complete excision. Destructive techniques include cold coagulation, diathermy or laser. Initial treatment has 95% success rate. Patients are followed up with a smear, usually after 6 months. Cervical cancer develops in under 1% of young women with carcinoma in-situ per year.

Investigations

Cervical cytology (smear test)
If a smear test is overdue, this can be performed. The screening programme uses liquid-based cytology to collect samples of cells from the cervix. Smears must be taken before taking any swabs or performing a vaginal examination, which may dislodge cells on the surface of the cervix. Using a Cusco's speculum the visible cervix is gently swept through 360° five times with a cervical Cytobrush (see Fig. 3.1). The sample is then placed into the fluid medium. Occasionally a smear test requires repeating due to inadequate cell sampling.

Colposcopy
Women with HPV-positive dyskaryosis or an abnormal looking to the cervix should be referred for colposcopy (see below) plus biopsy if required.

Specialist tests
Once a tissue diagnosis has been made the next step is to stage the disease. The staging has traditionally been clinical with the patients undergoing an examination under anaesthesia, a cone biopsy/LLETZ, and if there is still concern of disease extent, MRI and CT of the chest/abdomen/pelvis are performed.

Colposcopy
The colposcope is a binocular microscope enabling the surface epithelium of the cervix to be assessed under magnification and is usually performed as an outpatient. The patient is positioned in a modified lithotomy position and the cervix is exposed using a Cusco's speculum. The cervix is then viewed through the colposcope to identify any visible lesions. Two solutions are then applied:

- 5% Acetic acid solution – this is applied to the entire surface of the cervix and produces 'acetowhite' changes on abnormal epithelial cells due to coagulation of

proteins by the acetic acid. Areas of CIN appear as these distinct acetowhite lesions with demarcated edges.
- Iodine solution – this further highlights the squamocolumnar junction and areas of abnormalities as an orange colour.

The extent of lesions can be noted and any extension in to the cervical canal. All abnormal looking areas should be biopsied for further histological assessment.

CLINICAL NOTES

Suspicious features at colposcopy
- Intense acetowhite (5% acetic acid solution), pale on iodine staining
- Mosaicism and punctation due to atypical vessel formation
- Raised or ulcerated surface

Table 12.3 shows the staging of cervical cancer.

Treatment

The treatment of cervical cancer can be by surgery, radiotherapy and chemotherapy. Factors to take into consideration when planning management include patient age, disease stage, comorbidities and fertility concerns. Treatment options and decisions are usually made within a multidisciplinary team.

In stage I disease the treatment may need to be tailored to the patient's individual circumstances and desire for children.

Table 12.3 Staging of cervical cancer

Stage	Description
0	Carcinoma in-situ
I	Confined to the cervix
A	• Visible only under a microscope
A1	• <3 mm in depth
A2	• >3 mm in depth
II	Beyond the cervix
A	• No parametrial involvement
B	• Parametrial involvement
III	Spread to the pelvic side wall, or affecting the ureter, or spread to the lower third of the vagina
A	Lower third of vaginal
B	To pelvic wall/incolving ureters
IV	Spread to bladder/rectum or beyond pelvis
A	Involving the rectal or bladder mucosa
B	Beyond the true pelvis

Stage Ia1 (microinvasive disease) may be diagnosed on an LLETZ sample and if the lesion has been completely excised, no further treatment may be necessary. Stages IA2–IIA (early stage disease) can be treated with surgery or chemoradiation with equivalent results. It is advised that for tumours 4 cm or less radical hysterectomy with lymphadenectomy is preferred to chemoradiation, and for tumours larger than 4 cm, chemoradiation is preferred. If the woman wishes to preserve her fertility, a radical trachelectomy (surgery to remove the entire cervix) and lymphadenectomy may be considered, depending on the disease stage. Stages IIb and above are treated with radiotherapy combined with chemotherapy.

Prognosis

The cervical cancer survival rates have been improving over the last 40 years and continue to improve. When diagnosed at its earliest stage, around 95% of women with cervical cancer will survive their disease for over 5 years. Overall, the current 1-year survival rate is 83%, 5-year survival 67% and 10-year survival 63%. Younger age at diagnosis is associated with an improved prognosis. Approximately 1000 women per year die from the disease.

In the coming years data will become available regarding the HPV vaccine and the predicted reduction in cervical cancer diagnoses.

VULVAL CANCER

Background

Vulval tumours are rare, with an incidence of around 3 in 100,000 women per year. The peak incidence is from the ages of 63 to 65 years. Approximately 1000 new vulval cancers are diagnosed each year in the UK. About 55% of vulval cancer cases in the UK each year are diagnosed in females aged 70 years and over and incidence rates for vulval cancer in the UK are highest in females aged 90+ years. Around 90% of vulval tumours are squamous cell carcinomas. Nonsquamous cell tumours include melanoma, sarcoma, adenocarcinoma and basal cell tumours.

Predisposing factors include:

- history of CIN, vulval intraepithelial neoplasia (VIN) or HPV
- immunosuppression
- lichen sclerosus (Box 12.7)

CLINICAL NOTES

Lichen sclerosus is a benign skin condition, with white plaques and atrophy seen in a figure-of-eight pattern around the vulva and anus. Extragenital

---

plaques on the trunk and back might be seen. It is associated with autoimmune disorders (e.g., vitiligo). It can be classed as premalignant, as around 4% will go on to develop vulval squamous cell carcinoma.

Symptoms

The most common presenting symptoms are:

- pruritus
- lump/ulcer
- bleeding
- pain
- discharge

Urinary symptoms may be a feature or, indeed, there may be no symptoms at all. The most common sites are shown in Fig. 12.2, and the tumour may be multifocal on the vulva. Some elderly patients who are embarrassed to seek help may present late with advanced disease. Local spread occurs to the vagina, perineum, clitoris, urethra and pubic bone. Lymphatic spread is to the superficial inguinal, deep inguinofemoral and iliac nodes. Unless the tumour is central (i.e., within 1 cm of the midline) only the nodes on the affected side are involved.

RED FLAG

Consider a suspected cancer pathway referral (for an appointment within 2 weeks) for vulval cancer in women with an unexplained vulval lump, ulceration or bleeding.

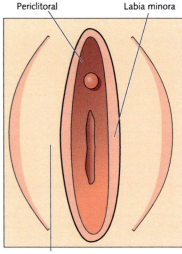

Fig. 12.2 Squamous cell carcinoma of the vulva.

Premalignant changes (VIN)

Similar to CIN, VIN is a premalignant condition that can progress to invasive carcinoma. If VIN is present, CIN is often seen too with HPV being the causal factor.

Paget's disease

Paget disease of the vulva is a malignant adenocarcinoma in cells of the intraepidermal layer, which has a characteristic appearance, initially appearing as a red or pink patch with scattered white islands of hyperkeratosis, progressing to plaque-like lesions. The presence of vulval Paget disease is associated with an adenocarcinoma elsewhere in the body in one in four cases, with the most common sites being breast, urinary tract, rectum and genital tract.

Investigations

Biopsy

A tissue diagnosis is obtained by taking a biopsy, and at the time of biopsy the vagina and cervix are thoroughly inspected for signs of involvement. All cases of suspected vulval cancer should have the diagnosis confirmed with a biopsy and reviewed by the specialist multidisciplinary team prior to radical treatment.

Specialist tests

Positive nodes may be detected by CT or MRI scan. Stages are shown in Table 12.4.

Treatment

As vulval cancers are rare, it is best practice for them to be managed in specialist centres. The aim of treatment is to excise the cancer and minimize the risk of recurrence while preserving as much function as possible. Women with high-grade VIN, VIN in the immunosuppressed or those with Paget disease should have regular specialist follow-up.

The management plan depends on the stage; early tumours are treated by wide local excision. Wide radical local excision

Table 12.4 Staging of vulval cancer

Stage	Description
I	Confined to vulva
A	<1-mm invasion
B	<2-cm diameter, no groin nodes
II	Confined to vulva, >2-cm diameter, no groin nodes palpable
III	Confined to vulva, suspicious nodes or beyond vulva with no suspicious nodes
IV	Obvious groin nodes or involving rectum, bladder, urethra or bone or pelvic or distant metastases

Table 12.5 Complications of treatment

Type of treatment	Complication
Vulvectomy	Haemorrhage Thromboembolism Infection – wound, urinary tract Wound breakdown
Radiotherapy	Erythema Necrosis of the femoral head or pubic symphysis Fistula formation (urethrovaginal, vesicovaginal or rectovaginal)

of the primary tumour with a minimum margin of 15 mm of disease-free tissue is often sufficient. Individual women who cannot be optimized to enable surgery can be treated with primary radiotherapy. Primary and recurrent vulval cancer does respond to chemotherapy, but responses are variable and toxicity may be a problem in this population of patients.

Complications of treatment are shown in Table 12.5. Because of the large area involved, wound breakdown is, sadly, relatively common. Some surgeons advocate performing skin grafts at the time of initial surgery. Plastic surgery involvement may be required for large defects and when radiotherapy has been used. The vulva is a challenging area for wound healing and faecal and urinary diversion is often required.

Prognosis

Stage I disease has a 92% 5-year survival rate, whereas advanced disease (stage IV) has only a 13% 5-year survival rate. Vagina and vulva cancer survival in England is highest for women diagnosed aged under 50 years (more than 8 in 10 women aged 15–49 years survive their disease for 5 years or more, compared with almost 6 in 10 women diagnosed aged 70–89 years).

VAGINAL CANCER

Background

Vaginal tumours are rare and are usually either primary squamous carcinoma or spread from vulval or cervical squamous cancers. Even rarer tumours include endodermal sinus tumours, rhabdomyosarcoma (both seen in children, but the latter also seen in older women), melanoma, clear cell adenocarcinoma and leiomyosarcoma. Approximately 250 new vaginal cancers are diagnosed each year in the UK. Almost half of vaginal cancer cases in the UK each year are diagnosed in females aged 70 years and over. Risk factors include:

- CIN
- HPV (63% positive)
- current/history of another gynaecological malignancy
- diethylstilbestrol in utero

Symptoms

The upper third of the vagina is the most common site, and women usually present at an early stage with abnormal bleeding, mass or lesion in the vagina.

INVESTIGATIONS

Biopsy

Staging is shown in Table 12.6 and requires biopsy for histological diagnosis.

Specialist tests

Examination under anaesthetic and assessment of the bladder and rectum for spread either at operation or on MRI. Chest X-ray is performed as part of the evaluation.

Table 12.6 Staging of vaginal cancer

Stage	Description
0	Vaginal intraepithelial neoplasia
I	Limited to the vaginal wall
IIA	Subvaginal tissue, but not the parametrium, involved
IIB	Parametrial involvement
III	Spread to the pelvic side wall
IV	Bladder/rectum involved or distant organ spread

Treatment

Almost a fifth of vaginal cancer patients receive major surgical resection as part of their cancer treatment. Treatment is otherwise a combination of external beam and intravaginal radiotherapy, with the complications being fistulae (as with vulval radiotherapy) and stenosis of the vagina and rectum.

Prognosis

About 70% of women who present have stage I or II disease, with 5-year survival rates of around 70%. More than half of women diagnosed with vaginal cancer in England survive their disease for 10 years or more.

● Chapter Summary

- Early diagnosis of all gynaecological cancers will result in improved prognosis. However, it is well-known that some of these cancers, such as ovarian cancer, typically present late.
- Screening programmes, such as the National Cervical Cytology Programme, have already improved early diagnostic rates and outcomes of cervical cancer. It is hoped that these rates will continue to improve since the introduction of the human papilloma virus vaccine.
- Red flag symptoms, particularly in the postmenopausal population, such as postmenopausal bleeding, abdominal distention or masses, should prompt urgent 2-week wait referrals to a gynaecology department.

Benign vulval disease 13

BACKGROUND

Prevalence

Disorders of the vulva and vagina are very common and cause considerable discomfort. Younger women are more likely to have an infectious cause, whereas vulval dystrophies and cancers are more likely in older women.

Symptoms

The vulva extends from the mons pubis anteriorly to the perineum posteriorly and the labia majora laterally (Fig. 13.1). The whole surface of the vulva up to the inner aspect of the labia minora is covered by stratified keratinized squamous epithelium with a superficial cornified layer.

Common signs and symptoms of benign vulval disease include pain, irritation and itching, known as 'pruritus vulvae'. Common skin changes include changes in texture and colour.

Itching is a common symptom with a varied aetiology (Table 13.1) including vulval dystrophy, dermatological conditions, infection, systemic illness and neoplasia (see Chapter 12).

DIAGNOSIS

History

The diagnosis of benign vulval disease is strongly reliant on a thorough history due to the varied possible underlying aetiology. It is important not to miss any signs or symptoms suggestive of neoplasia (see Chapter 12).

A full medical and gynaecological history should be taken, including age and menopausal status.

When did the vaginal discomfort or itching begin? Have you had any postmenopausal bleeding (PMB)? Acute onset of symptoms is more suggestive of an infective source compared with insidious onset. Any PMB should be managed as suspicious of malignancy.

Table 13.1 Differential diagnosis of pruritus vulvae

Type of cause	Description

Infection	Fungal
	  Candida
	  Tinea
	Parasitic
	  Trichomonas vaginalis
	  Enterobius (pinworm)
	  Pediculosis pubis
	Bacterial
	  Bacterial vaginosis/vaginitis
	Viral
	  Herpes simplex virus
	  Human papilloma virus

Vulval dystrophy	Lichen sclerosus Hypertrophic vulval dystrophy
Neoplastic	Vulval intraepithelial neoplasia Squamous carcinoma Paget disease of the vulva
Dermatological	Psoriasis Eczema Contact dermatitis

Fig. 13.1 The anatomy of the vulva.

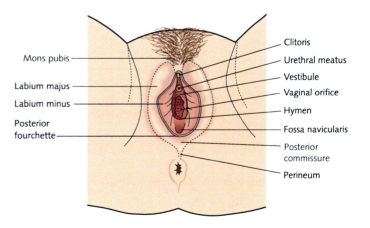

Mons pubis
Labium majus
Labium minus
Posterior fourchette

Clitoris
Urethral meatus
Vestibule
Vaginal orifice
Hymen
Fossa navicularis
Posterior commissure
Perineum

Do you have any vaginal discharge? Have you changed soap or washing powder? Abnormal vaginal discharge can suggest infection, and a detailed sexual history should be taken. The colour and odour of the discharge may suggest the underlying cause. Recent changes to soap or washing powder can cause contact dermatitis, as can overzealous hygiene and douching.

How long has the lesion been present? Was the onset sudden or gradual? Could it be related to trauma or another trigger? How did the lesion look when it first appeared? Is it different now? Does it come and go? The history and progress of any lesion are helpful in identifying its aetiology.

Do you have any existing dermatological conditions, allergies or chronic conditions? Existing dermatological conditions such as psoriasis can affect the vulva, so this information may be relevant. Chronic conditions such as diabetes mellitus or autoimmune conditions can also be responsible.

What prescribed or over-the-counter medications do you use? Have these helped? Self-treatment with emollients and antifungals is common and the response should be noted as this may be relevant.

> **RED FLAG**
>
> Consider malignancy if there are symptoms of postmenopausal bleeding, history of cervical intraepithelial neoplasia, previous vulval intraepithelial neoplasia or human papillomavirus infection, lymphadenopathy and immunosuppression.

Examination

General observations are important in the assessment. Is there any evidence of a dermatological condition? Assessment should be made of the face, hands, wrists, elbows, trunk and knees. Do they have any palpable lymph nodes? Inguinal lymphadenopathy can occur secondary to infection or malignancy.

An external genital examination, including the vulva, urethral meatus and perianal region, should be performed with patient's consent and a chaperone present. Are there any visible lesions, plaques, ulcers or erythema?

A Cusco's speculum can be used to examine the patient vaginally. Is there any visible abnormality of the vaginal tissue or cervix? Any vaginal discharge? Generalized vulvitis, discharge and ulcers suggest an infective cause, although ulcers can suggest possible malignancy.

INVESTIGATIONS

Bacterial swabs

These should be taken to exclude infection such as *Candida albicans* (thrush) and *Staphylococcus aureus*. Sexually active women should be screened for sexual transmitted infections.

Biopsy

Although some conditions can be identified by history and examination alone, the mainstay of diagnosis of these conditions is histological. Punch biopsies can be performed under a local anaesthetic in an outpatient setting or under a general anaesthetic if more extensive samples are required. If the diagnosis is uncertain or there are atypical features, this is advised (Fig. 13.2).

Blood tests

Where systemic disease is suspected investigations such as thyroid, liver and renal function should be performed. Investigation for autoimmune disease should be performed if clinically indicated, as it is often asymptomatic.

Transvaginal ultrasound scan

This should be performed in any postmenopausal woman complaining of bleeding to assess endometrial thickness and ensure a potentially malignant cause is not being missed.

Specialist tests

Patch testing is not commonly required and only indicated if allergy is suspected. This should be done only with dermatological input.

See Fig. 13.3 for investigative algorithm.

TYPES

The most common local causes of vulval skin disorders are lichen sclerosis, lichen planus, dermatitis and candidiasis. Common dermatological conditions involving the vulva include psoriasis and eczema. Infective causes include sexually transmitted infections, herpes and scabies. Systemic causes include diabetes, renal failure and Crohn disease (Table 13.1).

Infection

A history of vaginal discharge, vaginal irritation and warty or ulcerative lesions in a sexually active woman may highlight an infective cause (see Chapter 8).

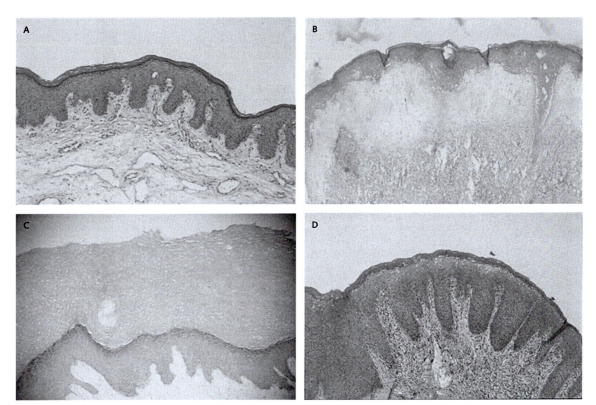

Fig. 13.2 Histology: (A) normal, (B) lichen sclerosus, (C) squamous hyperplasia and (D) dysplasia. From Llewellyn-Jones D: Fundamentals of obstetrics and gynaecology (9th edn), London, 2010, Mosby, with permission.

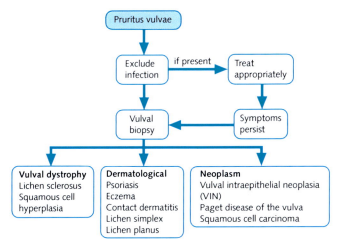

Fig. 13.3 Algorithm for the management of pruritus vulvae. From Llewellyn-Jones D: Fundamentals of obstetrics and gynaecology (9th edn), London, 2010, Mosby, with permission.

Lichen sclerosis

Lichen sclerosis is the most common vulval dystrophy, which usually develops in postmenopausal women. The aetiology is unknown, but there is evidence to suggest that autoimmune factors may be involved in its pathogenesis.

Symptoms include discomfort, introital narrowing leading to dyspareunia and itching, which can lead to skin spitting

and bleeding. The condition can affect the whole vulval and perianal region, with thinning of the skin and pale or white atrophic areas, known as 'leucoplakia'. Anatomical changes include shrinkage of the labia minora and midline fusion causing introitus narrowing. Purpura and fissuring are also common.

Diagnosis is based on the characteristic clinical appearance and histology findings of thinned epidermis with hyalinization and deep inflammation.

Treatment is aimed at managing the symptoms, and is usually intermittent as the condition is chronic and relapsing. Advice is short courses of potent topical steroids (e.g., Clobetasol propionate) and review after 3 months to assess progress. Alternative options include a potent topical steroid with antifungal agent (e.g., fucidic acid/betamethasone). Any complex disease or if it is not responding adequately should be referred to a vulval clinic.

Complications include dyspareunia and urinary issues secondary to anatomical changes. Women with lichen sclerosis should be reviewed yearly due a long-term 5% risk of developing squamous cell carcinoma.

Lichen planus

Lichen planus is a common skin condition that may occur anywhere on the body, predominantly the skin, genital and oral mucous membranes. It is an inflammatory condition of unknown aetiology, but is likely to be an immune response.

Symptoms include irritation, soreness, urinary symptoms and vaginal discharge, but it can be asymptomatic. Typical anogenital lesions are observed, most commonly flat-topped purpuric plaques with a fine white reticular pattern (Wickham striae).

Diagnosis is based on the characteristic clinical appearance and histology findings of irregular 'saw-toothed' acanthosis, an increased granular layer and basal cell changes.

Treatment options include potent topical steroid courses with maintenance treatment of a weaker steroid preparation. Vaginal corticosteroids are also used in more severe cases. In the case of complex disease, referral to a specialist is required, who may use oral ciclosporin, retinoids or oral steroids as management. Patients with active disease should be assessed for response to treatment every 3 months.

Complications include vaginal and vulval scarring, and a risk of development of squamous cell carcinoma is up to 3%.

Lichen simplex

Lichen simplex is a condition associated with vaginal itch and soreness. Aetiology is considered to be related to underlying dermatitis, systemic illness causing pruritis and environmental factors such as clothing rubbing, and there is also an association with psychiatric conditions such as anxiety and depression.

Lichenification is noted on examination with thickened or scaly skin and evidence of excoriation. Fissuring can be noted and pubic hair is often lost in the area of scratching.

Treatment options include avoidance of precipitating factor if identified and use of emollient substitute as soap. Topical corticosteroids for limited periods, combined with antifungal or antibiotic, are used if secondary infection is suspected. In some cases cognitive behavioural therapy may be helpful.

Dermatological

Vulval psoriasis

Psoriasis is a chronic inflammatory skin disease presenting with typically well demarcated, raised, erythematous scaly-topped plaques, which can occur on the vulval and natal cleft. The presence of psoriasis elsewhere suggests the diagnosis; it rarely is the only area affected. Symptoms include vulval itch, soreness and burning sensation.

If the diagnosis is unclear, it can be confirmed histologically. Treatment options include mild-to-moderate topical corticosteroids, coal-tar preparations or vitamin D analogues.

Vulval eczema

This is an uncommon presentation and is more commonly due to an allergic or irritant contact rather than in patients with existing atopic conditions. Symptoms include vulval soreness and itch, with clinical evidence of erythema, lichenification and excoriation. It is associated with a risk of secondary bacterial or fungal infection.

Treatment includes avoiding source of irritation, emollient soap substitute and often a course of topical corticosteroid, titrated depending on severity.

CLINICAL NOTES

The following general advice should be given to all women with vulval conditions:

- Avoid contact with soaps, shampoos and bath additives – use simple emollients as a substitute.
- Avoid tight-fitting underwear and trousers which can cause irritation.
- Avoid spermicide-lubricated condoms.
- Always give clear explanations of the patients' condition and written advice.

FEMALE GENITAL MUTILATION

Female genital mutilation (FGM) describes any procedure that involves partial or total removal of the external female genitalia or other injury to the female genital organs for nonmedical reasons (World Health Organization).

It is performed for a variety of reasons, predominantly the belief that it is beneficial. However, it is an illegal procedure with short-term complications such as haemorrhage and infection, and causes multiple long-term complications such as genital scarring, urinary tract complications, dyspareunia, genital infection, obstetric complications and psychological sequelae.

Female genital cosmetic surgery (FGCS), such as labiaplasty (labia minora reduction), is only appropriate if it is necessary for the patient's physical or mental health. All surgeons who undertake FGCS must be sufficiently trained, and ensure any surgery complies with FGM laws.

Prevalence

Worldwide it is estimated that over 125 million women and girls have undergone FGM (United Nations Children's Fund), and it is a traditional cultural practice in 29 African countries. It is almost exclusively performed on girls under the age of 15 years. In the UK it has been estimated that 137,000 women and girls, born in countries where FGM is practiced, have undergone FGM. About 3 million girls are thought to be at risk of FGM each year.

Diagnosis

FGM varies in extent and severity from genital cutting, to removal of the clitoris, removal of the labia or even abrasion and restitching of the labia majora leaving only a small vaginal opening.

Type 1: Partial or total removal of the clitoris and/or the prepuce (clitoridectomy).

Type 2: Partial or total removal of the clitoris and the labia minora, with or without excision of the labia majora (excision).

Type 3: Narrowing of the vaginal orifice with creation of a covering seal by cutting and appositioning the labia minora and/or the labia majora, with or without excision of the clitoris (infibulation).

Type 4: All other harmful procedures to the female genitalia for nonmedical purposes, for example, pricking, piercing, incising, scraping and cauterization.

RED FLAG

Female genital mutilation (FGM) is illegal as per the Female Genital Mutilation Act 2003 in England, Wales and Northern Ireland and the Prohibition of Female Genital Mutilation (Scotland) Act 2005:

- It is illegal to arrange, or assist in arranging, for a UK national or UK resident to be taken overseas for the purpose of FGM.
- It is an offence for those with parental responsibility to fail to protect a girl from the risk of FGM.
- If FGM is confirmed in a girl under 18 years of age, reporting to the police is mandatory and this must be within 1 month.
- Reinfibulation (resuturing of FGM) is illegal.

Management

Women with FGM should be managed by a multidisciplinary team of gynaecologists, obstetricians and midwives trained to identify and manage the condition. Consultations should be appropriately sensitive and nonjudgemental; it is crucial that the psychological consequences of FGM are considered. There must be an awareness of the techniques for management of FGM which adhere to the FGM act 2003, particularly in the event that clinical signs and symptoms suggest recent FGM or if the patient presents with pain, haemorrhage, infection and urinary retention.

Narrowing of the vagina due to type 3 FGM can prevent vaginal examination for smears and infection screens. Deinfibulation is a minor surgical procedure to divide the scar tissue sealing the vaginal introitus. It may be required prior to gynaecological procedures such as surgical management of miscarriage or prior to pregnancy. It is also recommended if there are issues with menstrual flow or sexual intercourse.

Chapter Summary

- Vulval disease is a common presentation, particularly in the postmenopausal population.
- It is associated with severe discomfort, itching, dyspareunia, anatomical changes with secondary complications including infection and risk of developing squamous cell carcinoma.
- Aetiology of vulval disease is varied and systemic conditions, infectious cause and neoplasia (see Chapter 12) must be considered as differentials.
- Female genital mutilation is an illegal practice with complex short- and long-term complications. All physicians should be trained to identify and sensitively manage the presentation.

Urogynaecology 14

PELVIC FLOOR PROLAPSE

Background

Definition

A prolapse is the protrusion of an organ or structure beyond its normal anatomical site. Pelvic floor prolapse involves weakness of the supporting structures of the pelvic organs due to which they descend from their normal positions. In the female genital tract the type of prolapse depends on the organ involved and its position in relation to the anterior or posterior vaginal wall. Table 14.1 defines and names the different types of prolapse.

Prolapse can occur to different degrees, ranging from first (uterine descent only within the vagina) to complete descent outside of the vagina (procidentia; Fig. 14.1).

Table 14.1 Diagnosing and defining type of prolapse

Organ that has prolapsed	Name of prolapse
Bladder	**Cystocoele:** Prolapse of the upper anterior wall of the vagina, attached to bladder by fascia.
Bladder and urethra	**Cystourethrocele:** A cystocoele extending into the lower anterior vaginal wall, displacing urethra downwards.
Rectum	**Rectocoele:** Weakness in the levator ani muscles causes a bulge in the midposterior vaginal wall which incorporates the rectum.
Small bowel	**Enterocoele:** True hernia of the pouch of Douglas. Prolapse of the upper third of the posterior vaginal wall and contains loops of small bowel.
Uterus and cervix	**Uterine descent:** Uterus descends within the vagina and may even lie outside it (called 'procidentia'). May be associated with a cystocoele and/or rectocoele. Graded according to the position of the cervix on vaginal examination: *First degree:* Cervical descent within the vagina *Second degree:* Cervical descent to the introitus *Third degree:* Cervical descent outside the introitus (procidentia)
Vaginal vault	**Vault descent:** After hysterectomy, the proximal end of the vaginal vault can prolapse within or outside the vagina.

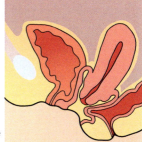

1st degree
descent within the vagina

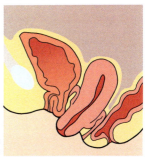

2nd degree
descent to the vaginal introitus

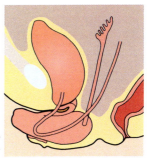

3rd degree/procidentia
descent outside the vagina

Fig. 14.1 Degree of prolapse.

Prevalence

Pelvic floor prolapse is common, particularly in older women. It is thought that 50% of women over 50 years of age have some symptoms of pelvic organ prolapse and by the age of 80 years more than 10% would have had surgery for prolapse.

Symptoms

The most common symptom that patients complain of is the sensation of a lump 'coming down', which may have an associated dragging discomfort or heaviness in the vagina. This tends to increase after periods of standing or exertion. Some patients may be able to feel or see a vaginal lump. If there is bladder prolapse (cystocele), patients may experience increased urinary frequency, feeling of incomplete bladder emptying or frequent urinary infections. If there is bowel prolapse (rectocele), they may complain of low back pain, constipation or incomplete bowel emptying. The prolapse may also cause discomfort during intercourse.

Some patients do not have symptoms at all and prolapse may be diagnosed incidentally at the time of a vaginal examination, for example, at the time of a smear test.

Anatomy

Knowledge of pelvic anatomy and the pelvic floor muscles is important to understand the physiology of pelvic organ prolapse and explain this to patients. It is weakness of the pelvic floor muscles, fascia and ligaments that results in descent of the pelvic organs.

The pelvic floor muscles consist of a series of forward sloping muscles that form a hammock consisting of the levator ani muscles, coccygeus, piriformis and obturator internus. The levator ani consists of a pubococcygeal part anteriorly and the iliococcygeal part posteriorly and is covered by pelvic fascia. The vagina and urethra pass through the urogenital aperture formed by the medial border of the levator ani. The rectum passes posteriorly with muscle fibres from the pubic bone uniting at the anorectal junction. Thus the muscles provide an indirect support for these structures (Fig. 1.4).

The pelvic fascia condenses to form strong ligaments which support the upper portion of the vagina, cervix and uterus. The transverse cervical (cardinal) ligaments support the cervix to the pelvic side wall and the uterosacral supports the cervix to the sacrum. The round ligament passes from the cornu of the uterus through the inguinal canal to the labia majora, and has a minimal role in support.

Aetiology

Pelvic floor prolapse is commonly acquired and worsened throughout life by situations that weaken the pelvic floor. Examples include obstetric factors, postmenopausal atrophy and raised intra-abdominal.

Pregnancy and childbirth are the most common causes of weakening of the pelvic floor, particularly in cases of macrosomia, instrumental (forceps/ventouse) delivery, prolonged labour and high parity. Care must be taken intrapartum to avoid increasing these risks and education should be provided regarding pelvic floor exercises.

The incidence of prolapse increases with age, particularly postmenopause, when the hypo-oestrogenic state leads to atrophy of connective tissues.

Any factors that chronically raise intra-abdominal pressure can lead to prolapse. This includes being overweight, chronic constipation, persistent coughing, prolonged heavy lifting or an intra-abdominal.

Prolapse can also be caused iatrogenically. Hysterectomy predisposes to future prolapse of the vagina by surgical division of the transverse cervical and uterosacral ligaments which support the upper vagina. This causes an integral weakness.

Women can also be born with a predisposition to prolapse, which is probably secondary to abnormal collagen production. Examples include spina bifida and connective tissue disorders.

Diagnosis

History

The diagnosis of pelvic floor prolapse can often be made from its typical presenting symptoms alone. However, it is important to not miss an alternative diagnosis as individual symptoms could be related to a different pathology.

A full medical and gynaecological history should be taken, including menopausal status.

Are you experiencing any vaginal discomfort or dyspareunia? Do you have any vaginal discharge or bleeding? As described earlier, local discomfort is the most common symptom. This is typically worse with prolonged standing and straining and relived by lying flat. A procidentia can cause discomfort by rubbing on a patient's clothing which can cause ulceration as well as a bloody or purulent discharge.

Do you have any dysuria or increasing urinary frequency? The patient may notice incomplete bladder emptying which in turn can cause urinary tract infection (UTI) and possible overflow incontinence. If there is descent of the bladder neck (urethrovesical junction), stress incontinence can be present.

Do you have any difficulty opening your bowels? As a result of difficulty opening bowels, some patients digitally push back the prolapse to allow emptying.

How does this affect your quality of life? Symptoms of prolapse can be very troubling to women and can affect their day-to-day life. It is important to consider this when deciding most appropriate management.

Examination

General observations are important in the assessment – for example, what is the patient's body mass index and general mobility?

On abdominal examination are there any scars from previous surgery? Are there any palpable abdominal masses?

A Cusco's speculum can be used to examine the patient vaginally with the patient's consent and a chaperone present. Alternatively, the patient can be examined with a Sims speculum in the left lateral position. With the posterior vaginal wall retracted, an anterior prolapse can be easily seen; conversely if the anterior wall is retracted, a posterior prolapse can be assessed. Does the cervix appear normal? Does the vaginal tissue appear healthy?

A bimanual pelvic examination should be performed. Is there uterine descent? Is there descent on straining or coughing? Is there urinary leakage on straining or coughing? A vaginal examination can be performed with the patient standing for a thorough assessment of descent.

Investigations

Few investigations tend to be required as prolapse is a clinical diagnosis. However, if the patient has urinary symptoms it is important to explore these symptoms.

Urine test

Perform a midstream urinary test to exclude UTI as a cause or contributing factor for the symptoms.

Urodynamics

In cases where the patient has a history that suggests stress or urge incontinence it is important to assess this fully. Urodynamics are a series of specialist tests that looks at how well the bladder, sphincters and urethra are storing and releasing urine by showing what happens to the bladder on filling and emptying.

Management

Prevention

As pelvic organ prolapse is such a common phenomenon, it is crucial that we educate women about the importance of preventative measures to strengthen the pelvic floor.

As the most common acquired cause is related to obstetric factors, it is important that efforts are made to minimize damage to the supportive pelvic structures. Appropriate management of labour should therefore include preventing prolonged first and second stages, and thorough advice on postnatal pelvic floor exercises.

Conservative

Lifestyle changes to treat the underlying cause of chronic raised intraabdominal pressure can make a considerable difference to symptoms, particularly those that only remain mild. These include losing weight if you are overweight, managing a chronic cough, for example, by stopping smoking, avoiding constipation and avoiding heavy lifting or high-impact exercise, such as using the trampoline.

Pelvic floor exercises may help to strengthen your pelvic floor muscles and therefore improve symptoms, in some cases considerably. It may be possible in some hospitals to refer patients for a course of treatment to a physiotherapist who specializes in prolapse.

In women who are postmenopausal, the presence of atrophic pelvic tissues may be contributing. Hormone replacement therapy, particularly topical vaginal oestrogen treatment, can help increase collagen content and reduce friability of atrophic tissue.

A pessary is a removable plastic or silicone device placed into the vagina that is designed to support areas of pelvic organ prolapse. There are various types and sizes that are chosen as per patient suitability, but the most commonly used type is a ring pessary. After a vaginal examination is performed and appropriate size is chosen, the pessary is passed into the vagina so that it sits behind the pubic bone anteriorly and in the posterior fornix of the vagina posteriorly, thereby enclosing the cervix. Fitting the correct size of pessary is important and may take more than one attempt. You do not want the pessary to be too small and risk falling out, but if it is too large it can cause discomfort or urinary difficulty. On occasions pessaries can cause local inflammation or bleeding and granulation tissues can develop. Pessaries should be changed or removed, cleaned and reinserted regularly to reduce this risk, ideally every 6 months. Oestrogen cream is used when changing the pessary, to minimize soreness. It is possible to have intercourse when a pessary is in-situ. A pessary insertion is a very good alternative to surgical options in situations where the patient is not medically fit for surgery, would prefer conservative management or if their family is not yet complete.

Surgical

Surgery should be considered with a severe degree, very symptomatic prolapse or if conservative management fails. The aim of surgery is to relieve symptoms whilst optimizing bladder and bowel function. It is not recommended if a woman has not yet completed her family. It is important to educate the woman about risks and benefits. A common risk is narrowing and shortening of the vagina which can potentially cause dyspareunia.

It is important to emphasize that no operation can be guaranteed to cure prolapse, but has a good chance of improving symptoms. Up to 30% of women having surgery for prolapse will develop another prolapse in the future, which can occur in another part of the vagina.

A pelvic floor repair can be performed if there is prolapse of the anterior or posterior wall of the vagina. An anterior repair (anterior colporrhaphy) is indicated for the repair of a cystocele. A portion of redundant anterior vaginal wall tissue mucosa is excised and the exposed fascia is plicated to support the bladder. This operation is done via the vagina without abdominal incisions. Postoperatively there is a risk of worsening urinary symptoms.

A posterior repair (posterior colporrhaphy) is indicated for the repair of a rectocele using a technique similar to an anterior colporrhaphy on the posterior vaginal wall. It is possible to perform anterior and posterior repairs concurrently.

A vaginal hysterectomy (removal of the uterus) can be performed for uterine prolapse and can reduce the risk of recurrence of cystocele or rectocele. Anterior or posterior repair can also be performed at the same time. At the time of hysterectomy, a McCall culdoplasty can be performed, which opposes the uterosacral ligaments to support the remaining vaginal vault.

Operations can also be performed to lift and support the vaginal vault. Sacrospinous fixation fixes the apex of

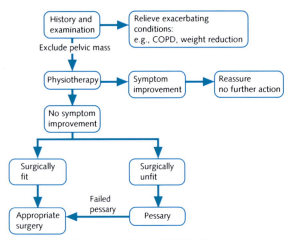

Fig. 14.2 Algorithm for prolapse. *COPD,* Chronic obstructive pulmonary disease.

the vault to the sacrospinous ligament via a transvaginal approach. Sacral colpopexy is an abdominal procedure that suspends the vaginal vault from the sacral promontory using strips of fascia or a synthetic mesh or suture. Complications can include nerve damage, bleeding and infection.

See Fig. 14.2 for management summary.

URINARY INCONTINENCE

Background

Definition

Urinary incontinence (UI) is the complaint of any involuntary leakage of urine. It is a common symptom that can affect women of all ages with a wide range of severity. The bladder has two major roles: the retention of urine and the expulsion of urine. Failure to retain urine or loss of normal voiding control are the two aetiologies of incontinence.

Stress urinary incontinence (SUI) is involuntary urine leakage on effort or exertion such as with sneezing, coughing or laughing and accounts for 50% of incontinence. Urge UI, or detrusor overactivity (DO), is involuntary urine leakage proceeded by a sudden compelling urge to urinate when the bladder is either unstable or overactive and accounts for 40% of incontinence.

Mixed incontinence is a combination of SUI and DO. Overactive bladder is urgency that occurs with or without incontinence and commonly with frequency and nocturia. It is suggestive of DO (Box 14.1).

Prevalence

The prevalence of UI increases with increasing age with 8.5% of women aged under 65 years, 11.6% over 65 years and 43.2% over 85 years affected.

Diagnosis

Stress incontinence

The bladder acts as a low-pressure reservoir. As the volume of urine increases, the bladder pressure rises slightly. Urethral closure pressure, produced by the passive effect of elastic and collagen fibres and active striated and smooth muscle, causes the urethra to remain closed at rest. In the resting state the urethral closure pressure is higher than the relatively low bladder pressure, and continence is maintained (Fig. 14.3).

Raised intra-abdominal pressure, such as when coughing or sneezing, increases the bladder pressure and bladder neck pressure. If the bladder neck and proximal urethra is above the pelvic floor, the positive pressure gradient and continence is maintained. However, if the bladder neck and proximal urethra are below the pelvic floor, then the positive pressure gradient is lost and incontinence occurs. Therefore SUI has an association with pelvic floor prolapse.

SUI increases with increasing age due to parity, postmenopausal status and as maximal urethral closing pressure decreases. Vaginal tissue atrophy and pelvic floor surgery are also associated.

Urge incontinence/detrusor overactivity

In women with DO the urethra functions normally, but if the uninhibited detrusor activity increases bladder pressure above maximal urethral closure pressure, urinary leakage can occur.

The majority of women with DO have idiopathic aetiology with no demonstrable abnormality, but it increases with age. However, causes can include surgery to the bladder neck and proximal urethra, such as surgery for SUI. Neurological conditions such as multiple sclerosis, autonomic neuropathy and spinal lesions lead to uninhibited detrusor contractions, causing detrusor hyperreflexia (Table 14.2).

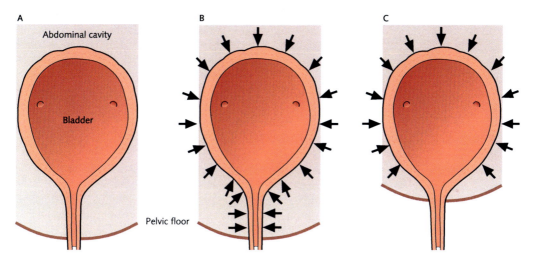

Fig. 14.3 Mechanism of stress urinary incontinence (SUI). (A) Bladder at rest; (B) intraabdominal pressure transmitted to the bladder and urethra (normal) and (C) intraabdominal pressure not transmitted to the bladder/urethra (SUI).

Table 14.2 Neurological causes of voiding difficulties (acute and chronic retention).

Type of lesion	Neurological cause of voiding difficulty
Central (suprapontine)	Cerebrovascular accident Parkinson disease
Spinal	Spinal cord injury Multiple sclerosis
Peripheral	Prolapsed intervertebral disc Peripheral autonomic neuropathies (e.g., diabetic)

Sensory urgency

Irritation of the bladder mucosa, due to acute infection, chronic infection, bladder stones or tumours can cause sensory urgency. The aetiology of primary vesicle sensory urgency is not well understood but accounts for almost 4% of incontinent women.

Voiding disorders

Voiding difficulties can present as acute or chronic urinary retention with overflow incontinence. Chronic overdistension of the bladder is then likely to be exacerbated, worsening symptoms with additional detrusor ischaemia and denervation.

Voiding difficulties can occur secondary to mechanical obstruction, medication or neurological conditions. Impaction of a pelvic mass, for instance, a fibroid uterus, bladder polyps or malignancy might obstruct the urethra. It is also common to have a temporary blockade caused by swelling following bladder neck surgery. Postoperative pain can cause reflex inhibition of micturition, as can severe inflammation of the bladder, urethra and vulva.

Central, spinal and peripheral neurological lesions can produce voiding difficulties. Approximately 25% of women with multiple sclerosis will present with acute urinary retention.

Medications can cause voiding difficulties, the most common example being epidural or spinal anaesthesia during labour. Tricyclic antidepressants, anticholinergic agents, α-adrenergic agonists and ganglion blockers can all impact voiding.

Fistulae

The most common cause of urogenital fistulae worldwide is obstructed labour, which is almost eradicated in the UK due to our care of prolonged labour. Fistulae can also occur secondarily to urogynaecological surgery, malignancy or pelvic radiotherapy. The can occur from the ureter, bladder or urethra to the vagina.

History

A detailed history is important as patients can present with multiple symptoms of varying degrees (Table 14.3). It is important to correlate the history with a bladder diary. History should be taken as per pelvic floor dysfunction history (see discussion earlier) with a full medical and gynaecological history. A medical history is important to identify possible neurological symptoms, such as those suggestive of multiple sclerosis.

The history of urinary symptoms should be extensive to highlight possible pathology.

Do you have any dysuria or increasing urinary frequency? Do you ever see blood in your urine? This may suggest excluding acute or recurrent UTI or may highlight an underlying pathology.

Do you experience urinary leakage? Is leakage small amounts or large volumes? The amount of leakage should

Table 14.3 Commonly used urogynaecological terms

Term	Definition
Cystometry	The measurement of bladder pressure and volume
Detrusor overactivity	An overactive bladder is one that is shown objectively to contract spontaneously or on provocation during the filling phase while the patient is attempting to inhibit micturition
High frequency of micturition	Voiding more than seven times per day
Stress urinary incontinence	The involuntary loss of urine when the intravesical pressure exceeds the maximum urethral pressure in the absence of detrusor activity
Nocturia	Voiding more than twice per night
Nocturnal enuresis	The involuntary passage of urine at night
Stress incontinence	Involuntary loss of urine associated with raised intraabdominal pressure
Urge incontinence	Urinary leakage associated with a strong and sudden desire to void
Urgency of micturition	A strong and sudden desire to void
Urinary incontinence	Involuntary loss of urine that is a social or hygienic problem and is objectively demonstrable
Uroflowmetry	The measurement of urine flow rate
Videocystourethrography	Combines radiological with pressure and flow studies

be classified. Is it triggered by coughing or laughing? Do you ever have a sudden strong urge to pass urine? Do you always manage to make it to the toilet? These questions may identify whether the patient is predominantly suffering from an SUI or DO.

How many times do you pass urine during the day? How many times do you pass urine at night? Nocturia is a common feature with DO.

Do you have good flow of urine? Do you have to strain to pass urine? Do you ever have the feeling of incomplete emptying? Do you suffer with continuous leakage? These may highlight an outflow obstruction, or, rarely, a fistula.

What is your body mass index? Do you smoke or have a chronic cough? What medications do you take? Information regarding general health and lifestyle is important as age, parity, obesity, smoking and medications can contribute to incontinence symptoms.

How much water do you drink in a day? Do you consume caffeine? When is the last time at night you have a drink? These are common lifestyle factors that can be adjusted to help reduce symptoms.

ETHICS

It is important to acknowledge the considerable psychosocial impact of urinary incontinence symptoms. Some hospitals have the benefit of a continence specialist nurse to provide additional support. Support groups are available, such as ERIC (https://www.eric.org.uk/) for children, and Bladder Health UK (bladderhealthuk.org) for adults.

Examination

Examination focusses on the same features as examined with pelvic floor prolapse (see earlier discussion).

Examine the external genitalia – are there signs of excoriation or chronic inflammation of the bladder? Are the vaginal tissues healthy or are there signs of tissue atrophy?

Whilst performing a pelvic examination assess for uterine descent – is there descent on straining or coughing? Is there urinary leakage on straining or coughing? A vaginal examination can be performed with the patient standing and often stress incontinence can be demonstrated by coughing with a moderately dull bladder.

If there is suspicion from the history of neurological cause of incontinence, a full neurological examination should be performed.

Investigations

Urine test
Perform a urinary dipstick to exclude UTI as the cause.

Bladder diary
This is a recording of times and volumes of urine passed, leakage and pad usage along with fluid intake, degree of urgency and degree of incontinence. It is recommended that this is kept for a minimum of 3 days on both working and leisure days. It will highlight triggers for incontinence episodes related to lifestyle that may be adjustable, such as high caffeine intake.

Urodynamic studies
This term encompasses tests that assess the function of the lower urinary tract, and therefore the ability to void.

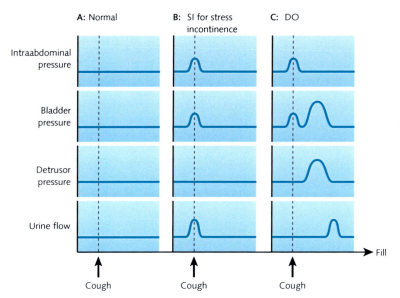

Fig. 14.4 Cystometry. (A) Normal bladder: no increase in detrusor pressure with filling or contraction with cough; (B) genuine stress incontinence – urine flow with cough seen and (C) detrusor overactivity (DO) – detrusor contracts after cough and urine flows with detrusor contraction.

Flow studies, using a flowmeter, assess the rate of flow of urine that normally should be above 15 mL/s. A low flow rate suggests poor action of the detrusor muscle, or an outflow obstruction.

Cystometry measures bladder pressure during filling and voiding using pressure catheters inserted in the bladder (intravesical pressure) and the rectum (intraabdominal pressure). The bladder pressure can be subtracted from the intraabdominal pressure to give the detrusor pressure. This can detect detrusor instability, contractility and outflow resistance (Fig. 14.4).

Video cystourethrography involves real-time radiological monitoring of the bladder during cystometry using contrast material in the bladder. This can concurrently help to identify anatomical anomalies – such as diverticula and fistula, stress incontinence or bladder neck descent – seen on coughing or outflow pathology visualized on voiding.

Cystoscopy

This is an investigation involving a narrow camera being introduced in the bladder via the urethra, which allows inspection of the bladder neck and internal bladder anatomy. It will enable identification of polyps, calculi, chronic inflammation and malignancies. However, it elicits no information regarding bladder function so has no role in the initial assessment of women with UI alone. Fig. 14.5 summarizes the investigation and diagnosis pathways.

Management

Conservative

Conservative or preventative management includes weight loss, fluid management and caffeine reduction. Stopping smoking and treating constipation and chronic cough can improve urinary symptoms.

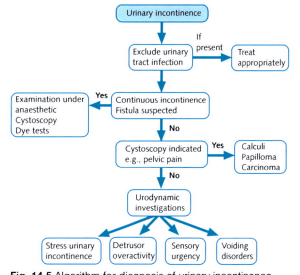

Fig. 14.5 Algorithm for diagnosis of urinary incontinence.

Physiotherapy and pelvic floor exercises can improve urinary control and symptoms in up to 60% of women with SUI. Techniques can range from simple muscular exercises to more complex therapy involving vaginal cones. However, symptoms can return if exercises are stopped.

Bladder retraining aims to improve bladder control in women with DO. Patients are taught how to 'reset' bladder function by micturating by the clock rather than by felling of need, gradually increasing voiding intervals. Offer a trial of supervised pelvic floor muscle training of at least 3 months' duration as first-line treatment to women with SUI or mixed incontinence. This may be successful in up to 80% of patients. Hypnotherapy and acupuncture have also been shown to be beneficial.

Medical

There is a strong placebo effect in the drug treatment of DO. Antimuscarinic medications act to increase bladder capacity by delaying initial desire to void, decreasing the strength of detrusor contractions and decreasing the frequency of detrusor contractions. The suggested preparations are oxybutynin (immediate release), tolterodine (immediate release) and darifenacin (once daily preparation). These medications can improve symptoms in many women, but can have unpleasant antimuscarinic side-effects such as a dry mouth (Table 14.4). It is therefore advised to prescribe the lowest recommended dose when starting a new treatment. Transdermal medications can be offered to women unable to tolerate oral medication. Mirabegron is recommended as an option for treating the symptoms of overactive bladder only for people in whom antimuscarinic drugs are contraindicated or clinically ineffective, or have unacceptable side-effects.

Duloxetine is an inhibitor of serotonin and noradrenaline re-uptake and increases the tone of the urethral sphincter. It is not recommended as a first-line treatment of SUI, but can be offered as a second-line therapy if women prefer pharmacological to surgical treatment or are not suitable for surgical treatment.

Topical oestrogen replacement can improve the symptoms of stress incontinence in postmenopausal women.

Surgical

The majority of women with SUI can be cured by surgery – lifting and supporting the bladder neck and urethra, restoring intraabdominal position. This is done by inserting a tension-free vaginal tape through a small vaginal incision over the mid-urethra. Long-term success rates are up to 90%, comparable to colposuspension (see earlier discussion).

Invasive options for improving DO include bladder wall injections with botulinum toxin A with good chance of a large reduction in symptoms. However, it is a treatment that wears off over time and has a risk of requiring temporary clean intermittent catheterization. If the patient does not respond or is not suitable, a specialist centre could suggest providing percutaneous sacral nerve stimulation to women. Surgical options include augmentation cystoplasty or urinary diversion, but these are major surgical procedures with potentially serious complications and life-long follow-up so must be carefully considered.

Acute urinary retention requires catheterization to both relieve the retention and avoid permanent bladder injury. Postoperative or postpartum retention usually resolves with free bladder drainage for 48 hours or so. If the bladder has an overdistension injury, then free bladder drainage is required until normal function returns. Chronic retention may require intermittent self-catheterization, a long-term indwelling catheter or a suprapubic catheter. However, there is an ongoing risk of infection and sepsis with these methods.

If a patient has a large fistula, closure by an experienced surgeon is required. However, it is possible for small fistulae to close spontaneously by continence-free drainage of the bladder.

Complications

Although incontinence itself is not life threatening, it does cause major psychosocial problems. Changes in lifestyle are common and occasionally symptoms are so severe to render the woman housebound. Continence pads can be a financial burden for patients. Excoriation and soreness of the vulva can cause great discomfort, and risk fungal infection and recurrent UTI with potential for damage to renal function.

Chronic overdistension of the bladder can cause denervation of the detrusor muscle and worsen ongoing voiding difficulties.

RED FLAG

Urgent referral for review is warranted in patients with macroscopic haematuria, microscopic haematuria over the age of 50 years, recurrent urinary tract infection with haematuria and suspected pelvic mass arising from the urinary tract, to exclude malignancy.

RECURRENT UTIs

UTIs are a common type of bacterial infection with up to 50% experiencing them as adults. Recurrent UTI is defined as three or more episodes of symptomatic UTI within a 12-month period, ideally culture-proven infections.

Recurrent infections suggest an underlying anatomical or functional pathology, therefore should be investigated. Renal tract ultrasound should be arranged and computed tomography scan of the kidneys, ureters and bladder should be considered with a history of renal colic. If there is any voiding dysfunction, urodynamics should be considered. Flexible cystoscopy should also be considered as up to 8%

Table 14.4 Antimuscarinic (atropine-like) side-effects

Type of side-effect	Description
Peripheral	Dry mouth
	Reduced visual accommodation
	Constipation
	Glaucoma
Central	Confusion

of women >50 years of age with recurrent infection will have significant abnormalities detected at cystoscopy, such as chronic inflammation.

Prophylactic low-dose antibiotic regimen treatment can be commenced for 6 months as data indicate that this can reduce rate of UTI. The choice of antibiotic used should be based on the most recent sensitivities when available, but it is important to remember that long-term antibiotic prophylaxis is strongly associated with the development of antimicrobial resistance.

● **Chapter Summary**

- Pelvic floor prolapse is a common condition caused by weakening of the pelvic floor by factors such as childbirth, postmenopausal atrophy and raised intraabdominal pressure.
- Urinary incontinence is the complaint of any involuntary leakage of urine. It is a common symptom that can affect women of all ages with a wide range of severity.
- Urogynaecological symptoms should be thoroughly investigated to achieve the correct diagnosis and to aid management options.
- It is important that treatment is determined by the underlying condition, the severity of the symptoms and crucially by the effect on the woman's quality of life.
- A sympathetic approach and detailed counselling is essential in imaging these patients.

BACKGROUND

Regular monthly periods in women of reproductive age are a manifestation of cyclical ovarian activity. This can be influenced by balances within the hormone profile, but can also be attributed to many other factors.

AMENORRHEA

Definition

Amenorrhoea is the absence of menstruation, therefore can be a physiological progress occurring in childhood, during pregnancy, during lactation and after the menopause. However, there are also multiple pathological causes of amenorrhoea and there may be an underlying disease or condition.

'Primary' amenorrhoea refers to when menstruation has not yet started by the age of 16 years in the presence of normal secondary sexual characteristics, or 14 years in the absence of other evidence of puberty.

'Secondary' amenorrhoea refers to absent periods for at least 6 months in a woman who has previously had regular periods, or 12 months if she has had oligomenorrhoea (bleeds less frequently than 6 weekly).

Prevalence

Primary amenorrhoea is relatively rare, occurring in approximately 0.3% of women. Secondary amenorrhoea is more commonly seen in approximately 4% of the population.

Causes

Physiological causes such as pregnancy, lactation or menopause must be excluded.

In primary amenorrhoea with normal secondary sexual characteristics, the most common causes are genitourinary malformations. Examples of this include an imperforate hymen, a vaginal septum, absent vagina or absent uterus.

If there are no secondary sexual characteristics with primary amenorrhoea, this would suggest an underlying chromosomal or hormonal cause, such as in Turner syndrome (45,XO) or hypothalamic–pituitary dysfunction.

If secondary amenorrhoea is not physiological, iatrogenic causes should be excluded, such as progestogen methods of contraception, radiotherapy or illicit drug use. De-novo genitourinary malformations such as cervical stenosis or Asherman syndrome should be investigated. Hormonal factors should be investigated, including hypothalamic dysfunction, premature ovarian failure, pituitary causes and thyroid disease (Table 15.1).

Diagnosis

History

History is crucial in diagnosing the cause of amenorrhoea as the aetiology can be so varied. By definition, menarche will not have occurred in women with primary amenorrhoea. Important areas to cover include:

- menstrual and pubertal history
- gynaecological and obstetric history
- preexisting medical conditions and symptoms
- general health

HISTORY

How old were you when you went through puberty? What are your periods like? The timing of any pubertal development will establish whether this is normal, precocious or delayed. Menstrual irregularity or oligomenorrhoea may suggest conditions such as polycystic ovarian syndrome. Cyclical pain may suggest a congenital or acquired outflow obstruction to menstrual fluid.

Do you have any gynaecology conditions? Ask about any known gynaecology diagnosis such as polycystic ovarian syndrome (PCOS), prior pelvic surgery and sexually transmitted infections and check smear tests are up-to-date. Procedures such as cervical surgery can cause stenosis.

Have you had any previous pregnancies? Take a full obstetrics history of pregnancy outcomes and mode of delivery, also ensuring you ask about previous miscarriages. Pituitary failure can occur after massive postpartum haemorrhage (Sheehan syndrome). Any cause for uterine curettage, such as surgical management of miscarriage, can result in intrauterine scarring (Asherman syndrome).

Do you have any medical conditions? Do you take any regular medications? Some chronic medical conditions such as thyroid dysfunction or diabetes mellitus can affect menstruation. Hirsutism and virilism can be due to congenital adrenal hyperplasia, PCOS or an androgen-secreting tumour. A full drug history should identify medications that can cause amenorrhoea. Hot flushes and vaginal dryness suggest premature ovarian failure. Antipsychotics can cause increased prolactin levels and illicit drug use such as cocaine and opiates can cause hypogonadism (Table 15.1).

How is your general health? What is your current weight? Any symptoms such as excess hair or production of breast milk? Any central nervous system symptoms such as headache or visual disturbance can suggest diagnosis such as a pituitary tumour. It is important to ask about emotional stress, weight loss from dieting or anorexia, as low body mass index can cause amenorrhoea.

Table 15.1 Prescribed drugs that can cause hyperprolactinaemia[a]

Types of drug	Drug class
Antipsychotic drugs	Phenothiazines Haloperidol
Antidepressants	Tricyclic antidepressants
Antihypertensive drugs	Methyldopa Reserpine
Oestrogens	Combined oral contraceptive pill
H_2 receptor antagonists	Cimetidine Ranitidine Metoclopramide and domperidone

[a] Do not forget chemotherapy for malignancy or immunological disorders.

Examination

A general examination should be performed. Measure height and body weight, and calculate body mass index (BMI).

The examination should be top-to-toe. Look for signs of excess androgens such as hirsutism, acne, weight gain and male pattern balding. Assess for signs of thyroid disease, diabetes and Cushing syndrome such as striae, buffalo hump and significant central obesity. Typical features of Turner syndrome include short stature, a webbed neck, shield chest with widely spaced nipples, wide carrying angle and scoliosis. Assess visual fields if a pituitary tumour is suspected.

Table 15.2 Tanner staging of puberty for females

Tanner stage	Breast development	Pubic hair
1	Prepubertal – no breast tissue	Prepubertal – no pubic hair
2	Breast bud stage with elevation of breast and papilla; enlargement of areola	Sparse growth of long, slightly pigmented hair, straight or curled along labia
3	Further enlargement of breast and areola; no separation of their contour	Darker, coarser and more curled hair, spreading sparsely over the junction of pubis
4	Areola and papilla form a secondary mound above level of breast	Hair adult in type, but covering smaller area than in adult; no spread to medial surface of thighs
5	Mature stage: projection of papilla only, related to recession of areola	Adult in type and quantity, with horizontal distribution

A full gynaecological examination is required. Examine the abdomen for any pelvic masses. Examine for secondary sexual development using the Tanner system (Table 15.2). This includes assessment of breast development as well as axillary and pubic hair. Absence of axillary and pubic hair with normal breast development suggests androgen insensitivity.

A pelvic examination should be performed with patient's consent and a chaperone present. This should be performed with particular sensitivity in young girls. Assess for clitoromegaly, a sign of virilization, and for vaginal patency. If a haematocolpos is present, you may see a bulging blue-coloured bulge at the introitus. In young girls who are not sexually active, ultrasonography should be performed to assess pelvic anatomy.

Investigations

Target investigations for amenorrhoea to a specific cause as highlighted by the history if possible (Figs 15.1 and 15.2 present a related summary).

Urine test

Perform a urinary pregnancy test to exclude pregnancy as the cause.

Pelvic ultrasound

This can identify polycystic ovaries if suspected with typical appearance of enlarged ovaries and multiple peripheral follicles. It can also be used to identify anatomical abnormalities (such as an absent uterus caused by androgen insensitivity) or outflow obstruction such as haematometra (blood within the uterus).

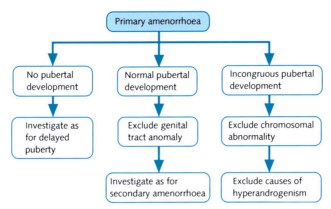

Fig. 15.1 Algorithm for primary amenorrhoea.

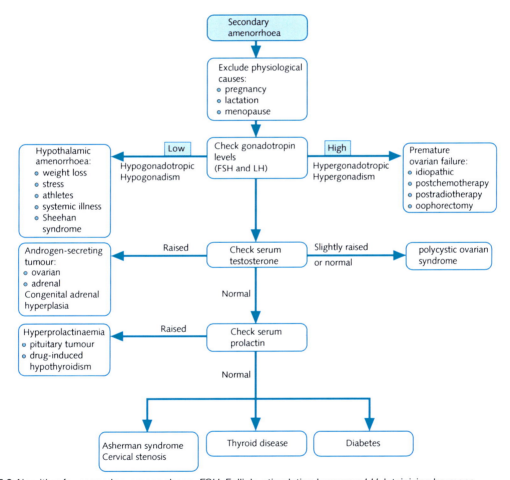

Fig. 15.2 Algorithm for secondary amenorrhoea. *FSH,* Follicle-stimulating hormone; *LH,* luteinizing hormone.

Blood tests

Serum gonadotrophins, luteinizing hormone (LH) and follicle-stimulating hormone (FSH), should be measured. In polycystic ovarian syndrome (PCOS) the LH-to-FSH ratio is usually greater than 2.5. Levels of both are greatly raised with ovarian failure, at both the lower limit with hypothalamic amenorrhoea and hypogonadotropic hypogonadism.

Serum testosterone levels might be normal or raised with PCOS, although free testosterone is usually raised. With very high testosterone levels an androgen-secreting tumour should be suspected.

Serum prolactin levels are important to exclude hyperprolactinaemia. However, probation levels can also be temporarily raised, for example, as a response to stress or following a breast examination. Thyroid-stimulating hormone and free thyroxine levels should be tested if dysfunction is suspected.

Specialist tests

Chromosomal analysis should be performed in unexplained primary amenorrhoea, primary ovarian failure or if there is suspicion of a chromosomal analysis such as Turner syndrome. If there is galactorrhoea or high prolactin level, consider cranial imaging such as magnetic resonance imaging (MRI) to assess for pituitary or central nervous system (CNS) tumour. If chronic illness is suspected, investigations should be guided by clinical findings.

Management of primary amenorrhea

Gonadal dysgenesis describes congenital developmental disorder of the reproductive system, which leads to underdeveloped gonads consisting of fibrous tissue (streak gonads). An example includes Turner syndrome (45,XO). Management involves hormone replacement therapy (HRT) to stimulate secondary sexual development in those not yet exposed to oestrogen and to protect against cardiac disease and osteoporosis. Women who carry a Y chromosome should have both gonads removed, because of the risk of malignancy.

If the cause is a genital tract anomaly such as haematocolpos, it can be surgically treated by excision of the persistent vaginal membrane and allow ongoing drainage of menstrual blood. Congenital conditions such as an absent vagina should be referred to a tertiary centre for vaginal reconstruction.

ETHICS

It is important to appreciate the psychosocial and psychosexual aspects of a diagnosis of conditions such as gonadal dysgenesis and absence of female reproductive organs. Patients receiving these diagnoses must be adequately supported and counselled.

Management of secondary amenorrhea

Polycystic ovarian syndrome

One of the key treatments for PCOS is weight loss. As the BMI approaches the normal range, spontaneous ovulation and regular menstruation often occur. Long-term protection of the endometrium can be provided using cyclical progestogens, the combined oral contraceptive pill (COCP) or the Mirena intrauterine device. There are COCP preparations available that work particularly well with symptoms

of PCOS due to the antiandrogen and progestogenic effect of cyproterone acetate or additional antimineralocorticoid activity (Dianette, Yasmin).

As insulin resistance is an important part of the disease process of PCOS, metformin, an oral hypoglycaemic agent, is being used as a management option. Women with PCOS on metformin find weight loss targets easier to achieve, and some may start to ovulate spontaneously.

Hyperprolactinaemia

Pituitary microadenomas are tumours less than 10 mm in diameter that can secrete hormones, but most are clinically inactive. Treatment is advised to reduce risk of osteoporosis. Dopamine agonists such as bromocriptine and cabergoline should be used and will lower serum prolactin levels. Side-effects include nausea, dizziness, hypotension and headache. Cessation of therapy is recommended in pregnancy, but any cessation likely causes reoccurrence of hyperprolactinaemia.

A pituitary macroadenoma over 10 mm may require surgical in addition to medical intervention, but medication alone can cause improvement of symptoms and tumour shrinkage. A transsphenoidal resection can be performed but has a risk of diabetes insidious, cerebrospinal fluid leak and tumour reoccurrence.

If hyperprolactinaemia is medication induced, then stopping the medication will resolve the prolactin levels and symptoms. However, if it is not suitable to stop the treatment, additional oestrogen may be advised to protect from osteoporosis.

Hormone-secreting tumours

Ovarian and adrenal hormone-secreting tumours should be surgically removed, preserving maximal ovarian tissues.

Asherman syndrome

Asherman syndrome is the presence of intrauterine adhesions. These can be divided hysteroscopically and temporary insertion of an intrauterine contraceptive device can help prevent redevelopment of adhesions. Cervical stenosis may require cervical dilatation.

Sheehan syndrome

Sheehan syndrome is a postpartum infarction of the pituitary gland, triggered due to massive obstetric haemorrhage. Oestrogen replacement would be required as COCP or HRT. In addition, replacement of all pituitary hormones may be required.

PRECOCIOUS PUBERTY AND DELAYED PUBERTY

Definition

Precocious puberty occurs when pubertal characteristics occur before the age of 9 years.

Delayed puberty is considered when there are no signs of pubertal development by age 14 years.

Prevalence

The overall prevalence of precocious puberty is estimated to be 1:5000 to 1:10,000 children. The exact prevalence of children with delayed puberty is unclear due to many variable factors such as variation in the mean pubertal age between different ethnic groups and genetic influence on the onset of puberty.

Causes

Aetiology of precocious puberty and delayed puberty are both varied and with multiple systemic causes. The majority of cases of precocious puberty have idiopathic causes, followed by ovarian causes such as oestrogen-secreting tumours. Delayed puberty has predominantly CNS-related aetiology, such as infection, tumours and head trauma, followed by idiopathic causes. Rarer causes include genetic and chronic illness (Figs 15.3–15.5).

Diagnosis

History

History is very important to establish the cause of delayed or precocious puberty as the aetiology for both can be so varied. The following history should be part of a comprehensive medical and gynaecological history.

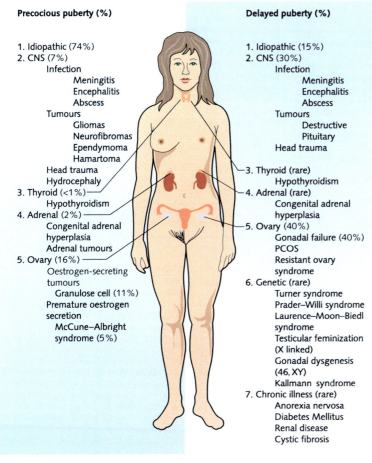

Precocious puberty (%)

1. Idiopathic (74%)
2. CNS (7%)
   Infection
       Meningitis
       Encephalitis
       Abscess
   Tumours
       Gliomas
       Neurofibromas
       Ependymoma
       Hamartoma
   Head trauma
   Hydrocephaly
3. Thyroid (<1%)
   Hypothyroidism
4. Adrenal (2%)
   Congenital adrenal
   hyperplasia
   Adrenal tumours
5. Ovary (16%)
   Oestrogen-secreting
   tumours
       Granulose cell (11%)
   Premature oestrogen
   secretion
       McCune–Albright
       syndrome (5%)

Delayed puberty (%)

1. Idiopathic (15%)
2. CNS (30%)
   Infection
       Meningitis
       Encephalitis
       Abscess
   Tumours
       Destructive
       Pituitary
   Head trauma
3. Thyroid (rare)
   Hypothyroidism
4. Adrenal (rare)
   Congenital adrenal
   hyperplasia
5. Ovary (40%)
   Gonadal failure (40%)
   PCOS
   Resistant ovary
   syndrome
6. Genetic (rare)
   Turner syndrome
   Prader–Willi syndrome
   Laurence–Moon–Biedl
   syndrome
   Testicular feminization
   (X linked)
   Gonadal dysgenesis
   (46, XY)
   Kallmann syndrome
7. Chronic illness (rare)
   Anorexia nervosa
   Diabetes Mellitus
   Renal disease
   Cystic fibrosis

Fig. 15.3 Causes of precocious puberty and delayed puberty. *CNS*, Central nervous system; *PCOS*, polycystic ovarian syndrome.

Fig. 15.4 Aetiology for precocious puberty. *CAH*, Congenital adrenal hyperplasia; *CNS*, central nervous system.

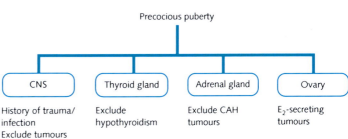

Precocious puberty

CNS	Thyroid gland	Adrenal gland	Ovary
History of trauma/ infection Exclude tumours	Exclude hypothyroidism	Exclude CAH tumours	E_2-secreting tumours

Fig. 15.5 Aetiology for delayed puberty. *BMI,* Body mass index; *PCOS,* polycystic ovarian syndrome.

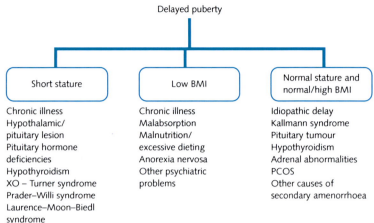

Delayed puberty

Short stature

Chronic illness
Hypothalamic/
pituitary lesion
Pituitary hormone
deficiencies
Hypothyroidism
XO – Turner syndrome
Prader–Willi syndrome
Laurence–Moon–Biedl
syndrome

Low BMI

Chronic illness
Malabsorption
Malnutrition/
excessive dieting
Anorexia nervosa
Other psychiatric
problems

Normal stature and normal/high BMI

Idiopathic delay
Kallmann syndrome
Pituitary tumour
Hypothyroidism
Adrenal abnormalities
PCOS
Other causes of
secondary amenorrhoea

HISTORY

Have your periods started yet? Have you developed breast, genital or hair growth? How old were you when you went through puberty? What are your periods like? Do you know the age of your mother at menarche? The timing of any pubertal development will establish whether this is normal, precocious or delayed.

Do you have any medical conditions or chronic illnesses? Are you aware of any chromosomal abnormalities? Have you recently had any infections? Do you take any regular medications? These questions may identify medical causes for the presentation.

How is your general health? What is your current weight? It is important to ask about emotional stress, weight loss from dieting or anorexia as low body mass index can cause amenorrhoea.

Examination

Examination should be a full physical examination as described in examination for 'amenorrhea' as above.

Investigations

Ultrasound pelvis and adrenals

This can identify features such as polycystic ovaries and congenital anomalies. If tumours are suspected, computed tomography (CT) or MRI scans are the gold-standard investigations.

Blood tests

A full endocrine profile should be performed including serum gonadotrophins LH and FSH, oestradiol, testosterone, sex hormone-binding globulin (SHBG), androstenedione, progesterone and dehydroepiandrosterone sulphate. This will highlight endocrinological causes.

Specialist tests

If other tests have not highlighted aetiology, bone age studies, chromosomal analysis and CT/MRI should be performed in unexplained precocious or delayed puberty. If chronic illness is suspected, investigations should be guided by clinical findings.

Management

Management of delayed puberty is aimed at treating the underlying cause.

Management of endocrine precious puberty is by suppression of oestrogen and androgen production by gonadotropin-releasing hormone analogues to reverse the physical changes. If the diagnosis is congenital adrenal hyperplasia (CAH), the treatment is with steroid replacement.

Congenital conditions will need paediatric and genetic team input. With conditions such as XY gonadal dysgenesis that may predispose to gonadal malignancy, the removal of gonads may be required. Similarly, medical conditions such as chronic illness or hypothyroidism need the appropriate medical team input. If a tumour is discovered, then this is usually dealt with surgically.

Psychological support and counselling are essential as these girls and teenagers will feel different from their peers, which could cause long-lasting issues.

VIRILISM

Definition

Virilism is a severe form of androgen excess characterized by hirsutism, voice deepening, temporal balding, amenorrhea, clitoromegaly and breast atrophy. It can be due to excessive endogenous or exogenous androgens, with endogenous production by the ovary being the most common source.

Hirsutism is the excessive growth of terminal hair in androgen-dependent areas (face, chest, lines alba). It can be due to increased androgen levels, but can be idiopathic.

Prevalence

Approximately 10% of healthy normal women have some degree of hirsutism, but without signs of virilism. True virilism is a rarer presentation.

Causes

See Figs 15.6 and 15.7 for summary.

Ovarian androgens

PCOS is the most common cause of ovarian androgens and hirsutism (90%), and occurs in 20% of women. Characteristically there are raised levels of circulating LH and sex steroids. Pituitary production of LH is raised in PCOS, causing increased ovarian androgen production and increased LH-to-FSH ratio. This leads to a reduced production of SHBG by the liver, and, as SHBG binds to circulating androgens, free testosterone levels increase (Fig. 15.8).

Androgens are converted to oestrogen in adipose tissue, raising oestradiol levels, which further stimulates pituitary production of LH. Obesity increases insulin levels, which stimulates further ovarian androgen production, but also reduces SHBG levels and increases the peripheral conversion of androgens to oestrogen.

Androgen-secreting tumours of the ovary are rare and include arrhenoblastomas and hilar cell tumours. Pregnancy luteomas are a rare source of excess ovarian androgen secretion that develop due to an exaggerated response by the ovarian storm to human chorionic gonadotropin.

COMMUNICATION

Polycystic ovarian syndrome (PCOS) is diagnosed by two of the three criteria: oligo/anovulation, clinical or biochemical signs of hyperandrogenism, polycystic ovaries (12+ peripheral follicles or increased ovarian volume).

It is possible to have polycystic appearances of the ovaries on ultrasound without a diagnosis of PCOS. It is important to explain to patients what the diagnosis means as there is often confusion, due to the name of the condition, with a diagnosis of ovarian cysts.

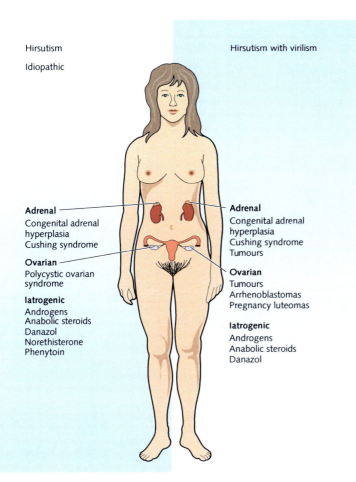

Fig. 15.6 Causes of hirsutism and virilism.

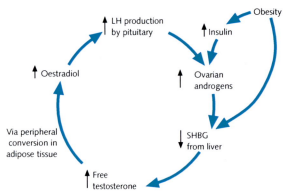

Fig. 15.7 Mechanism of increased androgen production in polycystic ovarian syndrome. *LH*, luteinizing hormone; *SHBG*, sex hormone-binding globulin.

Adrenal androgens

CAH describes a group of rare inherited disorders caused by mutations in genes that code for enzymes involved in hydroxylation of cortisol precursors in the adrenal glands. The most common enzyme defect, 21-hydroxylase deficiency, leads to excess circulating levels of cortisol precursors and androgens. These precursor steroids are similar to the male hormone testosterone, therefore there can be development of male characteristics and precocious puberty.

Excessive stimulation of the adrenal cortex, such as with an adrenal adenoma causes raised cortisol levels and is often associated with excess androgen production, as seen with endogenous Cushing syndrome. Adenoma and adenocarcinoma of the adrenal gland produce high levels of androgens but are rare.

Exogenous androgens

Androgens, like most hormones, have a normal concentration range with a circadian rhythm. Additional androgens and anabolic steroids can cause hirsutism and virilism depending on the amount and length of time taken. Certain medications have androgenic properties that can lead to these side-effects, including norethisterone, phenytoin and danazol.

Diagnosis

History

A full medical and gynaecology history should be taken and emphasis should be on the following questions to assess likely causation:

- onset of symptoms
- menstrual history
- medical history

HISTORY

When was the onset of your symptoms? Did they progress quickly? Rapid progression of hair growth may be due to androgen-secreting neoplasia, particularly when associated with virilization. However, polycystic ovarian syndrome typically presents with milder symptoms present since menarche.

What are your periods like? A detailed menstrual history is important. Irregularity (particularly oligomenorrhoea) may be due to anovulatory cycles in polycystic ovarian syndrome, nonclassic congenital adrenal hyperplasia or hyperprolactinaemia. Amenorrhoea could be associated with virilism.

What medications are you currently taking? Have you ever taken anabolic steroids? A careful drug history is crucial as over-the-counter and herbal medications could also affect androgen levels.

Does anyone else in your family suffer with hirsutism? Hirsutism in other family members suggests a genetic component as well as idiopathic hirsutism.

Examination

Examination should be a full physical examination as described in examination for 'amenorrhea' as above.

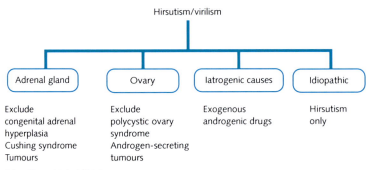

Fig. 15.8 Algorithm for hirsutism and virilism.

Levels of hirsutism can be objectively scored using scoring systems such as the visual scale Ferriman–Gallwey, which assesses nine areas of the body, and a nonaffected woman would usually score under 8. Women with idiopathic hirsutism usually have no other abnormal findings on examination. Signs of virilism such as temporal balding and breast atrophy should also be assessed. Marked symptoms of virilism suggest an androgen-secreting tumour.

Obesity is associated with increased androgen production and clearance rates. A pattern of fat distribution of truncal obesity associated with cervical fat pad, purple striae, thin skin and facial plethora indicates that Cushing syndrome should be considered. Obesity without cushingoid features and acanthosis nigricans (pigmented raised patches) is suggestive of PCOS. Severe CAH will have been diagnosed in childhood due to ambiguous external genitalia; milder late-onset forms of CAH have similar presentations to those of PCOS.

Palpation of an abdominal or pelvic mass in a hirsute woman is suggestive of androgen-secreting neoplasia, although the tumours are usually too small to cause palpable masses.

Investigations

Degree of necessary investigation is determined by the degree of symptoms experienced by the woman. For example, rapid onset of symptoms is more likely to suggest a serious pathology.

Pelvic ultrasound

This can identify polycystic ovaries if suspected with typical appearance of enlarged ovaries and multiple peripheral follicles, or be suggestive of an ovarian androgen-secreting tumour.

Blood tests

Serum gonadotrophins LH and FSH should be measured. With very high serum testosterone levels an androgen-secreting tumour should be suspected.

Specialist tests

It is possible for small tumours to be missed with ultrasound scanning, so if there is a level of suspicion, CT scanning should be performed. Investigations for CAH and Cushing syndrome should be performed if symptoms and clinical signs suggest these diseases.

Idiopathic hirsutism is a diagnosis made by excluding other pathology.

Management

Idiopathic hirsutism can be treated cosmetically using electrolysis or bleaching. Medical treatment of hirsutism with PCOS is most effective using a combination of ethinyloestradiol with an antiandrogen such as dianette (see management of PCOS above).

Androgen-secreting tumours should be surgically removed. Treating the cause of excess cortisol production in Cushing syndrome should normalize circulating androgen levels.

Glucocorticoid and mineralocorticoid replacement is the mainstay of treatment for CAH. Hirsutism and virilism respond to medical treatment, but sometimes there is a need to perform genital surgery reconstructive procedures.

CLINICAL NOTES

Women with gynaecological conditions requiring treatment with medications that have androgenic properties should be forewarned about the potential virilizing side-effects and the lowest therapeutic dose should be used.

Chapter Summary

- Regular monthly periods in women of reproductive age are a manifestation of cyclical ovarian activity.
- The hormones in the reproductive system are carefully balanced and can influence clinical presentation.
- It is important to exclude pathological causes to menstrual symptoms.

BACKGROUND

Definition

Fertility problems are estimated to affect one in seven heterosexual couples in the UK. Referral for clinical assessment and investigations for subfertility should be considered for women of reproductive age who have not conceived after 1 year of regular unprotected vaginal sexual intercourse, in the absence of any known cause of infertility.

Primary subfertility refers to couples who have never had any previous pregnancies, and secondary subfertility is if there has been previous gravidity.

In certain cases, it may be suitable for earlier referral for specialist assessment, such as a known clinical cause of infertility or a history of predisposing factors for infertility (e.g., pelvic infections) or age over 36 years.

Prevalence

Couples should be informed that over 80% in the general population will conceive successfully within 1 year if the woman is aged under 40 years and they are having regular unprotected vaginal sexual intercourse.

Of those who do not conceive in the first year, about half will go on to conceive within the second year (giving a cumulative pregnancy rate of over 90%).

Causes

There are multiple factors that can affect fertility, either from the male partner, female partner or both. To understand the causes and management it is important to understand what is necessary for conception (Fig. 16.1).

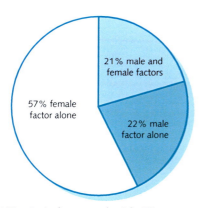

Fig. 16.1 Pie chart of causes of subfertility.

21% male and female factors

57% female factor alone

22% male factor alone

Natural conception requires XX and XY partners who have intercourse resulting in male ejaculation. The sperm must be of sufficient volume, count, progression and normal form to pass through the cervical mucus, uterine cavity and into the fallopian tube. The female must be able to ovulate, and the ovum be picked up by the fimbrial end of a patent fallopian tube and transported to meet the sperm, after which the fertilized embryo implants within the endometrium. Conception occurs in the 4 days around ovulation, sperm can survive for around 3 days and an egg can be fertilized for up to 1 day after ovulation.

Female fertility decreases with age, and factors such as body mass index (BMI), alcohol and smoking can also have a negative effect.

DIAGNOSIS

History – female

A thorough history from both male and female partners is crucial to suggest management and aid diagnosis of subfertility.

How long have you been actively trying to conceive for? How often are you having intercourse? Do you have any problems having intercourse? Current guidelines recommend intercourse every 2–3 days. Any issues with intercourse including vaginismus, dyspareunia or male erectile or ejaculatory dysfunction are relevant.

Have you had any previous pregnancies? Take a full obstetrics history of pregnancy outcomes and mode of delivery, also ensuring you ask about previous miscarriages and the gestation at which these occurred and any ectopic pregnancies which could suggest a tubal problem.

Do you have any gynaecology conditions? Ask about any known gynaecology diagnosis such as polycystic ovary syndrome (PCOS), prior pelvic surgery, sexually transmitted infections and check smear tests are up-to-date.

What are your periods like? Menorrhagia could suggest fibroids, dysmenorrhea could indicate endometriosis and oligo-amenorrhoea could suggest anovulation. Dyspareunia could also suggest pelvic inflammatory disease (PID) or endometriosis.

Do you have any medical conditions? Do you take any regular medications? Some chronic medical conditions such as renal disease, thyroid dysfunction and eating disorders can affect ovulation. Take a full drug history to identify any potentially harmful medications for pregnancy. Encourage women to take folic acid supplements (Table 16.1).

Table 16.1 Causes of female infertility

Problem	Cause
Ovulatory dysfunction	Chronic systemic illness
	Eating disorders
	Polycystic ovarian syndrome
	Hyperprolactinaemia
	Hypo/hyperthyroidism
	Cannabis use
	Nonsteroidal antiinflammatory diseases
Tubal factor	Pelvic inflammatory disease
	Previous tubal surgery
	Previous ectopic pregnancy
	Endometriosis
Uterine problem	Fibroid
	Uterine septa
	Congenital anomaly
	Asherman syndrome
Coital dysfunction	Vaginismus
	Dyspareunia

History – male

Have you ever fathered any pregnancies? If the answer is yes, this will suggest female factor infertility.

Have you ever had any injury or operations on your groin or testicles? Procedures such as inguinal hernia repairs, orchidopexy for undescended testes, previous testicular torsion and bladder neck surgery can all affect male fertility.

Do you have any medical conditions? Do you take any regular medications? Chronic conditions such as renal disease and diabetes can affect spermatogenesis, and cystic fibrosis can have agenesis of the vas deferens. Infections such as mumps orchitis and epididymo-orchitis can also cause obstruction or poor-quality sperm.

Does either partner smoke, drink alcohol or use any illicit drugs? Smoking, alcohol and drug use all reduce fertility and negatively affect sperm quality and quantity. Occupations that can cause raised testicular temperature such as prolonged driving, or exposure to metals, solvents or agricultural chemicals can lead to oligospermia.

Examination

General observations are important in the assessment – what is the patient's BMI [BMI = weight in kilogram/height in square metre (kg/m^2)]? Do they have appropriate secondary sexual characteristics? Evidence of hirsutism or acanthosis nigricans may suggest PCOS.

On abdominal examination are there any scars from previous surgery? The uterus may be enlarged and palpable, suggesting fibroids, or nonmobile due to adhesions or endometriosis. Large ovarian cysts can be palpated abdominally. In males is there evidence of prior inguinal hernia repair?

A Cusco's speculum should be used to examine the patient vaginally with patient's consent and a chaperone present. Is there an imperforate hymen or vaginal membrane visible? Does the cervix appear normal? Is there vaginal discharge suggestive of PID? If so, triple swabs should be taken. In males an orchidometer can be used to assess testicular size and the vas deferens should be palpated.

INVESTIGATIONS

Target investigations for subfertility to a specific cause as highlighted by the history if possible.

Blood tests

Hormone profiles may highlight anovulation, ovarian reserve or PCOS. Serum progesterone in the midluteal phase of their cycle (day 21 of a 28-day cycle) can confirm ovulation. Women with irregular menstrual cycles should be offered a blood test to measure serum gonadotrophins (follicle-stimulating hormone and luteinizing hormone). Antimüllerian hormone can highlight poor ovarian reserve. Prolactin should be assessed if the patient has irregular cycles or galactorrhoea to asses to possible prolactinoma. Thyroid function tests should be performed if there are any signs of thyroid disease. Testosterone levels can be performed in both males and females, for example if the man appears hypoandrogenic (nonhirsute, small soft testes) or if the woman is overly hirsute.

Semen analysis

This should be performed prior to any operative investigations on the female partner as it may identify the cause of subfertility and prevent unnecessary operations. The male partner should provide a specimen after 3 days of abstinence after a period of good health (systemic illness can reduce sperm quality). The examination should take place within 1 hour of production and is assessed for sperm volume, count, motility, progression and morphology. If the result of the first semen analysis is abnormal, a repeat confirmatory test should be offered ideally 3 months after the initial analysis to allow time for the cycle of spermatozoa formation to be completed (Box 16.1).

Transvaginal ultrasound

This can identify structural abnormalities of the pelvic organs such as fibroids, congenital abnormalities of the uterus and hydrosalpinx. It can also identify bulky ovaries with multiple peripheral follicles seen with polycystic ovaries. Total antral follicle count can give an impression of ovarian reserve.

Volume	>1.5 mL
Concentration	>15 million/mL
Progressive motility	32%
Normal forms	4%

Tubal investigations

Women who have comorbidities such as previous PID, previous ectopic pregnancy or endometriosis are at high risk of having tubal pathology, therefore it is advisable to have a laparoscopy (where pathology can be treated at the same time) and tubal dye test under general anaesthesia. This enables direct visualization of the pelvis to make diagnoses and provide appropriate treatment. Methylene blue is a dye introduced via the cervix through the uterus and can be seen to 'fill and spill' through the fallopian tubes at laparoscopy. No 'spill' into the pelvis indicates tubal occlusion.

If patients have no known risk factors for tubal disease, a hysterosalpingography (HSG) is an appropriate investigation (which avoids surgery). Radiopaque dye is introduced via the cervix through the uterus and an X-ray is taken to look for passage of the dye. Blockage can be caused by internal or external tubal factors or tubal spasm (Fig. 16.2). Hysterosalpingo-contrast-ultrasonography is an alternative to HSG performed using Doppler ultrasound to monitor the passage of fluid via the cervix through the uterus and tubes.

It is crucial to ensure the patient is not pregnant prior to tubal potency investigations, therefore they are usually performed at the beginning of the menstrual cycle. Infection

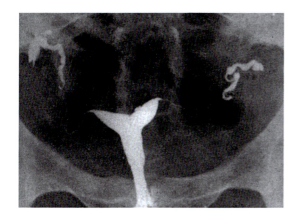

Fig. 16.2 Hysterosalpingogram. From Letterie GS: Management of congenital uterine abnormalities, *Reprod Biomed Online* 23:40–52, 2011. Elsevier, with permission.

screening for chlamydia and gonorrhoea is advised prior as tubal investigations could disseminate and worsen any existing sexually transmitted infections.

Hysteroscopy

If the transvaginal ultrasound highlights abnormality such as endometrial polyps or submucosal fibroids, this can be investigated and surgically treated. If there is history of previous uterine surgery (such as surgical management of miscarriage), this may identify uterine adhesions (Asherman).

TREATMENT

Treatment for subfertility should be aimed at the specific cause as identified by the investigations. However, many couples suffer from unexplained infertility and may go on to require in-vitro fertilization (IVF) treatment.

Female factor infertility – anovulation

Anovulation can be due to failure of the hypothalamo–pituitary–ovarian (HPO) axis [gonadotropin-releasing hormone (GnRH) deficiency], dysfunction of the HPO axis (PCOS) or ovarian failure. PCOS is the most common cause of anovulation.

Initial management to stimulate ovulation is to target general health: optimizing any chronic medical conditions, moderating BMI to 19–30 kg/m^2, decreasing high exercise levels, stopping smoking and moderating alcohol and caffeine intake.

Metformin has been shown to improve rates of ovulatory cycles in patients with PCOS and can be used in combination with other therapies. It can initially cause side-effects such as nausea and gastrointestinal symptoms.

Clomifene citrate is an antioestrogen that occupies oestrogen receptors in the hypothalamus, increasing GnRH release, which leads to increased release of luteinizing hormone and follicle-stimulating hormone. This induces follicular development and ovulation and should be given on days 2–6 of the cycle. Ovulation can be suggested by ovulation kits and raised day 21 progesterone. The dose can be titrated, but treatment should not be continued for longer than 6 months. There is a risk of multiple pregnancies whilst inducing ovulation; ultrasound follicle tracking can monitor for multiple follicles to ensure they are taking a dose that minimizes the risk of multiple pregnancy.

Second-line treatments include combined treatment with clomifene citrate and metformin or laparoscopic ovarian drilling.

If the ovulatory disorder is due to hyperprolactinaemia, the patient should be offered treatment with dopamine agonists.

Female factor infertility – uterine, tubal or pelvic problems

If there are known uterine abnormalities, such as fibroids, polyps or uterine septa, these can be removed hysteroscopically. They can impair fertility and cause miscarriage, therefore they are often removed to improve the chance of success with natural conception or IVF.

If there is known or suspected endometriosis (even if mild), they should be offered laparoscopic surgical ablation or excision of endometriosis plus laparoscopic adhesiolysis because this improves the chance of pregnancy. If they have endometriomas, laparoscopic cystectomy improves the chance of pregnancy.

If hydrosalpinges are identified, offer salpingectomy, as this improves the chance of a live birth with IVF. If there are proximal tubal blockages, salpingography plus tubal catheterization, or hysteroscopic tubal cannulation can be considered. However, tubal potency does not guarantee function and these patients are at risk of ectopic pregnancy.

Male factor infertility

Advice should be given regarding wearing loose underwear and reduction in alcohol and nicotine intake. Men with hypogonadotropic hypogonadism should be offered gonadotrophin drugs to improve fertility. Appropriate expertise should be considered to treat ejaculatory failure or for surgical correction of epididymal blockage. If semen analysis is persistently abnormal, assisted fertility should be considered, such as intrauterine insemination (IUI) or intracytoplasmic sperm injection (ICSI).

ASSISTED REPRODUCTION

Recent data suggest that just over 2% of all the babies born in the UK are conceived through IVF treatment. The number of IVF cycles performed each year has increased steadily since 1991. For people with unexplained infertility, mild endometriosis or mild male factor infertility, they should be advised to try to conceive for a total of 2 years prior to assisted reproductive techniques.

Intrauterine insemination

IUI is a technique where sperm are selected and introduced into the uterine cavity directly. The female partner can have stimulated ovulation or spontaneous. It is a technique option considered as an alternative to vaginal sexual intercourse in the case of physical disability or psychosexual problem, people in same-sex relationships or those using donor sperm. IUI is also used in cases when unprotected sexual intercourse is not recommended, such as with a human immunodeficiency virus (HIV) positive male parter, after 'sperm washing'.

Intracytoplasmic sperm injection

ICSI is an assisted fertility technique in which a single sperm is injected directly into an egg (Fig. 16.3). This technique is beneficial in patients with severe deficits in semen quality of low count. It should also be considered for couples in whom a previous IVF treatment cycle has resulted in failed or very poor fertilization.

In-vitro fertilization

IVF involves inducing ovulation followed by harvesting the oocytes and allowing them to fertilize in a laboratory using sperm from the partner or donor. The embryo is then transferred back into the patient in the hope of an ongoing pregnancy. The patients must be adequately educated about potential long-term health outcomes including the consequences of multiple pregnancy as well as potential small increased risk of borderline ovarian tumours. The absolute risks of long-term adverse outcomes in children born as result of IVF are low.

IVF techniques and protocols can vary, but generally involve the following steps:

- Downregulation of woman's own hormones using GnRH agonists to avoid premature luteinizing hormone surges in IVF.
- Controlled ovarian stimulation in IVF using an individualized starting dose of follicle-stimulating hormone for the lowest effective dose and duration of use.
- Using human chorionic gonadotrophin to trigger ovulation with ultrasound monitoring of ovarian response.
- Oocyte retrieval using transvaginal ultrasound under sedation and sperm retrieval.

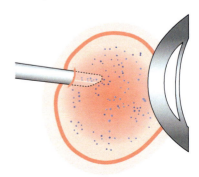

Fig. 16.3 Sperm injection into an egg.

- IVF of the oocytes with sperm and embryo transfer strategies.
- Luteal phase support with progesterone.

Donor sperm

It is appropriate to use donor semen and insemination in some cases, such as azoospermia or severe deficits in semen quality in those who do not wish to undergo ICSI. It can be considered if there is a high risk of transmitting a genetic or infectious disorder to the offspring.

Donor oocyte

In some cases it is appropriate to use a donor oocyte (egg), for example, in premature ovarian failure, gonadal dysgenesis such as Turner syndrome, bilateral oophorectomy and ovarian failure following chemotherapy or radiotherapy. It can be considered if there is a high risk of transmitting a genetic disorder to the offspring or in cases of IVF treatment failure.

CLINICAL NOTES

There has been a substantial increase in the number of patients freezing their eggs for future treatment; however, it still represents a small fraction of patients undergoing in-vitro fertilization. The most common reason was having no current male partner, with the most common age being 37–39 years. Success is affected by the age of the woman at the time of freezing and the live birth rate is lower than using fresh eggs or thawed frozen embryos. Since 2001 [as per Human Fertilisation and Embryology Authority (HFEA)] fewer than 60 babies have been born to patients storing and thawing eggs.

COMPLICATIONS

IVF has an association with multiple pregnancy and the high complication rate associated with this. Since 2009 the Human Fertilisation and Embryology Authority (HFEA) has introduced regulations to promote single embryo transfer only to minimize the risk of multiple births from IVF treatment. In IVF clinics the current regulated maximum multiple birth rate should be 10%.

Ovarian hyperstimulation syndrome (OHSS) is a serious systemic disease that occurs as a result of high levels of oestrogen during IVF treatment. The subsequent increased vascular permeability causes accumulation of fluid in the 'third space', such as the abdomen and chest, and intravascular fluid depletion.

In its mild form it can cause mild abdominal pain, but can lead to pronounced painful ascites and pleural effusions,

hepatorenal failure and respiratory distress syndrome. Treatment is conservative and symptomatic, ensuring thromboprophylaxis, careful fluid balance and ascitic or chest drains if required. If during IVF too many follicles have developed, it is safer to abandon the cycle than risk developing OHSS.

Multifollicular ovaries can have a dramatic increase in size during IVF treatment, and therefore there is a high risk of ovarian torsion.

ETHICS

Individual National Health Service (NHS) Clinical Commissioning Groups make the final decision about who can have NHS-funded in-vitro fertilization (IVF) in their local area. Common criteria to qualify for NHS funding include age <40 years, no previous children to either couple from current or previous relationships and body mass index <30 kg/m². It is important that when counselling your patients, you advise them early whether they may or may not qualify for NHS IVF if required.

PROGNOSIS

The age of the female partner is the most important prognostic factor in predicting IVF success. The chance of a live birth following IVF treatment falls with rising female age. Current data show that pregnancy rate per embryo transfer for patients receiving IVF treatment using their own eggs is over 44% under 35 years of age, but only up to 20% at age 40 years, and 2% if over 45 years of age. The chance of a live birth falls if the woman has never had a pregnancy or live birth and with the number of unsuccessful cycles.

Partners should be informed that maternal and paternal smoking, maternal caffeine consumption, BMI < 19 kg/m² or > 30 kg/m² and consumption of more than 1 unit of alcohol per day reduces the effectiveness of assisted reproduction procedures.

CLINICAL NOTES

Assisted reproductive technology is a rapidly developing and highly researched gynaecology subspeciality, with the aim to improve live birth rates with in-vitro fertilization. Recent advances include using a hyaluronan-enriched embryo transfer medium as a 'glue' to help embryo implantation and using time-lapse videography to monitor the cell division pattern of the embryos to select the embryos with the best potential.

● Chapter Summary

- Multiple factors can affect fertility from the male partner, female partner or both. Approximately 57% is linked to female factors, 22% to male and 21% mixed male and female.
- The key to subfertility treatment is to identify the underlying causative factor. This should be done by thorough history taking and then targeted investigations.
- Lifestyle factors impact greatly on fertility. Partners should be strongly advised to optimize body mass index and reduce or stop smoking and alcohol intake.
- The age of the female partner is the most important prognostic factor in predicting in-vitro fertilization success.

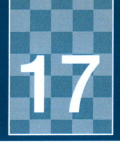

Menopause 17

BACKGROUND

Definition

'Menopause' is derived from the Greek words *Men* (month) and *Pausis* (cessation) and refers to the last menstrual period. The diagnosis can be made after at least 12 months of absent menstruation whilst not using hormonal contraception. Many women experience symptoms and irregular periods prior to the menopause, which is referred to as the 'climacteric' or 'perimenopausal' time. In women without a uterus, menopause is diagnosed based on physical symptoms.

The menopause generally occurs between the ages of 45 and 55 years with the average age in the UK of 51 years. 'Premature menopause' occurs in women under aged 40 years and can occur due to multiple reasons such as surgery or chemoradiotherapy.

Symptoms

In addition to the absent menstrual cycle, a variety of systemic symptoms occur. These include vasomotor symptoms, such as hot flushes and sweats, and musculoskeletal symptoms, such as joint and muscle pain. It can cause fluctuation in mood, including low mood and low sexual desire, and urogenital symptoms such as vaginal symptoms (Fig. 17.1).

Pathophysiology

After 45 years of age, as a result of successive menstrual cycles, only a few thousand oocytes remain. The depletion of the oocytes combined with their increased resistance to pituitary hormones follicle-stimulating hormone (FSH) and luteinizing hormone (LH) causes the cessation of menstruation. FSH and LH lose the function to regulate oestrogen,

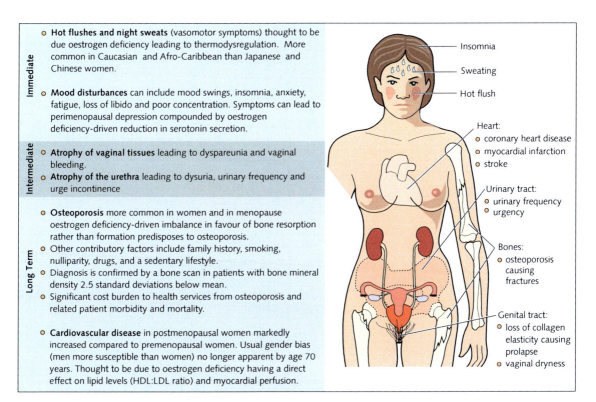

Immediate
- Hot flushes and night sweats (vasomotor symptoms) thought to be due oestrogen deficiency leading to thermodysregulation. More common in Caucasian and Afro-Caribbean than Japanese and Chinese women.
- Mood disturbances can include mood swings, insomnia, anxiety, fatigue, loss of libido and poor concentration. Symptoms can lead to perimenopausal depression compounded by oestrogen deficiency-driven reduction in serotonin secretion.

Intermediate
- Atrophy of vaginal tissues leading to dyspareunia and vaginal bleeding.
- Atrophy of the urethra leading to dysuria, urinary frequency and urge incontinence

Long Term
- Osteoporosis more common in women and in menopause oestrogen deficiency-driven imbalance in favour of bone resorption rather than formation predisposes to osteoporosis.
- Other contributory factors include family history, smoking, nulliparity, drugs, and a sedentary lifestyle.
- Diagnosis is confirmed by a bone scan in patients with bone mineral density 2.5 standard deviations below mean.
- Significant cost burden to health services from osteoporosis and related patient morbidity and mortality.
- Cardiovascular disease in postmenopausal women markedly increased compared to premenopausal women. Usual gender bias (men more susceptible than women) no longer apparent by age 70 years. Thought to be due to oestrogen deficiency having a direct effect on lipid levels (HDL:LDL ratio) and myocardial perfusion.

Insomnia
Sweating
Hot flush
Heart:
- coronary heart disease
- myocardial infarction
- stroke
Urinary tract:
- urinary frequency
- urgency
Bones:
- osteoporosis causing fractures
Genital tract:
- loss of collagen elasticity causing prolapse
- vaginal dryness

Fig. 17.1 Hormonal changes after the menopause. *HDL,* High-density lipoprotein; *LDL,* low-density lipoprotein.

Table 17.1 Hormonal changes with the menopause

Hormone	Levels during menopause
Follicle-stimulating hormone	↑↑
Luteinizing hormone	↑↑
Oestrogen	↓↓
Progesterone	↓↓

progesterone and testosterone, alongside a natural decline of oestrogen levels during menopause, causing the menopausal symptoms (Table 17.1).

DIAGNOSIS

History

The diagnosis of menopause can be made by history taking and examination due to the identifiable key features. However, it is important to not miss an alternative diagnosis as individual symptoms could be related to a different pathology.

Examination

A general examination including body mass index and blood pressure should be performed.

Examination should be tailored towards the history findings, for example, a bimanual pelvic examination, and Cusco's speculum performed if there are any urogenital symptoms (Table 17.2).

INVESTIGATIONS

A diagnosis of menopause should be made through history and clinical features. However, an elevated FSH level can be used to diagnose menopause in women aged 40–45 years with menopausal symptoms or change in menstrual cycle, or in women under 40 years of age with suspected menopause.

MANAGEMENT

Optimal management of the menopause should be tailored and adapted to the individual patient and their particular

Table 17.2 Investigating menopausal symptoms

Symptoms	Investigations
Urinary symptoms (dysuria, frequency, urgency)	Urine dipstick ± Urine microscopy, culture and sensitivities ± Urodynamic testing
Intermenstrual/postcoital bleeding	Cervical smear ± Colposcopy
Low-impact fractures/family history of osteoporosis	X-ray Dual-energy X-ray absorptiometry scan
Urogenital symptoms	Bimanual pelvic examination and speculum

symptoms. Options include hormone replacement therapy (HRT), nonhormonal treatments and nonpharmaceutical treatments.

Medical

Hormone replacement therapy

HRT reduces symptoms of the menopause and is the most effective and widely used treatment. It can contain oestrogen and progesterone, or oestrogen-only preparations. As oestrogen replacement alone can cause endometrial hyperplasia, it should only be used in women who have already undergone a hysterectomy. However, women who have a uterus must have progesterone added to protect the endometrium.

When prescribing HRT the lowest effective dose should be used. There are multiple routes of administration, which means treatment can be individually tailored to patients. These include oral tablets, transdermal patch, gels, implants, vaginal rings or pessaries. The Mirena intrauterine system can also be used as the progesterone component of HRT secreting local progestogen with low systemic levels. See Table 17.3 for advantages and disadvantages of different routes of administration. Oral preparations can be given continuously or in sequential preparations where patients will experience a monthly withdrawal bleed. Contraindications to initiating HRT are presented in Box 17.2.

Table 17.3 Route of administration for hormone replacement therapy

	Advantages	Disadvantages
Oral	Cheap, effective	First-pass metabolism Variable plasma levels Higher doses required
Transdermal (patch/gel)	Avoids first-pass metabolism Reduce risk of venous thromboembolism Continuous administration	Cost Skin reactions
Vaginal	Good for urogenital symptoms Minimal systemic absorption Licensed for 3 months' use without progesterone opposition (in the UK)	Unlikely to treat other symptoms
Mirena intrauterine system	Licensed for 4 years to provide the progesterone arm of hormone replacement therapy contraceptive	Only provides progesterone for endometrial protection Patients will still need oestrogen

CLINICAL NOTES

Contraindications to hormone replacement therapy:
- endometrial carcinoma
- breast carcinoma
- undiagnosed vaginal bleeding
- undiagnosed breast lumps
- severe active liver disease
- pregnancy (always rule out before starting therapy)
- personal history of venous thromboembolism – ORAL therapy is contraindicated but if benefits of treatment outweigh risks, then TRANSDERMAL preparations can be used

Common side-effects described with HRT include breast tenderness, leg cramps, nausea, bloating, irritability and depression. Unscheduled vaginal bleeding is common within the first 3 months of initiating treatment, but should be reported if ongoing. Review of patients on HRT should be made annually unless there are any clinical indications for an earlier review such as side-effects (Fig. 17.2).

In terms of other hormonal replacement options, testosterone supplements can be used for menopausal women with low libido.

CLINICAL NOTES

There has been much scrutiny and research into the long-term risks of hormone replacement therapy (HRT). The current advice from the National Institute for Health and Care Excellence (NICE) is:
- HRT with oestrogen is associated with little/no change in breast cancer risk. HRT with oestrogen and progesterone can increase risk of breast cancer, which reduces after stopping HRT.
- The risk of venous thromboembolism (VTE) is increased by oral HRT compared with baseline population risk, but standard doses of transdermal HRT do not increase VTE risk.
- There is no increased risk of developing type 2 diabetes.
- No increase in cardiovascular disease risk when started in women aged under 60 years or increase risk of dying from cardiovascular disease.

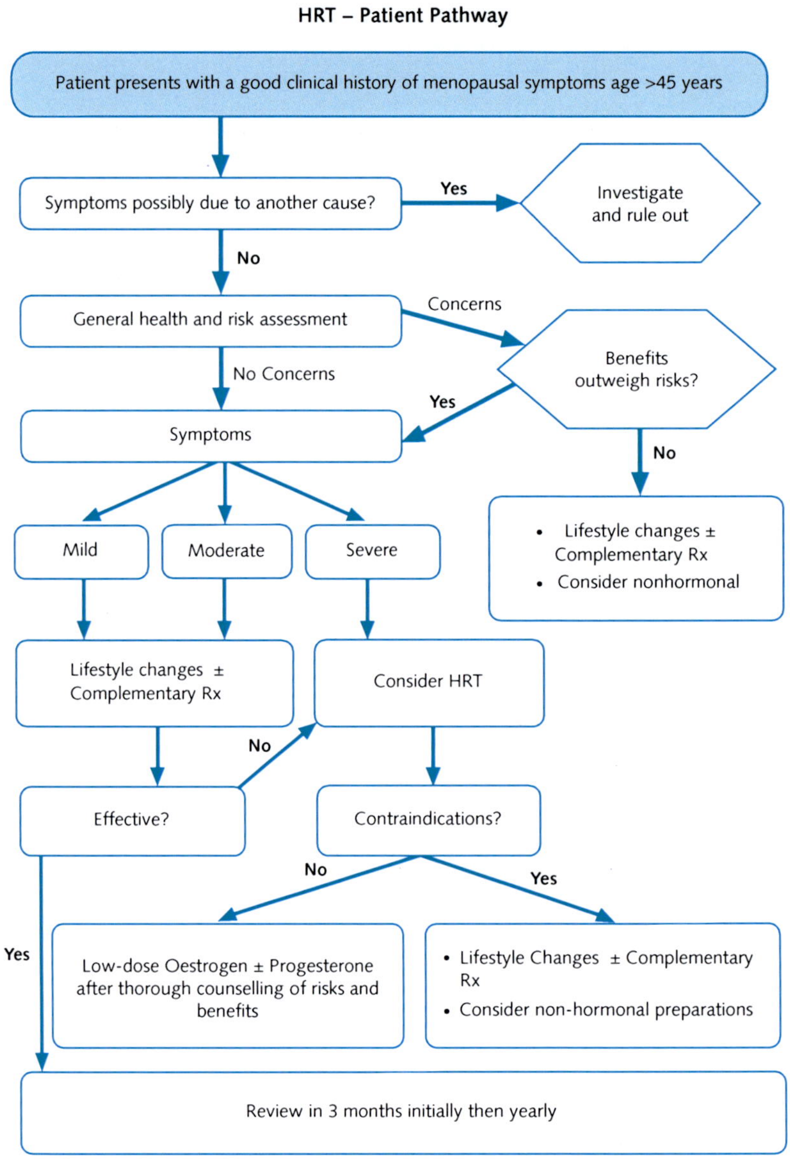

HRT – Patient Pathway

Patient presents with a good clinical history of menopausal symptoms age >45 years

Symptoms possibly due to another cause? → **Yes** → Investigate and rule out

No

General health and risk assessment → **Concerns** → Benefits outweigh risks?

No Concerns

Benefits outweigh risks? → **Yes** → Symptoms

Benefits outweigh risks? → **No** →
- Lifestyle changes ± Complementary Rx
- Consider nonhormonal

Symptoms → Mild / Moderate / Severe

Mild → Lifestyle changes ± Complementary Rx

Moderate → Lifestyle changes ± Complementary Rx / Consider HRT

Severe → Consider HRT

Lifestyle changes ± Complementary Rx → Effective? → **No** → Consider HRT

Consider HRT → Contraindications?

Contraindications? → **No** → Low-dose Oestrogen ± Progesterone after thorough counselling of risks and benefits

Contraindications? → **Yes** →
- Lifestyle Changes ± Complementary Rx
- Consider non-hormonal preparations

Effective? → **Yes** → Review in 3 months initially then yearly

Fig. 17.2 Hormone replacement therapy – patient pathway. Adapted from Panay N: Menopause. In Oxford desk reference: obstetrics and gynaecology, Oxford, UK, 2011, Oxford University Press. *HRT,* Hormone replacement therapy.

Vaginal oestrogen

Vaginal oestrogen preparations should be offered to women with urogenital atrophy, including those on systemic HRT to relieve symptoms. There is minimal systemic absorption and adverse affects are rare. Vaginal dryness can be helped with vaginal moisturisers and lubricants either in isolation or with vaginal oestrogen.

Nonhormonal pharmacological agents

If hormonal agents are contraindicated or not tolerated for vasomotor symptoms, nonhormonal treatments can be considered although are not routinely offered. Options include selective serotonin reuptake inhibitors, selective norepinephrine reuptake inhibitors and clonidine.

Conservative

Lifestyle changes

Lifestyle changes such as regular aerobic exercise, reduction in alcohol consumption and smoking are all beneficial for symptom control. Menopausal woman often find that certain food substances can trigger hot flushes.

Cognitive behavioural therapy

There is good evidence that cognitive behavioural therapy can alleviate low mood and anxiety as a result of the menopause.

Complimentary therapy

There are a variety of complimentary remedies believed to help menopausal symptoms. However, different preparations may vary, safety is not always certain and it is possible for medication interactions to occur. Isoflavones (phytoestrogens derived from beans) or black cohosh (a North American root) is thought to relieve vasomotor symptoms. There is evidence that St. John's Wort can relieve vasomotor symptoms in women with a history of or at high risk of breast cancer. However, it has potential serious interactions with other drugs including tamoxifen.

and a history of menopausal symptoms. Taking a thorough history is crucial as causes can include surgery, chemotherapy or radiotherapy, chromosomal defects and autoimmune disease. Formal diagnosis can be made with elevated FSH levels on two separate occasions taken 4–6 weeks apart.

Sex steroid replacement should be offered with combined hormonal contraception or HRT, unless contraindicated, which can continue until the age of natural menopause. Advice should be given about bone, cardiovascular health and managing symptoms.

Patients should be counselled about the need for in-vitro fertilization if they wish to conceive. However, it is important to remind patients that HRT does not act as a contraceptive and it is possible to have occasional ovulatory cycles with premature menopause, therefore natural conception can rarely occur.

ETHICS

It is important to fully inform women about the potential benefits and possible risks of hormone replacement therapy and the alternative therapies available when initiating treatment. This will enable them to make educated decision about their care.

COMMUNICATION

There can be both physical and psychosocial impacts of a diagnosis of premature menopause. It is important to acknowledge the impact of this and refer these women to healthcare professionals who have the relevant experience to manage the condition.

PREMATURE OVARIAN FAILURE

Approximately 1% of women experience 'premature menopause' or 'premature ovarian failure'. It is diagnosed in women under the age of 40 years with cessation of periods

---

● Chapter Summary

- The menopause can have a range of systemic symptoms including vasomotor, psychological and urogenital. It typically occurs between the ages of 45 and 55 years.
- Hormone replacement therapy (HRT) reduces symptoms of the menopause and is the most effective and widely used treatment. Women should be fully educated about the benefits, potential risks and alternative treatments available.
- Common side-effects with HRT include breast tenderness, leg cramps, nausea, bloating, irritability and depression.
- Conservative measures used to treat menopausal symptoms include cognitive behavioural therapy, lifestyle changes and complementary therapies such as isoflavones and St. John's Wort.
- 'Premature menopause' is a cessation of periods in women under 40 years old and occurs in approximately 1% of women.

MISCARRIAGE

Background

Definition
Early pregnancy is defined as the first 12 completed weeks of pregnancy. An 'early' pregnancy loss is therefore a pregnancy loss within this 12-week period. The recommended medical term for any pregnancy loss up to 24 weeks is a 'miscarriage'.

A miscarriage is confirmed with transvaginal ultrasound (TVUS) scan, and needs two clinicians to view the scan and confirm a definite miscarriage.

Recurrent miscarriage is defined as the loss of three or more consecutive pregnancies.

Different terms are commonly used to describe the type or stage of miscarriage, as outlined in Table 18.1.

Prevalence
Spontaneous miscarriage is the most common complication of pregnancy. Miscarriage occurs in approximately 20% of clinical pregnancies, and as a result, early pregnancy loss accounts for over 50,000 hospital admissions in the UK annually.

Recurrent miscarriage affects 1% of couples trying to conceive.

In the majority of cases it is not possible to identify the cause of miscarriage. Research suggests that up to 50% are due to spontaneous genetic or structural fetal abnormalities, which are incompatible with life and are unlikely to reoccur. However, there are other known risk factors for miscarriage and recurrent miscarriage (Table 18.2):

- maternal age >35 years
- previous miscarriages
- antiphospholipid syndrome
- infective factors
- maternal illness
- uterine cavity abnormalities

Miscarriage can be very distressing for the woman and family involved. It is very important to provide support and patient-centred care whilst managing a miscarriage.

COMMUNICATION

Charities such as 'The Miscarriage Association' (www.miscarriageassociation.org.uk) provide information and support for those experiencing a miscarriage. It is good practice to recommend resources such as these to our patients.

Table 18.1 Terminology of miscarriage

Terminology	Description	Scan findings
Viable intrauterine pregnancy	Ongoing pregnancy.	Normally sited gestational sac, fetal pole and cardiac activity.
Complete miscarriage	Miscarriage has occurred in a woman with previously confirmed pregnancy; she will have experienced bleeding. Cervical os may be open or closed.	No products of conception remaining within the uterus.
Incomplete miscarriage	Nonviable pregnancy in a woman who has experienced some bleeding that may or may not be ongoing. Cervical os may be open or closed.	Nonviable pregnancy tissue seen within the uterus (retained products of conception).
Missed/delayed/silent miscarriage	Nonviable pregnancy in asymptomatic woman. Cervical os is closed.	Nonviable pregnancy seen.
Threatened miscarriage	Currently ongoing pregnancy in woman presenting with bleeding or pain. Cervical os is closed.	Viable intrauterine pregnancy.
Inevitable miscarriage	Ongoing pain and bleeding. Cervical os is open.	Products of conception low in the uterus or within cervix.
Pregnancy uncertain viability	Scan findings suggest pregnancy may not be progressing normally.	Small sac without metal pole seen/fetus seen <6 mm without cardiac activity.
Pregnancy of unknown location	Positive pregnancy test without scan confirmation of intrauterine or extrauterine pregnancy.	No intrauterine or extrauterine pregnancy seen on scan.

Table 18.2 Aetiology of miscarriage and investigation of recurrent miscarriage

Aetiology	Examples	Investigation
Epidemiology	Maternal age and previous miscarriage are independent risk factors. Miscarriage rate increases more rapidly from age >35 years from 15% to 51% over 40 years.	–
Fetal abnormality	About 30%–57% of fetuses have genetic (e.g., trisomy) or structural (neural tube defect) abnormalities.	Karyotyping of both parents and pregnancy tissue.
Infection	Any severe infection that leads to bacteraemia or viraemia can cause sporadic miscarriage. *Toxoplasma* species, rubella virus, tuberculosis, *Listeria*, malaria, salmonella and cytomegalovirus are a few potential causes. Bacterial vaginosis (BV), where there is a change in the natural flora of the vagina, has been linked to second-trimester miscarriage.	A high vaginal swab can be used to screen for BV.
Maternal illness	Conditions such as diabetes, renal or thyroid disease are associated with miscarriage, particularly if poorly controlled. Thrombophilia is also implicated in recurrent miscarriage.	Women can be screened for inherited thrombophilias including factor V Leiden, factor II (prothrombin) gene mutation and protein S.
Antiphospholipid antibodies	Antiphospholipid antibodies are present in 15% of women with recurrent miscarriage, and is a treatable cause. They inhibit trophoblastic function and differentiation, can cause a local inflammatory response and cause thrombosis of placental vasculature.	Antiphospholipid antibody assays are performed on two occasions at least 6 weeks apart to account for false-positive or false-negative results.
Cervical weakness	The diagnosis of cervical weakness is a clinical one, therefore true incidence is unknown. Diagnosis is usually based on a history of second-trimester miscarriage preceded by spontaneous rupture of membranes or painless cervical dilatation.	Transcervical monitoring of cervical length is often practiced in subsequent pregnancies.
Uterine abnormality	The reported prevalence of uterine anomalies is from 2% to 38%. It appears to be higher in women with second-trimester miscarriages compared with first-trimester loss.	Transvaginal ultrasound scan can be used to assess the uterine cavity and ovaries. In suspected abnormality hysteroscopy and laparoscopy can be used to investigate further.

Symptoms

The most prevalent symptoms of miscarriage are vaginal bleeding and abdominal pain, although it is possible to miscarry without symptoms (missed miscarriage – see Table 18.1). It is important to also remember that pain and bleeding can be presenting symptoms of an ectopic pregnancy (see later this chapter) unless an intrauterine pregnancy (IUP) has been previously seen on scan.

Bleeding is the most common symptom, and can range from light 'spotting' to heavy bleeding with large clots. Occasionally women report passing products of conception (POC), or 'bits of tissue' with the clots that may be POC. It is important in your history to quantify the bleeding (see the following discussion).

Women typically describe cramping, central lower abdominal pain 'like period pain' or 'like contractions'. It often requires analgesia to help the pain. Concurrent presentation of vaginal discharge and loss of pregnancy symptoms are also common.

RED FLAG

A woman presenting with lower abdominal pain (with or without bleeding) and a positive pregnancy test must be managed as an ectopic pregnancy until ruled out.

COMMUNICATION

It is important to let women know that light vaginal spotting and abdominal pain are very common in early pregnancy and do not necessarily indicate a miscarriage or ectopic pregnancy. It is also important to emphasize that intercourse or exercise will not provoke a miscarriage.

Diagnosis

History

History is important to distinguish if the woman is experiencing a miscarriage or other differentials such as an ectopic pregnancy, or nonpregnancy-related conditions such as appendicitis or gastroenteritis.

HISTORY

Establish her presenting complaint focusing on any bleeding, pain and vaginal loss. Try to quantify amounts of bleeding – ask how large clots were (5p, 50p, palm-size), how many pads were used in the day, were they soaked through? This gives us an idea about the likelihood of inevitable miscarriage.

Have you had any fevers? Do you feel dizzy/nauseous/unwell? Establishing that the patient is systemically well will help aid our ongoing management.

Is this a spontaneous or in-vitro fertilization (IVF) pregnancy? Is this a planned pregnancy? Although all women can be very affected by a possible miscarriage, it is often those who have undergone IVF or planned a pregnancy who are most anxious and distressed.

Have you had a scan earlier in this pregnancy? This could conform an intrauterine pregnancy and rule out an ectopic as a differential diagnosis.

What is the first day of the last menstrual period (LMP)? LMP is important to calculate estimated gestation (how many weeks pregnant). It is important to establish whether the woman is sure of these dates and whether her periods are regular as this may alter the dates. We also need to know whether she was using contraception when she conceived – for example, if taking the oral contraceptive pill, her LMP would be a withdrawal bleed rather than a true period. In IVF pregnancy the patient will be able to inform you of an implantation date. The estimated gestation will help with interpreting a scan. For example, if she is by dates 9 weeks pregnant, we would expect to easily see a pregnancy on scan. However, if she was estimated 4 weeks, we may not yet see a fetal pole.

Tell me about your previous pregnancies? Do you have any gynaecology conditions? Take a full obstetrics and gynaecology history, ensuring you ask about previous miscarriages and the gestation these occurred, any ectopic pregnancies and any current contraception. Ask about any gynaecology diagnosis such as polycystic ovarian syndrome, pelvic surgery, sexually transmitted infections and check smear tests are up-to-date.

Do you have any medical conditions? Have you had any surgery on your abdomen? This is important background information and is also relevant if the patient requires any surgical intervention.

Examination

The first part of the examination is observation from the end of the bed. Does the patient look well or unwell? Is she pale and shocked? Are you able to see any bleeding externally? This first snapshot assessment will highlight a patient who may need urgent help.

Examining the abdomen, you are likely going to feel a soft abdomen. In early pregnancy <12 weeks the uterus is unlikely to be palpable unless, for example, the patient is known to have fibroids.

A Cusco's speculum should be used with consent, to examine the patient vaginally and with a chaperone present. The cervix should be visualized and determined whether the cervical os is open or closed. Try to establish whether there is any ongoing bleeding. POC may be visible within the external os. Care should be taken to remove these during the examination as products within the cervical canal can be a cause of cramping pain, bleeding and a vagal response.

Cervical swabs can be taken to assess for infection.

Investigations

Observations

The woman may be experiencing significant pain if the uterus is expelling clots or products and this can lead to elevated pulse and blood pressure. Products within the cervical canal can cause 'cervical shock', a vagal response to dilatation of the canal. This can cause low pulse, blood pressure and even fainting.

Urinary pregnancy test

This should have been performed on attendance to hospital to confirm that the patient is indeed pregnant.

Serum β-human chorionic gonadotropin

This can be helpful in combination with findings on ultrasound scan. A pregnancy may not be visible with β-human chorionic gonadotropin (bHCG) levels <1000. In an ongoing pregnancy bHCG levels would be expected to double every 48 hours.

Full blood count

Haemoglobin (Hb) levels are usually stable unless in cases of severe bleeding.

Group and save and blood group

If the patient has ongoing bleeding or may need surgical intervention, it is important to have two valid samples of group and save. Women who are Rhesus negative would require anti-D after an evacuation of retained products of conception (ERPC) if required, or in cases of miscarriage >12 weeks' gestation.

Transvaginal ultrasound

Transvaginal scans are the best modality for viewing the pelvis and early pregnancy (Fig. 18.1). The uterus is examined, looking for a gestational sac, fetal pole and fetal heartbeat (FH). FH can be seen from approximately 6 weeks' gestation. Once FH is seen there is a 90% chance of the pregnancy continuing.

It may be that nonviable pregnancy tissue is seen within the uterus as retained products of conception (RPOC). If the uterus is empty, the adnexa and ovaries are scanned to rule out an ectopic mass and the pouch of Douglas is examined for free fluid.

Management

Conservative

Following diagnosis of a nonviable pregnancy expectant management (allowing miscarriage to happen naturally) can be offered for up to 14 days. In the majority of cases the uterus will expel the POC spontaneously without requiring any additional intervention, but this may take several weeks and overall efficacy rates are lower compared with a surgical approach. The woman should be counselled and given written information about what to expect throughout the process, including the likely duration and severity of bleeding, advice on pain relief and where and when to get help in an emergency.

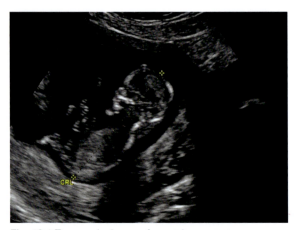

Fig. 18.1 Transvaginal scan of an early pregnancy.

Medical

Medical evacuation is an alternative technique with variable efficacy rates quoted as between 13% and 96%. Various methods using prostaglandin analogues have been described and misoprostol is most commonly used either vaginally or orally. Medical management can be undertaken as an inpatient or outpatient. Women must be advised of potential increase in pain and bleeding with medical methods.

Surgical

Surgical ERPC should be offered to women who prefer that option. If the woman is undergoing persistent excessive bleeding, haemodynamic instability, evidence of infected retained tissue or suspected gestational trophoblastic disease (GTD), it is advised to undergo ERPC. It is generally performed using suction curettage under general anaesthetic as a day case, although some units offer surgical evacuation techniques under local anaesthetic or sedation. Serious complications of this procedure occur in approximately 2% of cases, including uterine perforation and haemorrhage. Vaginal prostaglandin can be used prior to the procedure to help dilate the cervix and reduce chance of trauma. This procedure is also known as 'surgical management of miscarriage'.

Follow-up

POCs are sent to histology to ensure pregnancy tissue has been removed and molar pregnancy tissue is not present. After ERPC anti-D must be given if the patient is Rhesus negative.

No follow-up is required routinely following ERPC unless the patient is being investigated for recurrent miscarriage. Follow-up should be arranged with expectant/medical management if the symptoms are exceeding the period of expectant management or if a pregnancy test is positive after 3 weeks. It is crucial that women are given information of when and how to get help in an emergency.

Complications

Sepsis

RPOC within the uterus can be a site of infection and these patients are known to be undergoing a 'septic miscarriage'. They may present feeling systemically unwell, feverish, passing foul smelling vaginal loss or with elevated inflammatory markers. These patients would be encouraged to undergo an ERPC to remove the infective source. Antibiotics are not routinely used at the time of ERPC unless clinically indicated, such as in these cases.

Haemorrhage

Bleeding at the time of miscarriage can be heavy, and if there is RPOC, it can be increasingly heavy and prolonged. In the minority this can lead to haemorrhage and 'shock' as a result. All women should have an estimated blood loss calculated and careful observation of ongoing loss. If there are signs of haemodynamic instability (tachycardia, low blood pressure, feeling faint/unwell), they may require an ERPC urgently. All women presenting with miscarriage must have a baseline Hb and ensure a valid group and save.

Recurrent miscarriage

As mentioned recurrent miscarriage is the loss of three or more consecutive pregnancies, which affects 1% of couples. There are a number of known risk factors for recurrent miscarriage (Table 18.2).

Poor reproductive history is an independent predictor of future pregnancy outcome, and a previous live birth does not prevent a woman developing recurrent miscarriage. The risk of a further miscarriage increases after each successive pregnancy loss, reaching approximately 40% after three consecutive pregnancy losses. In addition, the prognosis worsens with increasing maternal age.

The experience of recurrent miscarriage can be traumatic for couples and ideally they should be assessed and counselled in a recurrent miscarriage clinic. If a patient is undergoing ERPC after a third consecutive miscarriage, the POC should be sent for karyotyping as well as for histology at the time and appropriate follow-up arranged. To investigate their risk factors, further investigations are also performed, as explained in Table 18.2.

ECTOPIC PREGNANCY

Background

Definition

An ectopic pregnancy is any pregnancy implanted outside of the endometrial cavity.

Approximately 97% of ectopic pregnancies occur in the fallopian tubes, specifically the ampullae or isthmic portions. Around 2%–3% occur as interstitial ectopic pregnancies.

Rarer locations include cervical, fimbrial, ovarian, caesarean section scar and peritoneal sites (Fig. 18.2).

A heterotopic pregnancy is an extremely rare occurrence of an IUP and a coexisting ectopic pregnancy.

Prevalence

In the UK, an estimated 11,000 ectopic pregnancies are diagnosed each year, an incidence of approximately 1 in 90 pregnancies.

Recent evidence has shown that the incidence of ectopic pregnancy diagnoses is currently static. Unfortunately, women can still die as a result of ectopic pregnancy; 0.2 per 100 cases lead to maternal death. Therefore it is crucially important to diagnose and manage the condition appropriately.

For the majority of women an ectopic pregnancy is a 'one-off' event. However, an ectopic pregnancy increases your chance of a subsequent ectopic pregnancy from just over 1% (in the general UK population) to 7%–10%.

One-third of ectopic pregnancies occur spontaneously, but the majority are caused by conditions that damage the fallopian tubes or their ciliary lining. Examples of this include pelvic inflammatory disease and tubal surgery, such as sterilization or reversal of sterilization. If pregnancy occurs following in-vitro fertilization (IVF), whilst using an intrauterine contraceptive device coil or the progesterone-only 'mini pill', there is increased risk of an ectopic pregnancy. Previous pelvic/abdominal surgery or pelvic conditions (e.g., endometriosis) also increase risk of ectopic pregnancy due to prevalence of adhesions. Women over the age of 40 years and smoking are independent risk factors.

Symptoms

Any presentation of lower abdominal pain (with or without bleeding) and a positive pregnancy test must be managed as an ectopic pregnancy until proven otherwise (such as with an IUP seen on TVUS).

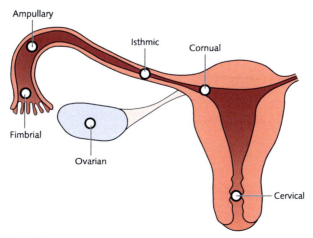

Fig 18.2 Implantation sites of ectopic pregnancy.

A high index of suspicion of ectopic pregnancy should be maintained with presentations of vaginal bleeding or lower abdominal pain with associated syncope, diarrhoea/vomiting and shoulder tip pain.

Similar to presentation of miscarriage, the most common symptom of an ectopic pregnancy is lower abdominal pain, although it is possible to be relatively asymptomatic in an early ectopic pregnancy.

Women typically describe a lower abdominal pain 'like period pain', which may locate to either the right or left iliac fossa, and typically is insidious in onset and worsening. In cases of a ruptured ectopic it can cause pain all over the abdomen, and irritation of the inferior diaphragm from blood can cause referred shoulder-tip pain. It often requires analgesia to help with the pain.

Blood in the pelvis can also cause irritability of the bowel, and therefore diarrhoea and vomiting can also be presenting symptoms. Any history of syncope, or dizziness that may indicate haemodynamic instability, must be considered. Cases of ectopic pregnancy presenting with gastrointestinal symptoms only have occurred, therefore all women presenting to accident and emergency with these symptoms must undergo a pregnancy test.

Vaginal bleeding is another common presenting symptom, and can range from light loss 'spotting' to heavy bleeding with large clots. It is important to note that having vaginal bleeding does not mean that the woman has an IUP.

Diagnosis

History
A thorough history must be taken as with presentation of possible miscarriage (see above).

Particular care should be taken in assessing current systemic symptoms (e.g., dizziness, syncope and gastrointestinal symptoms).

Past gynaecological history should focus on any relevant factors that may increase the possibility of an ectopic pregnancy (see above). Is this an IVF pregnancy? Have you ever had an ectopic pregnancy? Any history of tubal surgery, pelvic surgery or pelvic inflammation? This may increase your level of suspicion of an ectopic.

Past medical history is also important. If this is a confirmed ectopic pregnancy, the woman may require an operation, therefore it is important to establish possible anaesthetic fitness.

Examination
Similar to miscarriage examination, the first part of the examination is observation from the end of the bed. Does the patient look well or unwell? Is she pale and shocked? Is her pain under control? This first snapshot assessment will highlight a patient who may need urgent help.

Examining the abdomen, you may elicit localized tenderness in the right or left iliac fossa. Assess for guarding or peritonism. In ruptured ectopic pregnancy, the woman may have a generally tender abdomen with widespread peritonism.

A Cusco's speculum should be used to examine the patient vaginally with patient's consent and a chaperone present. The cervix should be visualized and determined whether the cervical os is open or closed. Try to establish whether there is any ongoing bleeding.

A vaginal examination should be performed and the adnexa should be examined. An ectopic pregnancy may cause fullness and tenderness on the affected side. Cervical excitation is severe pain occurring with movement of the cervix during examination and is often present with ectopic pregnancy.

Investigations

Observations
Reviewing the observations is crucial to assess whether the patient is haemodynamically stable. These must be reassessed regularly especially in the case of an ectopic pregnancy, as deterioration due to rupture can occur acutely and need to be managed as an emergency. An unwell patient with a ruptured ectopic pregnancy may have raised pulse and low blood pressure. Significant pain may also result in elevated pulse and blood pressure.

Urinary pregnancy test
To confirm pregnancy.

Serum bHCG
This can be helpful in combination with findings on ultrasound scan in planning the management of an ectopic pregnancy.

Full blood count
To assess current Hb levels. New anaemia may be indicative of a ruptured ectopic.

Group and save and blood group
Any patient with concern of ectopic pregnancy must have two valid samples of group and save. If the patient is haemodynamically unstable, a cross match of blood may be required.

Transvaginal ultrasound
TVUS is the diagnostic tool of choice for diagnosis of ectopic pregnancy. A TVUS should be performed as soon as possible unless the woman is haemodynamically unstable.

The majority of ectopic pregnancies will be visualized on the initial ultrasound examination. Most commonly an empty uterus is visualized, with an adnexal mass seen separately to the ovary. Some ectopic pregnancies are too small or too early to be visualized on the initial ultrasound examination. If no IUP or ectopic is seen, the patient will be classified as having a 'pregnancy of unknown location' (PUL – see later).

Management

Conservative

Conservative (expectant) management of ectopic pregnancy is an option available to clinically stable, asymptomatic women in some early pregnancy units. The woman must have a confirmed ectopic pregnancy without evidence of free fluid, be willing and able to attend for follow-up, have minimal pain and have low or declining serum bHCG levels. Lower initial bHCG and rapid decrease are a significant predictor of spontaneous resolution. They must be advised that up to 29% will require additional medical or surgical management and that ectopic rupture can occur with decreasing bHCG. The woman must present to hospital with any change to symptoms. Follow-up tends to be with bHCG and repeat TVUS at regular periods. Women who may be suitable for conservative management should also be offered medical or surgical management if preferred.

Medical

Medical management of ectopic pregnancy is an active management option for haemodynamically stable women with a diagnosis of ectopic pregnancy smaller than 35 mm, low serum bHCG, no pain and willingness for follow-up. The cytotoxic medication methotrexate is the most commonly used drug for medical treatment of tubal ectopic pregnancy, which acts to destroy the pregnancy tissue. It is usually given as a single-dose intramuscular injection dosed using body surface area of the patient. It is both cytotoxic and teratogenic medication, therefore the women must avoid contact with pregnant patients and avoid pregnancy for 6 months following completion of treatment. Women undergoing this management commonly experience side-effects, predominantly mouth ulcers, conjunctivitis, abdominal pain, nausea and vomiting.

Single-dose methotrexate has similar efficacy to surgical treatment in stable patients. Serum bHCG should be checked on day 4 and 7 – if bHCG falls less than 15%, they may need a repeat dose. In women who undergo medical management less than 10% go on to require surgical rupture, but 7% undergo tubal rupture during follow-up.

COMMUNICATION

Women undergoing conservative and medical management of ectopic pregnancy must be aware of the ongoing risk of ectopic rupture even in the event of a falling β-human chorionic gonadotropin. They must be given clear verbal and written advice and contact details in the event of an emergency.

Surgical

The majority of tubal ectopic pregnancies are managed surgically; laparoscopic (keyhole) surgery is offered as routine to all women with ectopic pregnancy.

Laparoscopic approach in the haemodynamically stable patient is preferable to laparotomy (open surgery). Laparoscopy has several advantages, such as shorter operation time, less intraoperative blood loss, shorter hospital stay, lower cost, lower analgesic requirements and less adhesion formation. However, management with haemodynamic instability, massive haemoperitoneum (blood in the pelvis) or dense adhesions should be by the quickest method, which may be laparotomy.

Salpingectomy (removal of the fallopian tube) on the affected side is how the ectopic pregnancy is routinely removed. Salpingotomy (removal of the ectopic pregnancy via an incision within the fallopian tube) should be considered with a history of contralateral tubal disease, such as previous salpingectomy (Fig. 18.3). Salpingotomy has higher rates of residual trophoblastic tissue being left within the tube.

Anti-D prophylaxis should be offered to Rhesus-negative women who have surgical management of ectopic pregnancy.

Prognosis

Following an ectopic pregnancy, risk of future ectopic pregnancy in subsequent pregnancies is 10%–20%, with up to 76% chance of subsequent IUP. Even with only one fallopian tube, chances of conceiving are only slightly reduced.

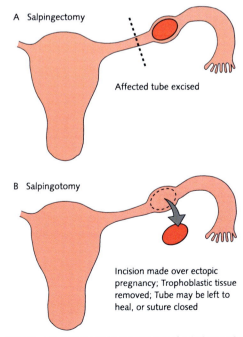

A Salpingectomy

Affected tube excised

B Salpingotomy

Incision made over ectopic pregnancy; Trophoblastic tissue removed; Tube may be left to heal, or suture closed

Fig. 18.3 Surgical options for treatment of tubal ectopic pregnancy.

Woman are advised to have an early scan in future pregnancies to locate the site of the pregnancy.

Complications

An ectopic pregnancy with tubal rupture is considered a gynaecological emergency. Because of advances in diagnosing ectopic pregnancies, currently >85% women are diagnosed prior to rupture. Tubal rupture can lead to haemoperitoneum, shock and even death. In the most recent confidential inquiry report (by the Centre for Maternal and Child Enquiries), six maternal deaths occurred because of ruptured ectopic pregnancies (2006–2008).

Complications of salpingectomy by laparotomy or laparoscopy include damage to surrounding organs, pain, infection and bleeding.

Both salpingectomy and salpingotomy can result in persistent trophoblastic tissue (incomplete removal of all pregnancy tissues, 4% vs. 8%). If this is the case, they may require further medical or repeat surgical treatment.

COMMUNICATION

Women should be advised of the advantages and disadvantages associated with each management option for ectopic pregnancy, and should participate in the selection of the most appropriate treatment.

Women should be made aware of how to access support via patient support groups, such as the Ectopic Pregnancy Trust, or local bereavement counselling services.

PREGNANCY OF UNKNOWN LOCATION

A PUL means there are no signs of either intrauterine or extrauterine pregnancy or RPOC in a woman with a positive pregnancy test.

This may be due to very early pregnancy not yet visible on scan, following miscarriage, or an undiagnosed ectopic pregnancy.

Up to 69% of PULs resolve spontaneously, but as many as 28% are subsequently diagnosed with ectopic pregnancy.

Above a certain serum bHCG level (between 1000 and 2000 depending on early pregnancy unit) the pregnancy should be visible on TVUS. Therefore, if no visible IUP is seen with high bHCG, these PUL patients should be managed carefully, as potentially undiagnosed ectopics.

Asymptomatic patients are managed expectantly, with a 48-hour serum bHCG plus repeat TVUS if required. Active intervention should be considered if the woman becomes

symptomatic of an ectopic or if there is a plateau in HCG. Intervention is required in 29% of diagnosed PULs.

Managing a PUL can be stressful and confusing for patients and it is crucial that the potential diagnoses and management strategies are clearly explained.

CLINICAL NOTES

Guidelines for managing ectopic pregnancy can be found in the Royal College of Obstetrics and Gynaecology 'Green-top guideline 21' entitled 'Diagnosis and Management of Ectopic Pregnancy.

MOLAR PREGNANCY

Background

Definition

Molar pregnancies (or GTD) are a group of conditions caused by abnormal fertilization, leading to abnormal formation of trophoblastic tissue. If GTD persists, it can act as a trophoblastic malignancy (gestational trophoblastic neoplasia [GTN]).

Complete molar pregnancies contain no fetal tissue. The majority arise when a single sperm or duplication of a single sperm fertilizes an 'empty' ovum, which contains no genetic material. This develops into a multivesicular mass of trophoblastic tissue (Fig. 18.4), which is described as having a 'bunch of grapes' appearance on TVUS.

Partial molar pregnancies can produce some fetal tissue. They are usually triploid, with two sets of paternal haploid

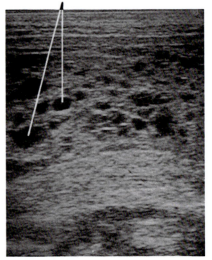

Vesicles

Fig. 18.4 Molar pregnancy.

genes and one set of maternal haploid genes. They usually occur with fertilization of a normal ovum.

Choriocarcinoma is an HCG-secreting tumour of trophoblastic cells that occurs when molar pregnancies are incompletely removed. It behaves like a cancer and can cause metastasis, particularly to the lung, liver and brain.

Prevalence

Partial moles occur more commonly than complete moles, with the incidence of GTD thought to be rare – approximately 1/700 live births. Women at the extremes of reproductive age, and those of Asian origin have a higher incidence. There is nearly 100% cure rate in the UK, with only 5%–8% of cases requiring chemotherapy. The need for chemotherapy following a complete mole is 15% and 0.5% after a partial mole.

Symptoms

Molar pregnancy tissues secrete HCG, therefore serum levels can be very high. This will classically lead to exaggerated symptoms of pregnancy. Woman may have irregular vaginal bleeding, severe hyperemesis, excessive uterine enlargement and early failed pregnancy.

Diagnosis

Definitive diagnosis of molar pregnancy can only be made with histologic examination of the POC. TVUS may be useful in a preevacuation diagnosis due to the classic appearance (Fig. 18.4) and likely assists in an earlier diagnosis. Serum HCG levels greater than two multiples of the median are also highly suggestive.

Management

Surgical

Molar pregnancies must be treated with surgical ERPC to remove the abnormal trophoblastic tissue. The POC must be sent to histology to confirm the diagnosis. Excessive vaginal bleeding can be associated with molar pregnancy, therefore the procedure should be supervised by a senior clinician.

Follow-up

There are several specialist centres in the UK that manage GTD and patients with confirmed molar pregnancies should be urgently referred for follow-up. Follow-up after GTD is individualized and monitored with regular repeats of serum bHCG to ensure it is falling. If bHCG has reverted to normal within 56 days of the pregnancy event, then follow-up will be for 6 months from the date of ERPC. If bHCG has not reverted to normal within 56 days of the pregnancy event, then follow-up will be for a more extended period.

If bHCG levels remain abnormal after 6 months, plateau or increase, chemotherapy is started. Women may be treated either with single-agent or multiagent chemotherapy depending on a risk scoring system (FIGO 2000 scoring system for GTN).

Women should be advisessd not to conceive until their follow-up is complete or from 1 year of completion of treatment. Reoccurrence rates are low (1/80) but all women should have bHCG levels measured 6–8 weeks after the end of the next pregnancy to exclude disease recurrence.

Chapter Summary

- Lower abdominal pain and vaginal bleeding can be presentations of both miscarriage and ectopic pregnancy.
- All unwell patients in early pregnancy must be treated as an ectopic until ruled out.
- Ectopic pregnancy can be a gynaecological emergency and patients may require urgent surgical management.
- Early pregnancy complications can cause distress to patients. Adequate support and information must be provided.

ANTENATAL BOOKING HISTORY

The antenatal booking appointment is arguably the most important visit a patient will make during their pregnancy. Ideally it occurs before the tenth week of pregnancy and is almost universally conducted by trained midwives. During this visit it is paramount to:

- take a thorough history to identify risk factors for the pregnancy
- educate the patient about key 'do's and don'ts' in pregnancy

Identifying a patient's risk factors allows their care to be tailored and any additional medications or investigations to be arranged. It is worth noting that during a booking visit, sensitive information may be disclosed. Therefore it is important to take the history in a sensitive and confidential manner.

Current pregnancy

An essential step in any booking visit is an accurate estimation of the gestational age. Most commonly this is calculated using the first day of the patient's last menstrual period and an obstetric wheel. The obstetric wheel will give both the current gestational age and an estimated date of delivery. Naegele's rule can also be used as an estimate.

HINTS AND TIPS

Naegele's rule. In situations where you do not have access to an obstetric wheel, using Naegele's rule is an easy way of estimating the due date. The rule assumes the patient has a 28-day cycle and the estimated date of delivery (EDD) is calculated by adding 7 to the first day of the last menstrual period (LMP) and deducting 3 from the month of the LMP. Finally add 1 to the year, for example, if a patient's LMP was April 5, 2012, then the EDD would be January 12, 2013.

However, national screening guidelines advise that all patients are offered an ultrasound scan between 11 and 14 weeks for the most accurate EDD, by measuring the fetal crown-rump length, as well as offering Down syndrome screening.

HINTS AND TIPS

An ultrasound scan between 11 + 4 and 14 + 0 weeks' gestation will:

- measure the crown-rump length to calculate the estimated date of delivery
- confirm a viable pregnancy
- diagnose multiple pregnancy and check chorionicity
- examine for fetal anomalies
- perform screening test for Down syndrome

The history includes whether or not it is a planned pregnancy and whether any fertility treatment was required to become pregnant. Patients who have undergone fertility treatment are at risk of multiple pregnancy (see Chapter 24) and/or may have had complications thus far such as ovarian hyperstimulation syndrome (see Chapter 16).

Obstetric history

A thorough enquiry about previous pregnancies and outcomes is essential as this may allow interventions in this pregnancy to reduce the risk of a further adverse outcome, for example, prescribing low-dose aspirin 75 mg daily for patients with a previous pregnancy complicated by pre-eclampsia.

When documenting previous pregnancies there is a widely accepted method of doing so using the letters G and P. G stands for 'gravidity' and refers to the number of pregnancies the patient has had including the current one. P denotes 'parity' and states the number of children the patient has delivered above 24 weeks of gestation. As an adjunct to this method, add the number of miscarriages or terminations a patient has had by documenting this after the parity.

HINTS AND TIPS

Catherine is 31 weeks in her third pregnancy; her first child was born at 38 weeks. Between these pregnancies, she had a miscarriage at 9 weeks. Therefore, her obstetric history is documented as G3 (this is her third pregnancy) P1 + 1 (she has had one child born after 24 weeks of gestation and one pregnancy ending before 24 weeks).

Medical history

Identification of co-existing medical problems is essential in pregnancy. For some disorders, early management plans may be appropriate to reduce the risk of adverse fetal and maternal outcomes (see Chapter 22). In some instances, it is better to initiate changes even before pregnancy and therefore some hospitals run preconception clinics. Optimizing conditions such as preexisting diabetes and epilepsy will improve outcomes. For example, many of the epilepsy medications are teratogenic and modification of the drug regimen may reduce this risk. With regard to diabetes, maternal serum HbA1c level at the time of conception is directly related to the risk of fetal abnormalities. Therefore excellent control of blood glucose levels preconception will reduce this risk. Another important group of medical problems in pregnancy is the mental health disorders – counselling must be given about the risks and benefits of remaining on medication during pregnancy, as well as planning care for the postnatal period.

Drug history and allergies

Enquiry should be made about what medications the patient may be taking including over-the-counter supplements. Folic acid should be recommended in the first trimester and specialist advice may be needed if the patient has been taking any potentially teratogenic medications. Any allergies must be highlighted.

Family history

Some diseases are relevant with regard to a family history, such as hypertension or diabetes. For example, a family history of type 2 diabetes in a first-degree relative confers an increased risk of developing gestational diabetes. These patients should be screened by way of a glucose tolerance test. Any genetic conditions that run through the family may prompt referral to a geneticist with or without invasive testing. This may be particularly important if the patient and her partner are related to each other.

Social history

Consideration should be given to the patient's occupation to minimize any risk she may be exposed to. For example, a nursery teacher who has not had chicken pox should be advised on how to minimize the risk and how to seek help should she come into contact with a child who has chicken pox. Other occupations to make note of are healthcare workers (infectious diseases), vets (toxoplasmosis) and chefs/butchers (food-borne infections such as listeria, salmonella and toxoplasmosis).

Smokers should be offered referral to a specialist smoking cessation clinic and educated about the risks to their pregnancy. In addition, alcohol abuse and illicit drug use should be identified with referral to the appropriate drug and alcohol service and education about the risks to pregnancy made as a priority. Social services may need to be informed so that appropriate postnatal care plans can be made for mother and baby. This may include those with a mental health history or teenage patients. Support is vital with a history of domestic violence.

EXAMINATION

At a booking visit the examination of a patient will generally be limited to measurement of the patient's blood pressure and recording their height and weight to allow calculations of their body mass index (BMI). A cardiovascular examination should be considered if the woman is newly arrived in the UK; this is to exclude conditions such as rheumatic heart disease that are more common in some developing countries, and may have a serious impact on health in pregnancy.

BOOKING INVESTIGATIONS

There is a nationally agreed set of investigations that should be offered to patients to allow screening for certain conditions to minimize their risk to mother and fetus, if present. A booklet has been produced by the UK National Screening Committee for patients to understand when they will be offered certain screening tests during their pregnancy and what the baby will be offered in the first few weeks after birth (see Further reading).

Full blood count

A full blood count is an important investigation as it allows for the detection of anaemia and assessment of the platelet count. There is a lower normal range for haemoglobin in pregnancy, due to the normal physiological changes that occur, with an increased circulatory volume. Anaemic patients need to be further investigated by measurement of their ferritin, folate and vitamin B12 levels if indicated.

The most common reason for anaemia is iron deficiency, which can be managed with iron supplements. Low platelets (thrombocytopenia) is more commonly gestational thrombocytopenia, again partly due to a dilutional effect. It may indicate an underlying issue such as idiopathic thrombocytopenia, which is an autoimmune condition that can affect the fetus. Severe cases may need specialist haematologist advice.

Haemoglobin electrophoresis

Haemoglobinopathies are disorders of haemoglobin structure and are more common in certain ethnic groups. Thalassaemia and sickle cell disease are screened for to allow identification of fetuses at risk of having the condition.

Both conditions are autosomal recessive, so for the individual to be affected they need to have two defective copies of the gene. Patients can be asymptomatic carriers of the condition without knowing. For example, in the UK there are estimated to be around 240,000 carriers of sickle cell.

Both conditions can render the patient anaemic and supplementation with iron and folate may be required if these levels are proven to be low. It is, however, important not to iron overload these patients.

Thalassaemia

The thalassaemias are denoted either α- or β- depending upon the affected haemoglobin chain. α-Thalassaemia is common in people of South East Asian descent and β-thalassaemia is common in people of Cypriot and Asian descent. During pregnancy, if the mother is found to be a carrier her partner should also be screened. Based on his results, invasive testing can be offered to make a diagnosis in the fetus.

Sickle cell disease

Sickle cell disease is also an autosomal recessive condition. People with one defective copy of the gene are referred to as sickle cell trait. Around 1:10 people of African-Caribbean descent have sickle cell trait and therefore screening can identify at-risk fetuses. Pregnant patients with sickle cell disease (i.e., two defective genes) should be managed in a specialist centre under a multidisciplinary team.

Blood group and antibody screen

Knowledge of a patient's blood group and antibody status is very important in pregnancy. Certain antibodies can cause haemolytic disease of the fetus and newborn, and therefore blood is screened at booking and again at 28 weeks to ensure antibodies have not developed. Patients who have these particular antibodies will need regular blood tests to quantify the levels and may require close surveillance in a fetal medicine unit if the levels rise. This is to exclude fetal anaemia caused by haemolysis.

The most common antibodies causing haemolytic disease of the fetus and newborn are the rhesus antibodies. Those that are rhesus negative will be offered anti-D prophylaxis.

HINTS AND TIPS

Rhesus blood group system and anti-D

The rhesus (Rh) blood group system is one of a number of systems and within it are many known antigens. In pregnancy the most important antigen is the D antigen. Those patients who have one or two copies of the Rh-D antigen gene will be Rh positive. Those patients who do not have copy of the gene will be Rh negative.

In pregnancy, if a Rh-negative patient has a partner who is Rh positive, their offspring may be Rh positive. During the pregnancy fetal blood may enter maternal circulation and cause antibodies to develop to the D antigen. If in a subsequent pregnancy the fetus is Rh negative, these antibodies may then cross the placenta and attack fetal red cells, causing anaemia and subsequent fetal hydrops with or without stillbirth.

In the last 1–2 years, patients who are found to be Rh negative at booking can be offered noninvasive prenatal testing – fetal DNA can be isolated from a maternal blood sample and therefore the fetal rhesus status can be determined. If the fetus is Rh negative, no treatment is needed. However if the fetus is Rh positive, the patient should be offered anti-D immunoglobulin, usually given at 28 weeks.

HINTS AND TIPS

Indications for anti-D if the fetus is rhesus positive:
- prophylaxis at 28 weeks
- postnatally
- if a potentially sensitizing event has occurred, that is, any event that may cause the passage of fetal cells into maternal circulation, such as abdominal trauma, bleeding in pregnancy after 12 weeks and amniocentesis.

Rubella

Since April 2016, antenatal screening for rubella is no longer advised by the National Screening Committee, because rubella infection in the UK is so rare and there have been high levels of uptake of the measles, mumps and rubella (MMR) vaccine in children. Women who have not been born in the UK are advised to discuss MMR vaccine with their general practitioner prior to planning a pregnancy so that they can receive the live vaccine if they are nonimmune.

Syphilis (*Treponema pallidum*)

Syphilis is a sexually transmitted infection that can be easily treated. Fetal infection can lead to nonimmune hydrops and stillbirth. The risk of transmission to the fetus can be dramatically reduced by treating the mother. Patients identified with syphilis should be referred to a genitourinary medicine clinic for:

- treatment with benzyl penicillin injections
- screening of other sexually transmitted infections
- contact tracing including partner

Hepatitis

Hepatitis B is a viral infection transmitted:

- sexually
- vertically (mother to fetus)
- via blood

The patient should be referred to a liver physician if she has not been seen previously and her liver function tests monitored in pregnancy and postnatally due to the chronic nature of the infection. Again, partner testing is recommended as well as testing any existing children she may have. They can be offered vaccination if found to be negative.

Postnatal vaccination of the fetus has been shown to reduce the risk of transmission. Patients who have the hepatitis E antigen (HBeAg) carry the highest risk of transmitting the infection to the fetus.

Hepatitis C is also a viral illness that is transmitted sexually, vertically (mother to fetus) or via blood. Current guidelines, however, do not recommend routine screening.

Human immunodeficiency virus

Human immunodeficiency virus (HIV) is a blood-borne virus transmitted sexually, vertically and by blood. Although incurable, modern advances in management have increased the life expectancy of affected individuals and significantly reduced the rate of vertical transmission (see Chapter 22).

Screening for HIV allows patients to commence on treatment if required and to assess how the patient should deliver. All cases should be managed by a multidisciplinary team involving obstetricians, HIV specialists and specialist midwives. Testing should be offered to the woman's partner and any children she has.

Urinary tract infections

Urinary tract infections may be symptomatic or asymptomatic. In untreated asymptomatic cases, there is a significant risk of pyelonephritis and preterm birth. Current guidelines recommend screening for asymptomatic bacteriuria in all pregnant women by means of a midstream urine culture.

ANTENATAL EDUCATION

For some patients, pregnancy can be a daunting time, especially those who are embarking on their first pregnancy or those who are very young. Therefore education at booking is a vital step and the provision of clear (often written)

information can be an invaluable tool to put patients at ease. Increasingly, online information is available in the form of phone apps for example.

Topics that should be covered include:

- Common symptoms in pregnancy (see Box 19.1).
- Maternity benefits.
- Working during pregnancy.
- Dietary information – advise a mixed diet with fruit, vegetables, fibre, lean meat, fish, lentils, starchy foods (bread/pasta, etc.) and dairy; foods to avoid and why are shown in Table 19.1.
- Smoking – discussion about smoking cessation is essential plus referral to specialist services if accepted.
- Alcohol consumption should be avoided completely in the first trimester and, ideally, throughout pregnancy. Those who choose to drink should be advised to drink no more than 1–2 units a week and to avoid binge drinking.

BOX 19.1 COMMON SYMPTOMS IN PREGNANCY

Nausea and vomiting/hyperemesis gravidarum

Mild symptoms usually resolve by 16–20 weeks and can be managed by eating little and often and with oral antiemetics.

If excessive and causing dehydration, it is called 'hyperemesis gravidarum' (see below).

Heartburn

Avoid large meals and lying supine soon after food. Reduce caffeine and foods with high fat content. Antacid preparations.

Constipation

Increase fibre in diet, avoid dehydration.

Haemorrhoids

Haemorrhoid creams, avoidance of constipation.

Varicose veins

Compression stockings can be helpful.
Elevation of legs.
Avoid prolonged periods of standing.

Backache

Advice on posture, massage and water exercising can help.

Symphysis pubis dysfunction

Physiotherapy referral for advice and consideration of pelvic support devices.

Table 19.1 Dietary precautions in pregnancy

Food product	Potential risks
Soft cheeses, unpasteurized milk/cheese, raw fish (sushi)	Infection with listeria, which can lead to miscarriage and stillbirth
Unwashed salad, fruit, vegetables, raw meats	Toxoplasmosis infection, which can lead to miscarriage, stillbirth or disability
Shellfish (oysters), raw eggs	Food poisoning
Caffeine	Limit intake to 300 mg per day

- Medications, vitamins and supplements: it is important to emphasize that most medications have insufficient data to be deemed 100% safe in pregnancy and therefore their use should be limited to occasions when they are absolutely necessary. Complementary medicines again have little or no safety data.
- Advise on the importance of taking folic acid (400 mcg od) during the first 12 weeks to reduce the risk of neural tube defects.
- Driving – appropriate positioning of the seatbelt, i.e., wearing it above and below the bump NOT over.
- Flying – flights more than approximately 4 hours are independently associated with an increased risk of venous thromboembolism. Therefore unless travel is essential it may be advisable to avoid it, especially when there are other risk factors such as raised BMI. Compression stockings have been shown to reduce this risk.
- Exercise – moderate exercise is safe in pregnancy, although patients should be informed of the risks with contact sports and other forms of vigorous exercise.
- Pets – there is a risk of toxoplasmosis from cat faeces and contaminated soil, therefore avoidance of handling cat litter and wearing gloves when gardening as well as handwashing should be advised.

Hyperemesis gravidarum

Nausea and vomiting in the first trimester is a common pregnancy symptom affecting 80% of pregnancies. Hyperemesis gravidarum affects up to 3.6% of pregnancies and is diagnosed by:

- >5% prepregnancy weight loss
- dehydration
- electrolyte imbalance

The cause is thought to be due to rising β-human chorionic gonadotropin (βHCG) levels, therefore trophoblastic or multiple pregnancies that are associated with higher βHCG levels can increase the severity of nausea and vomiting.

History and examination

Other causes of nausea and vomiting should be excluded by asking for symptoms of abdominal pain, urinary symptoms, infection, chronic *Helicobacter pylori* infection and by taking a drug history. A previous history of hyperemesis gravidarum should be sought as it can recur in subsequent pregnancy.

During the examination the following should be recorded:

- temperature
- pulse
- blood pressure
- oxygen saturations
- respiratory rate
- abdominal examination findings
- weight
- signs of dehydrations
- signs of muscle wasting

Investigations

Initial investigations include a urine dipstick to assess the degree of ketonuria and if leucocytes or nitrites are present, a sample of urine should be sent for microscopy, culture and sensitivities to rule out urine infection as a cause of symptoms.

A full blood count and urea and electrolytes need to be performed to rule out infection, anaemia, measure haematocrit and assess electrolyte imbalances, especially hyponatraemia and hypokalaemia. There is a structural similarity between thyroid-stimulation hormone and HCG, which can cause abnormal thyroid function test results. Hyperemesis gravidarum can cause deranged liver function tests with raised transaminases and bilirubin. Abnormal thyroid function tests and liver function tests normalize with treatment and resolution of hyperemesis gravidarum.

An ultrasound scan should be arranged to confirm a viable intrauterine pregnancy and exclude multiple pregnancy or trophoblastic disease.

Management

Hyperemesis gravidarum can be managed as an outpatient, in an ambulatory day care unit or as an inpatient depending on the severity of the nausea and vomiting.

Woman with mild nausea and vomiting can be managed in the community with oral antiemetics, oral hydration and dietary advice. Those who are not tolerating oral fluids can attend an ambulatory day care unit for intravenous (IV) fluids, antiemetics and vitamins, thus avoiding an admission to hospital. Inpatient management may be required if there is continued vomiting despite oral antiemetics, significant weight loss and ketonuria. The treatment involves IV antiemetics and fluids and replacement of B vitamins.

Initially, antiemetic treatment is with a single agent, but if nausea and vomiting are not controlled, then multiple agents can be used. Safe antiemetics to use in hyperemesis include cyclizine, metoclopramide (beware of extrapyramidal symptoms and oculogyric crisis as side-effects) and ondansetron. IV fluid replacement should be with 0.9% saline and supplemental potassium if required. Dextrose infusions should not be used as they can precipitate Wernicke encephalopathy.

If symptoms do not resolve, then a course of corticosteroid therapy can be considered after consultant review. IV hydrocortisone 100 mg twice a day is started and then converted to oral prednisolone on a reducing regime to the lowest dose to control symptoms. Corticosteroid treatment should continue until the gestation that hyperemesis should have resolved.

ONGOING ANTENATAL CARE

Depending upon the classification of risk, ongoing antenatal care in pregnancy may be delivered by general practitioners, midwives, obstetricians or a combination of all three. Generally, low-risk patients in their first pregnancy will have around 10 visits spread throughout their pregnancy and those who have had a baby before and are low risk will have 7 visits. In patients for whom issues have been identified, the schedule of care will need to be modified according to their individual needs.

SCREENING FOR CHROMOSOMAL ABNORMALITIES

National Screening Committee guidelines recommend offering all patients a screening test for Down syndrome (trisomy 21), Edward syndrome (trisomy 18) and Patau syndrome (trisomy 13). These three conditions increase in incidence with increasing maternal age. Informed consent must be obtained prior to testing, including the options for further testing and continuing care in pregnancy if the result is high risk.

Combined screening test

The recommended screening test in the first trimester for these three conditions is the combined test, ultrasound combined with maternal blood tests. Between 11 and 14 + 0 weeks' gestation, patients undergo an ultrasound assessment (Fig. 19.1), which measures the nuchal translucency (NT). They also have a blood test to measure maternal serum levels of βHCG and pregnancy-associated plasma protein A.

NT is an ultrasound observation and refers to the black space seen on ultrasound within the back of the fetus' neck. The width of this space is measured – on average, fetuses affected with Down syndrome have an increased NT. It should be remembered that not all fetuses with an increased NT will have Down syndrome.

Once the patient has undergone these tests, the results are combined to calculate a risk score, which denotes the risk of the fetus having Down syndrome, for example, 1 in 2000 (i.e. this is only a screening test). In the UK, guidance has recommended a cut-off of 1 in 150 for consideration as 'high risk' and these individuals are counselled about the option of invasive testing (i.e. do they wish to proceed with a diagnostic test).

Triple or quadruple test

For those patients who book late or have missed the cut-off for combined screening, a second-trimester screening in the form of the triple or quadruple test can be offered. These are also blood tests for placental hormones, following which a risk score is also generated. The triple test consists of α-feto-protein, oestriol and βHCG. The quadruple test is the same with the addition of inhibin-A.

Noninvasive prenatal testing

Noninvasive prenatal testing, also known as 'cfDNA (cell-free DNA) screening', is a blood test that looks at fetal DNA in maternal blood and gives the risk factor for conditions

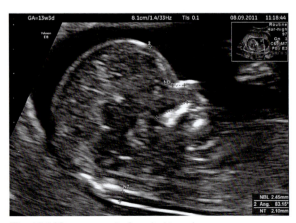

Fig. 19.1 Measurement of nuchal translucency.

such as Down syndrome. It can be done from about the 10th week of pregnancy, and offers a more accurate result than the routine 'combined screening' test. Again, it is not diagnostic, but large-scale studies show that the test has a detection rate of over 99%. Currently it is not available on the National Health Service (NHS), but it may be rolled out in 2018.

ULTRASOUND SCANNING FOR FETAL ABNORMALITIES

The dating ultrasound scan performed between 11+4 and 14 weeks can pick up some of the major fetal abnormalities such as acrania or exomphalos. According to National Screening Committee guidelines, all pregnant women in England with singleton and twin pregnancies should be offered an ultrasound scan between 18^{+0} and 20^{+6} weeks to check for structural fetal anomalies. If abnormalities are detected, then it may be appropriate to offer invasive testing and prenatal diagnosis with referral to a fetal medicine centre (e.g. if a cardiac anomaly is seen, the amniocentesis is offered for chromosomal abnormalities). In some situations, the woman will need follow-up scans and discussion with the neonatal team for delivery planning and a postnatal plan for the baby (e.g. gastrointestinal abnormalities such as gastroschisis involve scanning for fetal growth and planning delivery in a unit with neonatal surgery facilities).

PRENATAL DIAGNOSIS

The introduction of screening programmes and increased awareness of certain genetic conditions has led to the option of prenatal diagnosis becoming a common diagnostic tool. It is estimated that around 5% of pregnant patients are offered invasive prenatal diagnostic tests (30,000 patients in the UK).

As mentioned above, patients are offered screening for chromosomal abnormalities such as Down syndrome. These tests are NOT diagnostic and only offer a risk score. In individuals who are deemed high risk, prenatal diagnosis offers a way of establishing a diagnosis as to whether the fetus does indeed have the condition suspected by the screening. In addition, parents who are carriers for certain conditions (e.g. sickle cell disease) may wish to know whether or not their child is affected by the condition. Undergoing prenatal diagnosis allows the couple to be prepared for the needs of the child if they choose to continue with the pregnancy or indeed opt for a termination of pregnancy. Furthermore, it allows medical teams to modify antenatal care and to prepare for the delivery and needs of the baby once born.

Ultrasound

As mentioned above, ultrasound is used at a number of stages in pregnancy. The early scan at 11–14 weeks allows for the measurement of NT and later, the anomaly ultrasound scan (18–20 weeks) allows for a more detailed assessment of any structural anomaly. Although often not realized by patients, this indeed is a form of prenatal diagnosis. Some anomalies identified will prompt further diagnostic interventions such as amniocentesis or fetal blood sampling (FBS).

Chorionic villous sampling

Chorionic villous sampling (CVS) is a technique used to obtain a sample of chorionic villi from the fetal placenta. It can be carried out via the transabdominal route or less commonly, the transcervical route, and again is done under continuous ultrasound guidance (Fig. 19.2). CVS is usually performed between 11 weeks and 13 weeks + 6 days and should not be performed before 10 weeks due to concerns about increased loss rates and limb abnormalities.

The rate of miscarriage following a CVS is generally thought to be greater than that of an amniocentesis; however, data from specialist units where a large number of procedures are carried out have shown that the loss rates may actually be very similar (1%). As with an amniocentesis, there is a 0.1% chance of serious infection.

As CVS is performed earlier than amniocentesis, the patient has the choice of an earlier surgical termination if an abnormal result is confirmed, which patients may find more acceptable. However, there is the risk of placental mosaicism that can yield an inconclusive result requiring further testing.

Amniocentesis

The term 'amniocentesis' is derived from the Greek words *amnion* (referring to the amnion of the fetal membranes) and *kentēsis*, a puncture (i.e. a puncture of the amnion). The aim of the procedure is to obtain a sample of amniotic fluid from which fetal cells can be harvested. The fetal cells are then cultured and undergo testing to establish the fetal karyotype (the number and visual appearance of the chromosomes in the cell). Results take:

- 2–3 days using the polymerase chain reaction technique
- up to 2 weeks from a culture

Another use of amniocentesis is for diagnosis of suspected fetal infection where the amniotic fluid can be sampled and tested (e.g., cytomegalovirus infection).

The procedure is carried out after 15 weeks of pregnancy; those done prior to this are associated with a higher risk of fetal loss and limb abnormalities. Under ultrasound guidance, a needle is passed through the anterior abdominal wall into the amniotic cavity. Amniotic fluid is then aspirated and the needle withdrawn. Fig. 19.3 shows the technique.

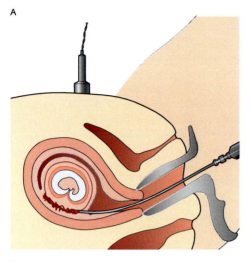

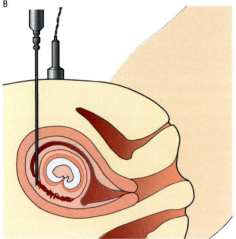

Fig. 19.2 Chorionic villous sampling: (A) transcervical; (B) transabdominal.

As with any medical procedure there are associated risks, therefore before undergoing the procedure it is essential that patients understand the risks and the benefits. This should include their potential options with a positive result. An amniocentesis carries a 1% risk of miscarriage and 0.1% risk of serious infection.

> **HINTS AND TIPS**
>
> Both an amniocentesis and chorionic villous sampling are considered a potentially sensitizing event and therefore the administration of anti-D immunoglobulin to rhesus-negative mothers is recommended.

Fetal blood sampling

FBS in prenatal diagnosis that involves the aspiration of fetal blood using a transabdominal approach under ultrasound guidance. It is important to recognize that this is very different to the FBS performed in labour when a sample of blood is obtained from the fetal scalp. The technique can be used to detect fetal anaemia or fetal thrombocytopenia. However, the use of middle cerebral artery Doppler assessment has largely replaced FBS for diagnosis of anaemia. This uses colour ultrasound to assess the dynamics of blood flow in the middle cerebral artery – if flow is faster than normal, this could be because the baby is anaemic. FBS also allows the transfusion of blood or platelets if required. However, the need for the procedure must be balanced against a miscarriage risk of 1%–2% in counselling a patient.

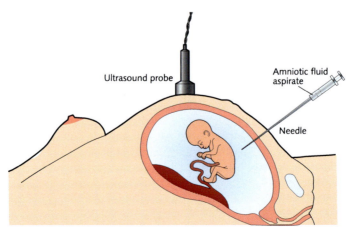

Fig. 19.3 Amniocentesis.

Chapter Summary

- The booking visit allows risks to the pregnancy to be identified and managed.
- Blood tests and ultrasounds scans are performed to screen for conditions and disorders.
- Antenatal screening tests that include the combined test, triple or quadruple test or noninvasive prenatal testing are offered to woman to identify those who are at high risk of having a baby with a chromosomal abnormality such as Down syndrome.
- Woman who are found to be high risk for chromosomal abnormalities during screening are offered diagnostic testing with chorionic villus sampling or amniocentesis.
- High-risk pregnancies are managed in a consultant-led clinic with regular growth scans at 28, 32 and 36 weeks.

FURTHER READING

Leslie, K., Papageorghiou, A., 2011. Invasive procedures in Oxford desk reference obstetrics & gynaecology. Oxford University Press, London, UK.

National Institute for Health and Care Excellence (NICE). NICE guidelines – Antenatal care for uncomplicated pregnancies 2017; Pregnancy and complex social factors 2010; Antenatal and post-natal mental health 2017. London, UK: NICE. Available at: guidance.nice.org.uk.

Nelson-Piercy, C., 2010. Handbook of obstetric medicine, 4th ed. Informa Healthcare, London, UK.

National Health Service (NHS) Fetal Anomaly Screening Programme. Available at: http://fetalanomaly.screening.nhs.uk.

Royal College of Obstetricians and Gynaecologists (RCOG), 2010. Amniocentesis and chorionic villus sampling: RCOG green top guideline no. 8. RCOG, London, UK.

UK National Screening Committee, 2013. Screening tests for you and your baby booklet. Available at: www.screening.nhs.uk/annbpublications.

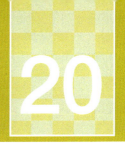

DEFINITION

Antepartum haemorrhage (APH) is defined as any bleeding from the genital tract that occurs after 24 + 0 weeks' gestation and before the birth of the infant.

HINTS AND TIPS

Antepartum haemorrhage (APH) is an important cause of increased maternal and perinatal morbidity and mortality. Up to 20% of very preterm infants are born in association with APH.

INCIDENCE

The incidence of APH is 3%–5%.

AETIOLOGY

A summary is shown in Table 20.1. Placenta praevia combined with placental abruption accounts for about 50% of the causes of an APH. In both cases, the bleeding comes from maternal vessels that are exposed as the placenta separates from the decidua (i.e. it is not fetal blood).

RED FLAG

With any bleeding in pregnancy, do not forget ABC – assess the patient's airway, breathing and circulation including the estimated blood loss and resuscitate.

HISTORY

When taking a history, it is important to elicit certain points including:

- amount of bleeding
- association with abdominal pain and/or contractions
- association with mucoid discharge

The presence or absence of constant abdominal pain is particularly important to differentiate between placenta prae-

Table 20.1 Aetiology of antepartum haemorrhage[a]

Source of haemorrhage	Type of haemorrhage
Uterine source	Placenta praevia Placental abruption Vasa praevia Circumvallate placenta
Lower genital tract source	Cervical ectropion Cervical polyp Cervical carcinoma Cervicitis Vaginitis Vulval varicosities
Unknown origin (approximately 50%)	

[a] Bloody mucoid vaginal loss may be the 'show' or cervical mucus plug associated with the onset of labour.

via and a placental abruption. With the latter, there may also be uterine contractions as the myometrium is infiltrated with blood that makes the uterus irritable.

There may be an obvious trigger event, for example, recent sexual intercourse can cause bleeding from a cervical ectropion. The date of the patient's last smear test is relevant to exclude a cervical cause for the bleeding. The patient should be asked about fetal movements.

COMMON PITFALLS

Do not forget to ask about the patient's smear history: when was the last smear? Was the result normal? Although rare, cervical disease can present for the first time in pregnancy.

HINTS AND TIPS

The presence of abdominal pain typically distinguishes placental abruption from placenta praevia.

EXAMINATION

The aim is to assess maternal and fetal wellbeing. This includes the following:

Maternal wellbeing:

- pulse/blood pressure/respiratory rate
- pallor
- abdominal palpation for uterine tenderness/contractions
- speculum examination for cervical abnormalities
- digital examination in the presence of contractions to assess cervical change, but only if placenta praevia has been excluded

Fetal wellbeing:

- abdominal palpation for lie/presentation/engagement
- auscultation of fetal heart to determine viability
- cardiotocograph (CTG) if >26 + 0 weeks' gestation to confirm fetal wellbeing

INVESTIGATIONS

Box 20.1 lists the investigations appropriate for the patient with an APH.

Blood tests

Blood should be cross-matched if the bleeding is significant and ongoing (e.g. major placenta praevia). Blood group must be checked – anti-D immunoglobulin should be given if the patient is rhesus negative, to prevent haemolytic disease of the fetus or newborn in a future pregnancy (see Chapter 19). A Kleihauer test examines the maternal blood film for the presence of fetal blood cells, suggesting fetomaternal haemorrhage. This can be seen with placental abruption.

If the patient also presents with hypertension, then liver and renal function tests can be performed and if they are deranged, pre-eclampsia should be considered as a cause (see Chapter 21)

Fetal monitoring

A CTG should be done to confirm fetal wellbeing after 26 + 0 weeks' gestation. It may also show uterine irritability or established contractions.

BOX 20.1   INVESTIGATIONS FOR A PATIENT WITH AN ANTEPARTUM HAEMORRHAGE

- Full blood count
- Group and save/cross-match
- Coagulation profile
- Kleihauer test
- Renal function tests
- Liver function tests
- Cardiotocograph
- Ultrasound scan

Ultrasound scan

The placental site is checked at the routine 20-week anomaly scan. If it is low lying, a diagnosis of placenta praevia is suspected and a repeat scan should be arranged at 36 weeks. The diagnosis of placenta praevia should be confirmed by trans-abdominal and trans-vaginal ultrasound scans. In the majority of patients, as the lower segment begins to form and the upper segment enlarges upwards, the placenta appears to move up away from the cervical os. A transvaginal scan is safe and may improve accuracy over the transabdominal mode, particularly with a posterior placenta.

An abruption is usually diagnosed on clinical grounds. A small retroplacental clot may not be seen on ultrasound scan, and so a normal scan does not exclude the diagnosis. A large retroplacental clot that can be seen on scan is likely to be obvious clinically, with abdominal pain and bleeding.

Women who present with recurrent unexplained APH should be classified as high risk and transferred to consultant-led care. Serial ultrasound assessment for fetal growth should be performed as these pregnancies are at risk of intrauterine growth restriction.

PLACENTA PRAEVIA

Definition

The placenta is wholly or partially attached to the lower uterine segment. The degree of attachment is classified as either minor, where the leading edge of the placenta is in the lower uterine segment but not covering the os, or major, where the placenta lies over the internal os.

Incidence

Placenta praevia occurs in 0.4%–0.8% of pregnancies; this figure has altered with routine use of ultrasound scanning. The incidence is increased with the following risk factors:

- previous caesarean section including previous placenta praevia
- advanced maternal age
- multiparity
- multiple pregnancy
- presence of a succenturiate placental lobe
- smoking

It is associated with a maternal mortality rate of about 0.03% in the developed world. However, both maternal and fetal morbidity are substantially higher in developing countries due to complications such as haemorrhage and prematurity.

Particularly with increasing numbers of caesarean sections, there is an increased incidence of placenta accreta. This is a condition found in up to 15% of those with placenta praevia, in which the placenta is morbidly adherent to the uterine decidua and may even penetrate through the myometrium to invade surrounding organs. Magnetic resonance imaging (MRI) scan is thought to be helpful to aid diagnosis of this complication.

> **HINTS AND TIPS**
>
> • Placenta praevia usually presents as painless vaginal bleeding.

History

Bleeding from a placenta praevia is usually unprovoked and occurs in the third trimester, in the absence of labour.

Examination

General observations including maternal pulse and blood pressure must be performed. On abdominal palpation, the uterus is soft and nontender. The low-lying placenta may displace the presenting part from the pelvis so that a cephalic presentation is not engaged, or there is a malpresentation.

With a minor degree of bleeding, a speculum can be passed to exclude a lower genital tract cause for the APH. A digital examination should be avoided because it may provoke massive bleeding.

RED FLAG

Do not perform a digital examination to assess cervical dilatation unless you have excluded placenta praevia.

Diagnosis

As described earlier, the placental site is localized as part of the routine 20-week ultrasound scan. If a low-lying placenta is noted, then a follow-up scan in the third trimester is usually performed to make the diagnosis of placenta praevia.

Investigations

These are outlined in Box 20.1. Blood should be sent for haemoglobin, and group and save. Anti-D is indicated if the patient is rhesus negative. If the bleeding is heavy, cross-matching blood for transfusion is indicated and a baseline clotting screen is performed. Renal function tests are important if the urine output is poor secondary to hypovolaemia. A CTG should be performed to check fetal wellbeing. An ultrasound scan should be performed if the placental location is unknown. An MRI scan may be indicated if there is a high index of suspicion about placenta accreta.

Management

Management depends first on assessing the severity of the bleeding and resuscitation of the patient. Immediate delivery by caesarean section may be appropriate if there is either maternal or fetal compromise.

Expectant management depends on the severity of bleeding, the gestation of the pregnancy and the placental site. If the placenta remains at or over the cervical os, massive bleeding is likely to occur if the patient goes into labour and the cervix starts to dilate. Therefore in-patient management is appropriate towards the end of the third trimester with immediate recourse to caesarean section if necessary. Steroids to improve fetal lung maturity should be considered following liaison with the paediatricians, in case preterm delivery is needed. Caesarean section is usually advised if the placenta is encroaching within 2 cm of the internal cervical os. A consultant obstetrician and consultant anaesthetist should be present for this. If the head of the fetus becomes engaged (i.e., it passes below the leading edge of the placenta), then vaginal delivery may be possible.

Complications

Placenta praevia is associated with an increased risk of post-partum haemorrhage (PPH; see Chapter 31) regardless of the mode of delivery. The lower uterine segment where the placenta is sited is less efficient at retraction following delivery of the placenta compared to the upper segment. Thus occlusion of the venous sinuses is less effective, resulting in heavier blood loss. This may be further complicated by the presence of placenta accreta. Therefore preparations should be in place for potential PPH. This includes cross-matching blood and both consultant obstetrician and anaesthetist input. The patient should be given adequate counselling regarding the possible need for medical and surgical measures to control bleeding including hysterectomy.

Future pregnancy

Placenta praevia has a recurrence rate of 4%–8% with an increased risk of placenta accreta in each pregnancy.

RED FLAG

Placenta accreta is defined as a morbidly adherent placenta that penetrates through the decidua basalis and myometrium. It is should be suspected with a history of repeated caesarean sections or previous placenta praevia. It is diagnosed by ultrasound scanning and magnetic resonance imaging can help to confirm its presence. Placenta accreta should be considered when any part of the placenta is low lying under the previous caesarean section scar.

Management should be with a multidisciplinary approach involving an anaesthetist, obstetrician and gynaecologist, as there is an increased risk of caesarean hysterectomy.

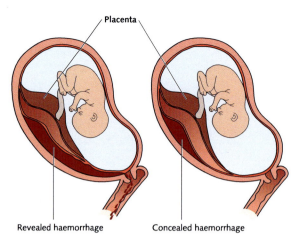

Placenta

Revealed haemorrhage   Concealed haemorrhage

Fig. 20.1 Types of placental abruption.

PLACENTAL ABRUPTION

Definition

The placental attachment to the uterus is disrupted by haemorrhage as blood dissects under the placenta, possibly extending into the amniotic sac or the uterine muscle.

Incidence

Placental abruption occurs in about 1% of pregnancies in the UK. In the majority of cases the cause is unknown, but it is associated with:

- previous abruption
- advanced maternal age
- multiparity
- maternal hypertension or preeclampsia
- abdominal trauma (e.g., assault, road traffic accident)
- cigarette smoking
- cocaine use
- lower socioeconomic group
- external cephalic version

HINTS AND TIPS

Placental abruption usually presents with vaginal bleeding associated with abdominal pain.

History

The patient can present at any stage of pregnancy with a history of bleeding and constant abdominal pain, which is usually unprovoked. There may be associated uterine contractions.

As maternal blood escapes from the placental sinuses, it tracks down between the membranes and the uterus and escapes via the cervix; this is known as a 'revealed haemorrhage'. Sometimes, the blood remains sealed within the

uterine cavity such that the degree of shock is out of proportion to the vaginal loss; this is known as a 'concealed haemorrhage' (Fig. 20.1).

HINTS AND TIPS

Preeclampsia is associated with placental abruption, so the patient should be asked if she has experienced symptoms including headache, blurred vision, nausea, epigastric pain and oedema. She should have the blood pressure measured and urinalysis performed to exclude proteinuria.

Examination

The general maternal condition, including pulse and blood pressure, should be assessed. On abdominal palpation the uterus is typically tender. As bleeding extends into the uterine muscle, a contraction can occur, making the uterus feel hard. Fetal parts are therefore difficult to palpate. If the placental site is known (i.e. if placenta praevia has been excluded) a digital examination is appropriate in the presence of uterine contractions to diagnose the onset of labour.

Maternal hypertension and proteinuria must be excluded due to the association between abruption and pre-eclampsia. If there is hypertension, liver tenderness, hyperreflexia and clonus should be excluded (see Chapter 21).

Investigations

These are outlined in Box 20.1. Blood should be sent for haemoglobin, and group and save. Anti-D is indicated if the patient is rhesus negative. If the bleeding is heavy or if the patient is shocked, cross-matching units of blood for transfusion is indicated and a baseline clotting screen is performed. A Kleihauer test should be requested to diagnose fetomaternal haemorrhage, which occurs in an abruption.

Renal function tests are necessary if the urine output is poor or in conjunction with liver function tests if pre-eclampsia is suspected. Urinalysis should be done to exclude proteinuria; if present, a protein-to-creatinine ratio or a 24-hour urine protein level may be helpful to determine the degree of renal involvement (see Chapter 21).

A CTG should be performed to check fetal wellbeing. A sinusoidal pattern can be seen with fetomaternal haemorrhage and is suggestive of fetal anaemia. The CTG will also monitor uterine activity, either contractions or a uterus that might simply be irritable with irregular activity.

An ultrasound scan is of limited value because only a large retroplacental haemorrhage will be seen. The diagnosis of abruption is usually made on clinical grounds.

Management

As for placenta praevia, management of a placental abruption must start with assessment of the severity of the symptoms and prompt resuscitation. Immediate delivery of the fetus may be necessary as a life-saving procedure for the mother, regardless of gestation.

In a situation where the patient is clinically well and the fetus is not compromised, expectant management might allow the symptoms to resolve. Again, steroids should be considered to aid fetal lung maturity if pre-term delivery is required.

Complications

Accurate assessment of blood loss is necessary to assess the risks of developing disseminated intravascular coagulation and renal failure. PPH occurs in 25% of cases, which rarely leads to Sheehan syndrome (pituitary necrosis secondary to hypovolaemic shock – see Chapter 31).

Future pregnancy

Women who have had a previous placental abruption are at increased risk in their next pregnancy. The risk of recurrence is about 8%.

VASA PRAEVIA

This is a rare cause of APH, 1 in 2000–6000 pregnancies. There is a velamentous insertion of the cord and the vessels lie on the membranes that cover the internal cervical os, in front of the presenting part. When the membranes rupture, either spontaneously or iatrogenically, the vessels can be torn and vaginal bleeding occurs. Unlike placenta praevia and placental abruption, this blood is fetal blood and the fetus must be delivered urgently before it exsanguinates.

If the diagnosis is unclear, a Kleihauer test can be performed on the vaginal blood loss to test for the presence of fetal red blood cells. However, this may delay delivery inappropriately and should only be considered if the CTG is normal.

CIRCUMVALLATE PLACENTA

This type of placenta develops secondary to outward proliferation of the chorionic villi into the decidua, beneath the ring of attachment of the amnion and chorion. This does not interfere with placental function, but it is associated with antepartum and intrapartum haemorrhage.

UNEXPLAINED ANTEPARTUM HAEMORRHAGE

In up to 50% of cases of APH, no specific cause is found. A history should be taken as described above including date of last smear test. The cervix should be visualized with a speculum examination and referral to colposcopy considered if any abnormality is seen.

However, overall, perinatal mortality with any type of APH is double that of a normal pregnancy, suggesting that placental function might be compromised. Therefore, with recurrent APH, it is appropriate to perform serial ultrasound scans to monitor fetal growth and to consider delivery at term, by inducing labour.

● Chapter Summary

- There are many causes of antepartum haemorrhage and by taking a good history and performing an examination a diagnosis can be made.
- Use an airway, breathing, circulation (ABC) approach when assessing a woman who presents with bleeding.
- Commonest causes of antepartum haemorrhage are placenta praevia and placental abruption.
- Placenta praevia usually presents with painless vaginal bleeding.
- Placental abruption usually presents with abdominal pain with or without bleeding.

FURTHER READING

Royal College of Obstetricians and Gynaecologists (RCOG), 2011. Antepartum haemorrhage: RCOG green top guideline no. 63. RCOG, London, UK. Available at: www.rcog.org.uk.

Royal College of Obstetricians and Gynaecologists (RCOG), 2011. Placenta praevia, placenta praevia accrete and vasa praevia: diagnosis and management: RCOG green top guideline no. 27. RCOG, London, UK. 2011. Available at: www.rcog.org.uk.

Hypertension in pregnancy 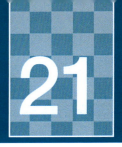 21

INTRODUCTION

Management of hypertensive disorders in pregnancy forms a large part of antenatal care as they affect 10%–15% of all pregnancies with pre-eclampsia occurring in 3%–5%. Accurate diagnosis with prompt treatment is essential to ensure a good outcome for both mother and fetus as hypertensive disorders are a leading cause of fetal and maternal morbidity and mortality. Maternal mortality from hypertensive disorders is reducing in the UK, with fewer than one death for every million women giving birth (see Chapter 32). 1 in 20 (5%) of still births are associated with pre-eclampsia (see Chapter 30). Hypertension is defined as blood pressure >140/90 mmHg in pregnancy. Hypertensive disorders fall into three main categories:

- Preexisting or chronic hypertension: patients may have a known history of hypertension or be found to be hypertensive at booking or at <20 weeks. Pre-pregnancy counselling allows review of medications that may cause fetal morbidity. Fetal monitoring for growth and maternal monitoring to enable prompt treatment of raised blood pressure are important.
- Gestational or pregnancy-induced hypertension (PIH): hypertension presenting after 20 weeks of the pregnancy with no proteinuria.
- Proteinuric hypertension or pre-eclampsia [pre-eclamptic toxaemia (PET)]: hypertension presenting after 20 weeks with significant proteinuria. The risk factors for PET are shown in Box 21.1 and, once identified at booking, consideration should be given

---

BOX 21.1 RISK FACTORS FOR PREECLAMPSIA

High risk

- previous pre-eclamptic toxaemia (PET)
- chronic kidney disease
- diabetes (type I and type II)
- systemic lupus erythematosus, antiphospholipid syndrome

Moderate risk

- primips
- age >40 years
- body mass index >35 kg/m^2
- family history of PET
- twins

---

to prescribing aspirin 75 mg daily from 12 weeks' gestation until delivery to reduce the risk. The aetiology of PET is still not fully understood, but it is thought that failure of the normal trophoblastic invasion of myometrial spiral arteries leads to a high-resistance circulation and uteroplacental underperfusion. This process then results in the release of antiangiogenic factors into maternal circulation causing vasoconstriction (hence hypertension) and endothelial damage causing morbidity such as proteinuria. It is therefore a multisystem disorder.

HISTORY

Presenting complaint

Hypertensive patients may be asymptomatic and a high blood pressure reading might only be picked up as part of the routine antenatal check. Therefore accurate blood pressure measurement is very important.

Symptoms and signs of preeclampsia are shown in Fig. 21.1. However, it is important to ask specifically about:

1. headache (secondary to cerebral oedema)
2. visual disturbance (typically in the form of flashing lights)

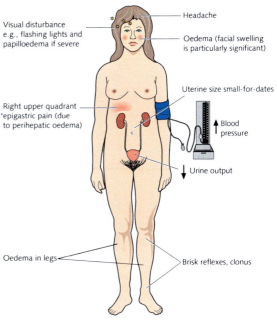

Fig. 21.1 Signs and symptoms of preeclampsia.

3. right upper quadrant or epigastric pain (due to oedema of the liver capsule)
4. vomiting
5. swelling of the face, hands or feet

Gynaecological history

A history of high blood pressure when taking the oral contraceptive pill indicates a susceptibility to high blood pressure in pregnancy.

Obstetric history

Hypertensive episodes in previous pregnancies should be discussed (see Chapter 2). Features of the history that are of significance include the gestation period during which hypertension was diagnosed, if treatment was required and duration of treatment postnatally. Pre-eclampsia does not always recur with every pregnancy; it is more common in primigravidae or in the first pregnancy with a new partner.

Medical history

Those with a history of pre-existing hypertension are very unlikely to have normal blood pressure in pregnancy and may even have evidence of end-organ damage at the start of pregnancy if it has previously been poorly managed. Conditions that predispose to hypertension include diabetes, renal and cardiac disease.

Family history

Pre-eclampsia is familial, with the strongest association being a sister affected in her pregnancy. The more severe the pre-eclampsia and the earlier it occurs in pregnancy, the more likely it is to be familial.

Drug history

Patients with pre-existing hypertension might already be on medication. Common antihypertensives, such as diuretics, are contraindicated. Others are teratogenic including angiotensin-converting enzyme inhibitors and angiotensin II receptor blockers. If a woman becomes pregnant whilst taking these medications, they should be discontinued as soon as possible and an alternative drug should be started.

EXAMINATION

Examination begins with a general inspection. Any facial oedema should be noted and if it is not obvious to the physician, the patient or her partner may be asked to confirm its presence. If it has not been done already, the patient's blood pressure should be taken.

HINTS AND TIPS

Blood pressure should be measured with the patient sitting or lying at 45 degrees. The arm should be at the same level as the heart, and when auscultating, one should observe the point at which the sounds disappear rather than muffle, as the cut-off for the diastolic. It is essential that the correct size of cuff is used; if a small cuff is used for an obese woman, the blood pressure will be artificially (and worryingly) high and vice versa for large cuffs in small women.

Abdominal palpation should then be performed to elicit liver tenderness followed by palpation of the uterus to ascertain if the symphysiofundal height is appropriate for the gestational age. A small-for-dates fetus may be a sign of intrauterine growth restriction as a result of poor placental function in pre-eclampsia.

Brisk reflexes should be assessed and the presence of any clonus noted as these can be a sign of pre-eclampsia. Fundoscopy should be performed to look for papilloedema, which can occur in pre-eclampsia, or retinopathy, which is a complication of severe pre-existing hypertension.

INVESTIGATIONS

Investigating hypertension in pregnancy is aimed at establishing which of the three categories the patient falls into and the severity of the disease.

RED FLAG

When seeing a pregnant woman with raised blood pressure, one of your first questions must be 'Is there any proteinuria?' The presence of proteinuria should always raise the suspicion of pre-eclampsia.

Urinalysis

The presence of proteinuria is very important when differentiating between PIH and PET. Therefore, in all cases, the urine should be tested using a urinary dipstick to provide a rapid bedside assessment.

The presence of protein may be due to PET, but may also be the result of contamination with blood, liquor (if the membranes have ruptured), vaginal discharge or a urinary tract infection (UTI). A UTI should be suspected if the proteinuria is associated with the presence of nitrites, leucocytes and/or blood. However, PET must still be suspected until a UTI is excluded by sending a mid-stream sample for microbiology testing.

Proteinuria assessed as ≥1+ on urinary dipstick should be quantified by sending samples to the laboratory for evaluating protein-to-creatinine ratio (PCR) or 24-hour urinary protein collection. These will help to distinguish between contaminants giving a false-positive and true proteinuria. A PCR > 30 mg/mmol or a level of more than 0.3 g of protein in 24 hours should be regarded as significant.

Blood tests

In patients with pre-existing hypertension, baseline investigations (full blood count, urea and electrolytes and liver function tests) should be performed at booking as they will be an important reference point later in the pregnancy if the hypertension gets worse and/or the patient develops PET. During pregnancy, hypertension is investigated with blood tests shown in Table 21.1.

COMMON PITFALLS

Because of the physiology of pregnancy, the normal ranges of some blood tests will change. For example, due to an increased glomerular filtration rate in pregnancy, there is a higher creatinine clearance. Hence a normal serum creatinine level in pregnancy will be lower than that of the normal adult range. Therefore a creatinine level which would be considered normal in an average adult can be significantly abnormal in pregnancy. Another example of this is the liver enzyme alkaline phosphatase, which is raised in pregnancy due to placental production. Therefore a high level in pregnancy does not usually indicate the liver disease, which may be seen in pre-eclamptic toxaemia.

Ultrasound

Essential hypertension, if poorly controlled, may affect fetal growth. Therefore in these cases serial ultrasound scans for fetal growth, liquor volume and dopplers should be requested at 28, 32 and 36 weeks' gestation. Some units offer ultrasound assessment of uterine artery dopplers at around 22 weeks in an attempt to predict those who may go on to develop pre-eclampsia. A renal tract ultrasound scan may also be considered antenatally for those women with chronic hypertension to assess end-organ damage.

PET may cause intra-uterine growth restriction, oligohydramnios and abnormal dopplers secondary to placental insufficiency. Therefore ultrasound scans for fetal growth, liquor volume and dopplers are also indicated at the aforementioned gestations.

TREATMENT

Pre-existing/essential hypertension

Those with pre-existing hypertension should ideally be seen pre-pregnancy and have their blood pressure optimized with a drug safe for pregnancy such as labetalol (Table 21.2). Any potentially teratogenic medications should be changed (see the 'Drug history' section).

HINTS AND TIPS

In a young person who is being diagnosed with hypertension for the first time it is important to exclude an underlying disease such as coarctation of the aorta, renal artery stenosis, Conn syndrome, Cushing syndrome or a phaeochromocytoma.

Table 21.1 Blood tests in the patient with hypertension

	Chronic hypertension	Pregnancy-induced hypertension	Preeclamptic toxaemia
Full blood count	Normal	Normal	↓ Platelets ↑ Haematocrit
Urea & electrolytes	Normal[a]	Normal	↑ Creatinine
Liver function tests	Normal	Normal	↑ Alanine aminotransferase (ALT)/aspartate aminotransferase (AST)
Clotting screen[b]	Normal	Normal	Can be deranged
Lactate dehydrogenase[b]	Measured if there are concerns regarding haemolysis[c]		

[a] Chronic hypertensives may have an element of preexisting renal impairment and therefore baseline renal function tests should be sent at booking to compare with later tests in pregnancy.
[b] Done only if indicated by clinical picture or low platelets.
[c] HELLP syndrome haemolysis elevated liver enzymes and low platelets is a severe variant of preeclamptic toxaemia, which is named after its features.

Table 21.2 Antihypertensives.

Drug	Description
Labetalol	α- and β-Blocker – regarded as first-line treatment. Has direct cardiac effects and also lower peripheral vascular resistance. Should be avoided in asthmatics.
Nifedipine	Calcium channel blocker which causes arterial vasodilatation. Can cause headaches.
Methyldopa	α-Agonist which prevents vasoconstriction. It has been used for many years with a good safety profile. Should be stopped within 2 days of delivery and changed to another agent due to the risk of postnatal depression.
Hydralazine	Intravenous drug which causes vasodilatation. Can cause rapid hypotension, so is often given after a bolus of colloid.

The aim of treatment in this group is to maintain blood pressure readings below 150/100 mmHg. Those with evidence of end-organ damage (renal or retinal) may need even tighter control, below 140/90 mmHg. The risks of uncontrolled hypertension in this group are cerebral haemorrhage and other end-organ damage. Low-dose aspirin (75 mg daily) from 12 weeks' gestation until delivery has been shown to be beneficial in this group for reducing the risk of developing PET.

Pregnancy-induced hypertension

PIH presents after 20 weeks of pregnancy in patients with no history of hypertension and in the absence of proteinuria. The risks of uncontrolled blood pressure are those described above, and therefore monitoring with blood pressure measurement, urine dipstick testing and blood tests is very important:

- Mild hypertension (i.e., between 140/90 and 149/99 mmHg) does not always require treatment; blood pressure and urine should be checked weekly.
- Moderate hypertension (i.e., between 150/100 and 159/109 mmHg) should be treated (Table 21.2) and monitored twice weekly.
- Severe hypertension (i.e., >160/110 mmHg) requires inpatient treatment and close monitoring.

Both pre-existing hypertensives and those with PIH are at an increased risk of developing pre-eclampsia, so continued monitoring is very important. Early delivery before 37 weeks of gestation is not usually indicated unless the blood pressure is very difficult to control or there are signs of fetal compromise. In those who require delivery before 37 weeks a course of steroids should be administered to aid fetal lung maturity.

Pre-eclampsia

Pre-eclampsia is defined as new hypertension developing after 20 weeks with significant proteinuria. The pathophysiological process of PET can only be ended by delivery of the placenta. Therefore, when treating PET, there is a fine balance between continuing pregnancy (to allow more time for fetal maturity) and risks to the mother (of worsening liver and/or renal symptoms or risk of cerebral haemorrhage).

Again, the severity of hypertension will influence whether or not antihypertensives are commenced:

- Mild PET (140/90–149/99 mmHg) does not always require antihypertensives.
- Moderate PET (150/100–159/109 mmHg) requires treatment (Table 21.2).
- Severe PET > 160/110 mmHg requires urgent treatment and if not responsive to first-line oral treatments, may require intravenous antihypertensives.

In severe cases where there is a risk of eclampsia (seizures), intravenous magnesium sulphate ($MgSO_4$) has been shown to be beneficial as prophylaxis. It is usually used if the mean arterial pressure (Box 21.2) remains above 125 mmHg despite initial treatment, as well as other features including:

- headaches
- visual disturbance
- epigastric pain
- brisk reflexes or clonus (>3 beats)
- deranged blood tests such as low platelets, rising alanine aminotransferase (ALT) or creatinine

Blood tests (Table 21.1) should be performed frequently to assess any deterioration when a woman requires $MgSO_4$. Strict fluid input/output measurement is essential, with fluid restriction to prevent fluid overload. This is accepted as 1 mL/kg/h, and therefore 85 mL/h is used unless the patient is very underweight or overweight. Using $MgSO_4$ generally means the clinical picture necessitates delivering the baby once the mother is stable and/or steroids have been

BOX 21.2   CALCULATION OF MEAN ARTERIAL BLOOD PRESSURE (MAP)

Mean arterial pressure (MAP) can be estimated using the following formula:

$$MAP = \frac{(2 \times Diastolic\ BP) + Systolic\ BP}{3}$$

Or

$$MAP = \frac{Systolic\ BP - diastolic\ BP + diastolic\ BP}{3}$$

given (if required; see Chapter 25). The MgSO$_4$ should continue for 24 hours postdelivery as the woman is still high risk for eclampsia.

Eclampsia

Eclampsia is defined as the occurrence of seizures in pregnancy on a background of PET. Eclampsia affects 1 in 2000 pregnancies with around 40% of seizures occurring postnatally (usually within 48 hours of delivery). Seizures presenting for the first time in pregnancy should always be assumed to be eclamptic seizures until proven otherwise. The differential diagnosis includes:

- epilepsy
- meningitis
- cerebral thrombosis
- intracerebral bleed
- intracerebral tumour

The management of eclampsia is detailed in Fig. 21.2. As always, the initial management of eclampsia should always follow the airway, breathing, circulation (ABC) approach. Stabilization of the mother is paramount and should be ensured before any consideration is given to the fetus.

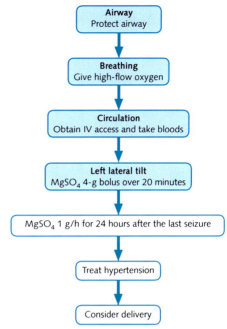

Fig. 21.2 Management of eclampsia. *IV*, Intravenous; *MgSO$_4$*, magnesium sulphate.

HELLP

HELLP syndrome is a life-threatening disorder thought to be a severe variant of pre-eclampsia.

It is characterized by:

Haemolysis
Elevated Liver enzymes (raised ALT)
Low Platelet count

Patients may present with the symptoms of pre-eclampsia (see Fig. 21.1). Investigations include a lactate dehydrogenase level and reticulocyte count to assess for haemolysis (see Table 21.1). The treatment for HELLP syndrome is delivery at a timely manner for mother and baby, as with PET. The complications of HELLP syndrome include subcapsular liver haematoma, liver rupture and disseminated intravascular coagulation.

POSTNATAL CARE

Following delivery women need to have a period of monitoring for up to 4–5 days in hospital, as blood pressure levels may reduce and medications may need to be amended accordingly. Those on methyldopa antenatally should be changed to an alternative drug due to the association with postnatal depression (Table 21.2). Antihypertensive drugs should be continued on discharge if required and follow-up in the community with the general practitioner should be arranged including a medical review at the 6-week postnatal check. This should include advice on a yearly blood pressure check as PET patients have been shown to be at increased risk of hypertension in later life. The risk of PET in a future pregnancy depends on the severity and gestation in the recent pregnancy, and aspirin may be advised next time from 12 weeks.

● Chapter Summary

- Pre-existing/chronic hypertension is defined as hypertension of >140/90 mmHg diagnosed at booking or <20 weeks' gestation.
- Gestational/pregnancy-induced hypertension is defined as hypertension >140/90 mmHg diagnosed after 20 weeks' gestation without proteinuria.
- Pre-eclampsia is defined as hypertension >140/90 mmHg associated with proteinuria >0.3 g in 24 hours.
- Treatment includes anti-hypertensives to control the blood pressure and in severe cases of pre-eclampsia treatment is with magnesium sulphate and planning of delivery.
- Pre-eclampsia can present in the postnatal period and women are at risk of eclampsia for up to 5 days postnatally.

FURTHER READING

Magpie Trial Follow-Up Study Collaborative Group, 2007. The Magpie Trial: a randomised trial comparing magnesium sulphate with placebo for pre-eclampsia. Outcome for women at 2 years. *BJOG*. 114 (3), 300–309. https://doi.org/10.1111/j.1471-0528.2006.01166.x.

National Institute for Health and Care Excellence (NICE), 2010. NICE guidelines – Hypertension in Pregnancy. NICE, London, UK.

Nelson-Piercy, C., 2015. Handbook of obstetric medicine, 5th ed. Informa Healthcare, New York, NY.

Royal College of Obstetricians and Gynaecologists (RCOG). The investigation and management of the small-for-gestational-age fetus: RCOG green-top guideline no. 31 (2nd ed.). London, UK: RCOG. February 2013 (minor revisions – January 2014).

Medical disorders in pregnancy

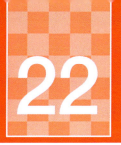

22

INTRODUCTION

Medical disorders in pregnancy can have a significant effect upon the outcome for both the mother and the fetus. Early optimization of certain conditions (ideally pre-pregnancy) can help to minimize the adverse effects and ensure a good outcome for both. The aim of this chapter is to highlight common medical problems that complicate pregnancy and discuss their management. Hypertension in pregnancy is covered in Chapter 21.

HAEMATOLOGY

Anaemia

The term anaemia comes from the Greek word *anaimia*, meaning lack of blood. Anaemia is a very common problem to encounter in pregnancy. The normal physiological changes in pregnancy result in an increased plasma expansion and because haemoglobin (Hb) levels are expressed as a concentration, it therefore follows that an increase in circulating volume results in a decrease in the concentration of Hb. Despite an increase in gastrointestinal absorption during pregnancy, iron requirements increase almost threefold.

As part of booking investigations all patients should have a full blood count (FBC) performed and repeated at 28 weeks. Treatment should be advised with Hb levels:

- <11 g/dL at booking
- <10.5 g/dL at 28 weeks

Some individuals may have preexisting anaemia, which is most commonly due to iron deficiency. Iron deficiency can be caused by lack of dietary iron, heavy periods, gastrointestinal bleeding or, indeed, as a result of a recent pregnancy and it is these individuals that need thorough treatment. It is also important to note whether or not the patient has a haemoglobinopathy (e.g., sickle cell anaemia, beta-thalassaemia), which can be responsible for their anaemia. In these patients, measurement of serum ferritin levels is vital to prevent iron overload. Partner testing needs to be considered in cases of haemoglobinopathy to assess the risk of the fetus being affected.

Folate and B12 deficiency can also be responsible for anaemia, and therefore estimation of serum haematinics may need to be performed to allow correction of the depleted factor.

Iron supplements are known to cause constipation that often leads to patients discontinuing therapy. Vitamin C has been shown to increase its absorption from the gut and patients should be advised to take orange juice or a similar vitamin C-containing juice. Tannins found in tea and coffee reduce absorption so should be avoided.

During pregnancy patients who complain about fatigue, dizziness or collapsing should be investigated for anaemia in addition to the routine screening that occurs at booking and 28 weeks.

> **RED FLAG**
>
>
> Correction of anaemia is essential as it has been linked with low birth weight and preterm delivery. In addition, patients with adequate haemoglobin levels are less likely to need a blood transfusion following delivery.

Thromboembolism

Venous thromboembolism (VTE) is one of the leading direct causes of maternal death and so all clinicians must be alert to the signs, symptoms, investigations and treatment.

The normal physiological adaptations to pregnancy mean that it is a prothrombotic state, increasing the risks of VTE. These include:

- increase in certain clotting factors
- increase in fibrinogen levels
- decrease in fibrinolytic activity
- decrease in protein S and antithrombin (endogenous anticoagulants)
- increased venous stasis in lower limbs (left > right)

Risk factors

Risk factors for VTE are given in Box 22.1. Risk assessments for VTE should be performed at the booking appointment and again at 28 weeks. Consideration should be given to prophylactic anticoagulation if there are multiple risk factors present.

Thromboprophylaxis

Given the increased risk of VTE in pregnancy, the Royal College of Obstetricians and Gynaecologists (RCOG) recommend that all patients undergo a risk assessment in early pregnancy to identify those at high risk who might benefit from prophylactic anticoagulation.

Obstetric patients admitted to hospital should undergo a risk assessment and be offered prophylactic low-molecular-weight heparin (LMWH), especially if they are going to be immobile for a period of time. Most patients should be offered graduated compression stockings.

A key point to remember is that the risk of VTE is not abolished once the fetus is delivered, but remains high until 6 weeks post delivery. Therefore, any prophylactic measures should continue up until this point. In fact, the puerperium is regarded as a particularly high-risk period. Delivery by caesarean section poses a significant risk of VTE and all patients (except those who have an uncomplicated elective operation with no risk factors) are offered 10 days of LMWH. If further risk factors are present, then the duration of thromboprophylaxis is increased to 6 weeks.

Symptoms and signs

Deep vein thrombosis (DVT) may present with pain, swelling and redness of the calf. Pulmonary embolism (PE) can present with shortness of breath, chest pain (pleuritic), collapse, cough or haemoptysis.

Patients found to be tachypnoeic, tachycardic, dyspnoeic or hypoxic [reduced saturations on pulse oximetry or low partial pressure of oxygen (PO_2) on arterial blood gas (ABG)] need to have a PE ruled out.

RED FLAG

In all cases of suspected deep vein thrombosis or pulmonary embolism, a high index of suspicion is advised and treatment must be initiated until the diagnosis is ruled out.

Investigations

Investigation of a DVT usually starts with a clinical examination followed by venous Dopplers. It is important to bear in mind that the thrombosis may be located higher than the calf (propensity for ileofemoral DVT in pregnancy compared with popliteo-femoral DVT), and therefore imaging should include this area. This kind of DVT can present with abdominal pain.

PE investigations usually begin again with a thorough examination followed by an electrocardiogram (ECG), ABG, FBC and chest X-ray (CXR). On the ABG the patient may be hypoxic and hypercapnic, the ECG may reveal a sinus tachycardia and the CXR is important to rule out other potential causes of the symptoms, such as infection or pneumothorax.

If the CXR is normal, the patient may proceed to a ventilation/perfusion scan. This may identify an area of underperfusion indicating a PE. If the CXR is abnormal, a computed tomographic pulmonary angiogram (CTPA) may be indicated. This is very sensitive at diagnosing a PE but involves high doses of radiation.

COMMON PITFALLS

A D-dimer test is not performed as part of the investigations as it is usually positive in pregnancy. However, a negative D-dimer would be very reassuring in ruling out a deep vein thrombosis or pulmonary embolism.

Treatment

With a confirmed DVT or PE, patients require anticoagulation with therapeutic doses of LMWH. Warfarin is generally avoided as it crosses the placenta and is known to be teratogenic, as well as carrying the risk of fetal intracranial bleeding. In the puerperium patients can be converted to warfarin even if they are breastfeeding as it is regarded as safe. Treatment should continue until the end of the pregnancy and for at least 6 weeks postnatally and until at least 3 months of treatment has been given in total.

Cerebral vein thrombosis

A cerebral vein thrombosis is an uncommon yet fatal problem encountered by obstetricians. It is more common in the puerperium and presents with headaches, seizures, vomiting, photophobia, reduced consciousness or even focal neurology. It is usually diagnosed with a magnetic resonance imaging (MRI) venous angiogram and treatment is usually with hydration and anticoagulation.

RESPIRATORY

Asthma

Asthma is frequently encountered in antenatal clinics and affects up to 7% of females of a childbearing age. The course of asthma in pregnancy varies and symptoms can improve, worsen or remain the same throughout the pregnancy. Those with the most severe asthma should be closely monitored.

New diagnoses of asthma in pregnancy, although not common, should be considered in patients complaining of cough, shortness of breath, wheezing or chest tightness. Classically these symptoms will be worse at night or associated with certain triggers like dust, exercise or pollen.

For known asthma sufferers, a detailed enquiry should include:

- current treatments
- peak flow record
- previous hospital admissions (especially those requiring admission to intensive care)

The peak expiratory flow rate trend will form an important part of monitoring in pregnancy, and therefore its importance should not be underestimated.

Some patients may discontinue their therapy due to fears over the effect they may have on the fetus. They can be reassured and encouraged to continue, to prevent any deterioration in their condition. The cessation of smoking and avoidance of trigger factors should also be emphasized.

ENDOCRINE

Diabetes

Management of diabetes in pregnancy forms a major part of antenatal care, so much so that most units have specialist joint multidisciplinary diabetic antenatal clinic, including obstetricians, endocrinologist, diabetic specialist nurses/midwives and dieticians, to optimize care. Patients can either have preexisting diabetes or develop gestational diabetes which, left untreated, can have severe ramifications for both mother and fetus.

Glucose metabolism is altered during pregnancy such that pregnancy itself is a state of impaired glucose tolerance, especially as it advances towards term. A major contribution to this is made by hormones secreted by the placenta:

- glucagon
- cortisol
- human placental lactogen

These effects are to some extent offset by increased insulin secretion. However, those who have an insufficient response will develop gestational diabetes. For the same reason, patients with pre-existing type 1 diabetes will require an increase in the amount of insulin they administer. Those with type 2 diabetes may need conversion to insulin from oral hypoglycaemics as pregnancy progresses.

Pre-existing diabetes

Pre-conception

Care of patients with pre-existing diabetes, either type 1 or type 2, should ideally start pre-conception, including:

- optimizing glycaemic control by monitoring glucose pre-meals and post-meals
- educating the patient about diabetes in pregnancy and the risks (Box 22.2)
- educating the patient about the risks of hypoglycaemia
- prescribing folic acid at the higher dose of 5 mg daily (pre-conception until 12 weeks)
- screening for nephropathy and retinopathy

Patients suffering with nephropathy and/or retinopathy may warrant specialist review prior to pregnancy to identify their risks, including review of hypertension and any medication.

Dietary advice regarding a low sugar, low fat and high fibre intake as well as the benefits of exercise and weight loss if their body mass index is $>27 \, kg/m^2$ should be discussed.

Ultrasound scans

Patients with pre-existing diabetes have a higher rate of miscarriage, and therefore may request an early ultrasound scan. In addition, there is an increased risk of congenital anomalies, so nuchal translucency and a detailed anomaly scan including detailed assessment of the fetal heart should be arranged. Poor glycaemic control can lead to fetal macrosomia and increased liquor volume (see Chapter 23), therefore diabetic patients are advised to have serial growth scans in the third trimester.

Antenatal care

Patients should be seen more frequently than the suggested antenatal care pathway with reviews occurring every

---

BOX 22.2   RISKS OF DIABETES IN PREGNANCY

- Miscarriage.
- Congenital anomalies, in particular, cardiac.
- Fetal macrosomia and/or polyhydramnios.
- Induction of labour.
- Caesarean section.
- Birth trauma.
- Shoulder dystocia.
- Stillbirth.
- Neonatal hypoglycaemia.
- Obesity/diabetes in the baby (later in life).

2–3 weeks in a multidisciplinary diabetic antenatal clinic. Patients should be encouraged to self-monitor their capillary blood glucose levels regularly to allow good glycaemic control. Target blood glucose levels are ≤5.3 mmol/L when fasting and ≤7.8 mmol/L 1-hour postmeals.

Both diabetic retinopathy and diabetic nephropathy can worsen during pregnancy. Patients should have their eyes checked at booking and at 28 weeks, as well as undergo regular blood pressure checks and assessment of proteinuria. Aspirin 75 mg daily is advised because of the increased risk of development of pre-eclampsia.

In the event of complications such as pre-eclampsia or growth restriction, the patient may require early delivery and may be offered steroids for fetal lung maturation. This commonly requires admission and an insulin sliding scale because administration of steroids will worsen glycaemic control.

Delivery and postnatal care

In the absence of complications, the timing of delivery needs to be carefully planned with the risks of prematurity and induction of labour against the risk of stillbirth (the rate of which is increased in diabetic mothers, as is the rate of caesarean section). Glucose control with a sliding scale is usually needed in labour. In addition, macrosomic babies have an increased risk of shoulder dystocia, so senior assistance must be available at delivery.

Immediately following delivery the fetus will be at risk of hypoglycaemia as it is no longer in a hyperglycaemic environment, although fetal insulin levels will still be high. Close monitoring and early feeds are important. Furthermore, once the placenta has been delivered, maternal requirements of insulin will fall and the doses of insulin should return to pre-pregnancy levels or slightly less than pre-pregnancy levels if breastfeeding.

Gestational diabetes

Gestational diabetes is described as a condition leading to impaired glucose metabolism first recognized in pregnancy. This will, therefore, include those patients who had unknown pre-existing diabetes, who will be found to have a high blood sugar level at booking.

Diagnosis

In the UK, the gold standard for diagnosis is widely accepted as the 75-g oral glucose tolerance test (OGTT). The World Health Organization (WHO) defines frank diabetes as a fasting glucose level of >7 mmol/L or a 2-hour level of >11.1 mmol/L. Gestational diabetes is defined as a fasting glucose level of >7 mmol/L or a 2-hour level > 7.8 mmol/L.

Screening for gestational diabetes is offered to 'at-risk' groups. Risk factors for gestational diabetes are shown in Box 22.3 and patients with one or more risk factors should be offered an OGTT at around 26–28 weeks. Patients who have had gestational diabetes in a previous pregnancy will be offered an earlier OGTT (usually 16–18 weeks), and if this is negative, it will be repeated at 28 weeks.

BOX 22.3   RISK FACTORS FOR GESTATIONAL DIABETES

- Body mass index >30 kg/m^2.
- Previous macrosomic baby weighing >4.5 kg.
- Previous gestational diabetes.
- First-degree relative with diabetes.
- Country of family origin:
  - South Asian
  - Black Caribbean
  - Middle Eastern

HINTS AND TIPS

When undergoing an oral glucose tolerance test the patient is asked to starve the night before the test and will then have a venous blood glucose level measured. Following this they will be asked to drink a glucose load (75 g) and have a second glucose level taken 2 hours later.

Antenatal care

Risks of gestational diabetes to both the mother and fetus are similar to pregnancies in patients with pre-existing diabetes (Box 22.2) with the exception of miscarriage and congenital anomalies, as this period has passed. Patients should be seen in a multidisciplinary diabetic antenatal clinic and advised to self-monitor with regular pre-meal and post-meal capillary blood glucose levels. They may respond to changes in diet (consider referral to a dietician) and exercise alone. If these measures are insufficient, oral hypoglycaemic agents with or without insulin may be required. They should have serial growth scans to look for macrosomia with or without polyhydramnios.

Delivery and postnatal care

The planning of delivery is not always as rigid as in those with pre-existing diabetes as the risk to the fetus may be less. Each case should be assessed individually taking into account any complications that may have developed.

Postnatally patients can discontinue their hypoglycaemic agents and should have a fasting plasma glucose test between 6 and 13 weeks after delivery. If the postnatal fasting glucose is normal, then they should be offered an annual HbA1c due to their increased risk of developing type 2 diabetes. The fetus will still be at risk of hypoglycaemia in the immediate period postdelivery, and therefore early feeds and close monitoring are advised. Patients with gestational diabetes mellitus should also be advised regarding weight loss and maintenance of a healthy diet with exercise and told of the high possibility of recurrence in future pregnancies.

Thyroid disease

Thyroid disorders again are commonly encountered in antenatal clinics. Pre-conception counselling and close monitoring reduce the impact on both mother and fetus.

Hypothyroidism

Hypothyroidism affects around 1% of pregnancies and is more common in those patients with a family history. Symptoms in pregnancy are similar to the nonpregnant patients:

- lethargy
- tiredness
- weight gain
- dry skin
- hair loss

These may be confused with normal pregnancy symptoms (cold intolerance, slow pulse rate and slow relaxing tendon reflexes are said to be discriminatory features in pregnancy). A goitre may also be present and should be carefully assessed when examining the patient.

In cases of known hypothyroidism pre-conceptual optimization of thyroid hormone levels with replacement therapy is very important as hypothyroidism itself can lead to subfertility. Up until 12 weeks the fetus is entirely dependent upon maternal thyroid hormones, and therefore if left untreated, there is an association with miscarriage, reduced intelligence, neurodevelopmental delay and brain damage.

Most cases of hypothyroidism encountered in pregnancy are due to either autoimmune (Hashimoto/atrophic) thyroiditis or treated Graves disease, but it can also be due to drugs or following treatment for hyperthyroidism.

In patients who are adequately treated, it is usual to continue the current dose of thyroxine and check levels in each trimester. Those who require modifications of their dosing will need more frequent thyroid function tests (TFTs). When interpreting TFTs, it is important to use pregnancy-adjusted values (Table 22.1). The importance of compliance with medication to minimize the impact on the fetus should be emphasized to all patients.

Hyperthyroidism

Hyperthyroidism, although less common than hypothyroidism, still affects around 1 in 800 pregnancies. Approximately 50% of those suffering with the disease will have a family history of thyroid disease.

Symptoms of hyperthyroidism are the same as in the nonpregnant population and again can mimic normal pregnancy symptoms. These include sweating, palpitations, heat intolerance and vomiting. When examining the patient, look for the following signs:

- tachycardia
- tremor
- eye signs (exophthalmos)
- goitre
- palmar erythema

The presence of the first three signs are said to help distinguish hyperthyroidism from normal pregnancy symptoms.

About 95% of hyperthyroidism encountered in pregnancy is due to Graves disease, a condition where thyroid receptor antibodies stimulate thyroid hormone production. It can also be due to:

- drugs
- multinodular goitre
- thyroiditis

Again, if untreated patients may have difficulty conceiving, pre-conceptual counselling and optimization are vital, as untreated hyperthyroidism is associated with miscarriage, pre-term labour and growth restriction.

Patients with hyperthyroidism should have their TFTs measured in each trimester and assessed using pregnancy-specific values (Table 22.1). Antithyroid drugs such as propylthiouracil should be continued and carbimazole can be used from the second trimester onwards. β-Blockers may be required to improve symptoms of sweating, tachycardia and palpitations, and rarely surgery may be required, especially if obstructive symptoms from the goitre are present.

About 1% of fetuses or neonates can suffer from neonatal thyrotoxicosis due to transplacental passage of thyroid antibodies. The condition should also be considered in fetuses or neonates of patients who are now hypothyroid as a result of thyroid treatment for Graves disease. Fetuses will exhibit signs of tachycardia, growth restriction and possibly a goitre, whilst neonates may present with jaundice, failure to gain weight, irritability or in severe cases heart failure.

Table 22.1 Pregnancy-specific thyroid hormone values

Hormone	Nonpregnant	First trimester	Second trimester	Third trimester
Thyroid-stimulating hormone	0–4	0–1.6	0.1–1.8	0.7–7.3
Free T$_4$	11–23	11–22	11–19	7–15
Free T$_3$	4–9	4–8	4–7	3–5

CARDIOLOGY

Cardiac disease is the leading indirect cause of maternal deaths (see Chapter 32) and so the management of cardiac disease in pregnancy is of upmost importance.

Congenital heart disease

Congenital heart disease includes patent ductus arteriosus, atrial septal defects and ventricular septal defects. The incidence of these in pregnancy is increasing as these women have undergone corrective surgery, and therefore can go on to have children themselves.

Following corrective surgery these heart defects cause little problem in pregnancy. These women should have consultant-led care and have an examination of the cardiovascular system at their first antenatal visit. If new symptoms arise during the pregnancy, such as tachycardia, chest pain or palpitations, they should be investigated with an echocardiogram and/or 24-hour ECG monitoring. Referral to a cardiologist may be necessary.

Acquired heart disease

The most common acquired heart disease in pregnancy is rheumatic fever, which is contracted in childhood and causes damage to one or more of the heart valves. It is more common in the migrant population and very rare in British-born women. All women from a migrant population should have an examination of their cardiovascular system during their early antenatal care.

Mitral stenosis

Mitral stenosis is the most common presentation of rheumatic heart disease seen in pregnancy. These women require an echocardiogram in pregnancy to assess severity of their disease. They may require treatment with β-blockers in pregnancy. The physiological changes in pregnancy can cause a deterioration in their condition. If there are any new signs or symptoms in pregnancy such as tachycardia, they will require reassessment.

Acute coronary syndrome

As women delay having children until their late 30s and early 40s, it is becoming increasingly more common to see myocardial infarctions and coronary artery disease in pregnancy. Coronary artery dissection and embolus are the more common causes in pregnancy than atherosclerosis. Box 22.4 presents the risk factors for ischaemic heart disease.

Acute coronary syndrome (ACS) is more common in the third trimester, intrapartum or postpartum and may not present with the usual symptoms of chest pain, but more atypical symptoms such as epigastric pain and nausea.

BOX 22.4   RISK FACTORS FOR ISCHAEMIC HEART DISEASE

- Obesity.
- Diabetes.
- Hypertension.
- Smoking.
- Hypercholesterolaemia.
- Multiparous.
- Age >35 years.
- Family history of ischaemic heart disease.

The management of ACS is the same in pregnancy as it is out of pregnancy. β-Blockers, aspirin, nitrates and heparin should be commenced. Thrombolysis and coronary angiography with stenting if required can be performed in pregnancy.

Aortic dissection

The risk of aortic dissection is increased in pregnancy and it is associated with a high mortality rate. It commonly presents with chest pain radiating between the scapulae and jaw pain. There may be a difference in the blood pressure readings from the left and right arm.

Diagnosis involves various imaging modalities including a CXR looking for mediastinal widening or confirmation of dissection on echocardiography.

Once the diagnosis of aortic dissection has been made the blood pressure needs to be controlled; plans to deliver the baby by caesarean section need to be made before cardiac surgery to replace the aortic root can take place.

NEUROLOGY

Epilepsy

Epilepsy affects around 1 in 200 women of childbearing age and is one of the most common neurological conditions in pregnancy. Similar to diabetes, the management of epilepsy should, ideally, begin pre-conceptually with the counselling of patients about the risks to the mother and fetus. It is very important that epileptic women who are of a childbearing age and who do not want to conceive be offered effective contraception.

Pre-conception and antenatal care

Preconception counselling should include review of antiepileptic drugs (AEDs) to reduce the exposure to teratogenic agents, such as sodium valproate, and minimize polytherapy after evaluating the risks and benefits to mother and baby. It is recommended that all epileptic women take folic acid 5 mg daily. As AEDs are known to be teratogenic, many patients are often concerned about the fetus, opting to discontinue therapy. The patient should be carefully counselled against doing so and warned about the risk of status epilepticus and sudden unexpected death in epilepsy.

The aim of treatment of epilepsy in pregnancy is to maintain a seizure-free status with monotherapy at the lowest possible AED dose. The approximate risk of congenital malformation for one AED appears to be around 6%, which is double the background rate. In addition, data on sodium valproate appear to show a significant increased risk of congenital malformations, whereas lamotrigine and carbamazepine monotherapy have the least risk. Box 22.5 lists the known complications of AED use in pregnancy.

BOX 22.5   FETAL AND NEONATAL COMPLICATIONS OF ANTIEPILEPTIC DRUG USE IN PREGNANCY

- Orofacial clefts.
- Neural tube defects.
- Congenital heart disease.
- Haemorrhagic disease of the newborn.

Therefore, patients should undergo a detailed ultrasound scan with particular attention to:

- cardiac function
- neural tube status
- skeletal condition
- orofacial structures

The course of epilepsy is variable; as seizure frequency can improve or worsen, approximately two-thirds of woman will not have any seizure deterioration. Levels of antiepileptic drugs can decrease during pregnancy due to increased hepatic metabolism and renal clearance. Seizures may therefore be difficult to control and dose increases may be required.

RED FLAG

If a pregnant woman presents with a seizure in the second half of pregnancy with no clear history of epilepsy, then she should be treated for eclampsia until a diagnosis can be made (see Chapter 21).

Delivery and postnatal care

There is an increase in the risk of seizures around the time of delivery and the following 24 hours and women should be advised to continue their AED medication. This risk is sufficient enough to recommend that patients deliver in hospital. Women with well-controlled epilepsy and no other risk factors can go on to have an uncomplicated labour and vaginal delivery. However, triggers for seizures, that is, insomnia, stress, pain, should be minimized in labour.

The neonates of women taking enzyme-inducing AEDs should receive 1 mg of vitamin K intramuscularly to prevent haemorrhagic disease of the newborn.

Breastfeeding is generally regarded as safe and should be encouraged. Postnatal education about safety measures should be given to all epileptic mothers such as the avoidance of excessive tiredness, changing the baby on the floor to prevent falls if a seizure occurs and also bathing the baby with another adult present, again in case of seizures.

ETHICS

The general driving restrictions that apply to epileptics also apply to pregnant women with epilepsy. Therefore they should be informed that if they were to stop or reduce their antiepileptic drugs, they may experience a deterioration in their seizure control and this can affect their driving privileges.

GASTROINTESTINAL DISORDERS

Obstetric cholestasis

Obstetric cholestasis (OC) is a condition in pregnancy that presents with itching especially of the palms and soles; it is associated with deranged liver function tests (LFTs) and occurs in the second half of pregnancy.

OC affects around 0.5% of pregnancies in the UK and is more common in certain ethnic groups (1.2%–1.5% Indian or Pakistani origin and up to 5% in the Araucanian, South American Indians). The cause is not clearly understood, but a susceptibility to the cholestatic effects of oestrogen and progesterone is thought to be key. Given that a family history of the condition is often found (35%) genetic factors are thought to play a role.

Diagnosis

OC is a diagnosis of exclusion, made in patients complaining of the characteristic symptoms of itching especially over the palms and soles; classically there is no rash, but excoriations from excessive scratching may be present. LFTs are abnormal with raised alanine transaminase (ALT) levels and bile acids. In some cases there may be dark stools, pale urine, anorexia and steatorrhoea. All other causes of deranged LFTs should be excluded including hepatitis, gallstones and autoimmune conditions by performing various blood tests and an abdominal ultrasound to assess the liver and biliary tract. Occasionally patients may present with characteristic symptoms, but have normal LFTs. These patients should have LFTs repeated every 1–2 weeks.

Treatment

Treatment of the condition is usually with chlorphenamine (Piriton), aqueous creams and ursodeoxycholic acid (UCDA) for symptom control. UCDA is unlicensed in pregnancy but no adverse effects have been reported. It works by altering the bile acid pool balance by reducing the number of hydrophobic bile acids, which are thought to be hepatotoxic. Symptoms of itching and abnormal LFTs results resolve after birth.

Antenatal care

Once diagnosed, patients need to be monitored with weekly LFTs until delivery. Bile acid levels of >40 mmol/L are associated with pregnancy and labour complications:

- stillbirth
- preterm delivery
- passage of meconium
- fetal anoxia
- postpartum haemorrhage

Fetal surveillance with cardiotocograph monitoring (although lacking evidence) is often offered to ease anxiety. Vitamin K supplementation should be provided for those with abnormal clotting.

Delivery and postnatal care

Discussion about induction of labour after 37 + 0 weeks should take place, although this is associated with an increased rate of caesarean section. Those patients with severe derangements of their bile acids and LFTs have a greater indication for intervention.

Once delivered it is important to ensure LFTs have normalized (after at least 10 days). Patients should be warned of the likelihood of recurrence in a future pregnancy and advised to avoid oestrogen-containing contraceptive pills as these may trigger cholestasis.

Acute fatty liver of pregnancy

Acute fatty liver of pregnancy (AFLP) is a rare (1 in 20,000), potentially fatal condition, which needs prompt recognition and management. Although the aetiology is poorly understood, a disorder of mitochondrial fatty acid oxidation may play a role. Risk factors include:

- primips
- those carrying male fetuses
- multiple pregnancy

BOX 22.6   ACUTE FATTY LIVER OF PREGNANCY BLOOD RESULTS

- ↑ Alanine transaminase.
- ↑ Alkaline phosphatase.
- ↑ Bilirubin.
- ↑ White cell count.
- Hypoglycaemia (severe).
- ↑ Uric acid.
- Coagulopathy.

The condition may be the same spectrum as pre-eclampsia and it may be difficult to distinguish from HELLP [*hae*molysis, *el*evated liver enzymes (raised ALT), *l*ow *p*latelet count] syndrome. It is a reversible condition, which affects both the liver and the kidneys.

Patients may present with nausea, vomiting, anorexia, malaise, abdominal pain or polyuria. Jaundice, ascites, encephalopathy and mild proteinuric hypertension may also be present. The haematological and biochemical derangements are shown in Box 22.6.

Confirmation of the diagnosis with imaging is not always possible as changes may not be seen on ultrasound, computed tomography or MRI. Liver biopsy may be considered, but in practice is not usually done due to the coagulopathy.

Patients diagnosed with AFLP need multidisciplinary input and urgent delivery. Supportive measures with fluids, correction of hypoglycaemia and correction of coagulopathy are important and patients may need intensive care and dialysis. In severe cases, liver transplant may be necessary.

INFECTIOUS DISEASES

Human immunodeficiency virus

Human immunodeficiency virus (HIV) is a chronic condition caused by infection with the virus via:

- sexual intercourse
- injecting drug use
- blood transfusion
- mother to fetus or neonate vertically during pregnancy or breastfeeding

Infection with the virus leads to immunosuppression and individuals become susceptible to infections and certain malignancies. However, advances in modern medicine and the production of antiretroviral drugs [antiretroviral treatment (ART)] have led to a significant decline in the morbidity and mortality from the illness.

Screening

In the UK all women are advised to have screening for HIV infection as part of their booking investigations.

Identification of HIV-infected individuals then allows appropriate care to improve maternal health and reduce the risk of transmission to the fetus from approximately 25% to less than 1%. The implementation of routine antenatal HIV screening has made mother to child transmission a rare occurrence in the UK.

Additional interventions for HIV-positive women include screening for hepatitis C, offering vaccinations against hepatitis B and screening for genital infection in the first trimester and at 28 weeks.

Testing for the patient's partner and any other children should be offered.

ETHICS

A major barrier to compliance with testing and treatment is the fear of stigmatization and patients should be reassured regarding confidentiality. It is good practice to ensure the patient's partner is aware of the diagnosis, as there may be health implications to them that need to be addressed. Patients with a new diagnosis should be encouraged to inform their partner.

Antenatal care

Care for patients with HIV should be given by a multidisciplinary team composed of HIV specialists, obstetricians, specialist midwives and paediatricians. The use of ART has been shown to dramatically reduce the risk of vertical transmission; therefore if a patient falls pregnant whilst taking ART, she should continue to do so. Patients who are not on ART but require it (following assessment) should commence treatment as soon as possible. Patients who are not on ART (i.e., that do not require treatment after assessment) should commence ART regardless from 20 weeks onwards until delivery.

HINTS AND TIPS

Patients on certain antiretroviral treatment should be screened for gestational diabetes due to their association with impaired glucose tolerance.

Delivery and postnatal care

A plan for mode of delivery is usually confirmed at 36 weeks of gestation. Patients will have their viral load measured and if <50 copies/mL, a vaginal delivery will be offered.

RED FLAG

When the patient is in labour, to reduce the risk of transmission, invasive procedures such as fetal blood sampling or attaching a fetal scalp electrode should be avoided.

Patients who have a high viral load will be offered a planned caesarean section with zidovudine cover (an antiretroviral) commenced 4 hours prior to delivery and continued until cord clamping).

In resource-rich countries the avoidance of breastfeeding is recommended (to prevent transmission) and formula milk is used as an alternative. It is, however, not always possible in developing countries.

Once delivered all neonates are treated with antiretrovirals as soon as possible (ideally within 4 hours). The neonate will be tested at regular intervals and, if not breastfed, a negative test at 18 months ensures the child is not affected.

HINTS AND TIPS

Three steps known to reduce rates of vertical transmission of human immunodeficiency virus:
- antiretroviral medication
- elective caesarean section
- avoidance of breastfeeding

PSYCHIATRIC ILLNESS

Identifying psychiatric illnesses in pregnancy is a vital part of assessing risk. Early specialist referral and multidisciplinary management are very important as psychiatric causes are a major contributor to maternal deaths, which can have a huge impact on a family.

Depression

Depression is one of the most common mental health problems that occur during pregnancy and in the postnatal period. Up to 25% of women will experience depression. It is important to identify risk factors and provide support for these women as depression can be associated with suicide. Symptoms of low mood, anxiety, loss of appetite, insomnia, low self-esteem, lack of energy, failure to find enjoyment and suicidal ideation should be actively enquired about.

Risk factors for depression are shown in Box 22.7.

Any patient with a history of depression or who is currently suffering with depression should be referred for specialist counselling, usually in the form of a perinatal mental health team. Both pharmacological and non-pharmacological (cognitive behavioural therapy) treatments may be required.

Patients with a history of depression outside or during pregnancy are at risk of postnatal depression (PND). PND can present as 'baby blues', which are usually short lasting (24–72 hours) and begin around the fifth day after delivery. Tearfulness, labile mood and irritability are possible symptoms. In more severe cases, especially with signs of neglect and suicidal ideation, prompt specialist intervention is important.

Puerperal psychosis

Puerperal psychosis is a serious disorder that affects around 1–2 in 1000 births. It usually starts abruptly around 2 weeks postnatally and presents with mania, delusions and hallucinations (both auditory and visual). Patients appear agitated and may exhibit disinhibited behaviour.

Puerperal psychosis is more common in patients with bipolar disorder (BD) or if they have had previous puerperal psychosis. Treatment invariably involves admission to hospital for both the safety of the mother and baby, ideally to a specialist mother and baby unit to prevent separation. Antipsychotic medications such as haloperidol may be required. Organic causes of psychosis (infection, drug withdrawals, etc.) must be excluded.

Schizophrenia

Schizophrenia affects around 1 in 100 women of childbearing age and again needs specialist management in pregnancy. As well as caring for the mother's health, an assessment must be conducted to identify any potential difficulties the patient may have in caring for the child and what risks an acute episode may pose.

Hallucinations, delusions or an abnormal affect may be encountered and should prompt specialist help. Antipsychotic medications may be indicated during the pregnancy, although the evidence regarding their safety is not clear. In practice, the lowest dose is used with a reduction in the dose towards term to prevent toxicity in the neonate. Breastfeeding on antipsychotics is not advised.

Bipolar disorder

BD is a condition characterized by episodes of acute illness mixed with periods of relative normality. Many of the drugs used to treat BD are teratogenic, and therefore careful assessment must be made to balance the risk of harm from a relapse in pregnancy against the risk of damage to the fetus. Lithium use is associated with cardiac defects. Again, management by specialist perinatal mental health teams is advised and particular attention needs to be paid to the puerperium when acute episodes are common.

Substance abuse

Substance abuse in pregnancy poses a risk to the health of the mother and the fetus. This risk is both direct (i.e., from the abused substance itself) and indirect (i.e., from risk allied to drug use like the transmission of infection from injecting drug use).

Booking assessments should be used as an opportunity to screen for substance abuse. Early cessation will help to minimize risk and enable implementation of other care such as screening for infection. This particular group may represent a challenge as their attendance for antenatal care may be poor, therefore care from specialist midwives may improve engagement as continuity of care is provided.

Cocaine abuse is associated with growth restriction, placental abruption, stillbirth and neonatal death. Opiates are associated with growth restriction, preterm labour and neonate dependence.

Alcohol abuse is known to cause fetal anomalies and fetal alcohol syndrome. Safe amounts of alcohol intake are the subject of much continuing debate and most people would recommend no alcohol at all, especially in the first trimester. Patients who wish to continue drinking alcohol should not exceed 1-2 units once or twice a week and binge drinking should be strongly discouraged.

Referral to drug and alcohol treatment services is important and patients should be offered a detoxification program where appropriate.

Smoking cessation advice should be offered at every visit and when accepted, appropriate referral made. Smoking is associated with growth restriction, placental abruption, cot death and childhood asthma, and therefore educating patients about the risks posed by both active and passive smoking is very important.

It is important to arrange serial growth scans for these women as the risk of intrauterine growth restriction is high.

Chapter Summary

- As woman are delaying their pregnancies until a later age, we are encountering more pregnancies complicated by medical disorders.
- In ideal circumstances the medical disorder should be managed prior to conception so that treatment can be optimized in terms of using nonteratogenic agents as well as maintaining good maternal health.
- A multidisciplinary approach should be used when managing woman with complex medical disorders.
- Pregnancies complicated by medical disorders require more frequent consultant-led antenatal visits and monitoring with additional scans.

FURTHER READING

'Anaemia', 2016. Collins English Dictionary – Complete & Unabridged (10th ed). HarperCollins, New York, NY.

De Swiet, M., 2002. Medical disorders in obstetric practice, 4th ed. Blackwell Publishing, London, UK.

Dhanjal, M., 2011. Thyroid and parathyroid disease. In Oxford desk reference obstetrics & gynaecology. Oxford University Press, Oxford, UK.

Murphy, V., Namazy, J., Powell, H., et al., 2011. A meta-analysis of adverse perinatal outcomes in women with asthma. *BJOG*. 118 (11), 1314–1323. https://doi.org/10.1111/j.1471-0528.2011.03055.x.

National Institute for Health and Care Excellence (NICE), 2008. Guidelines – Antenatal care. NICE, London, UK.

National Institute for Health and Care Excellence (NICE), 2008. Guidelines – CG63 diabetes in pregnancy: full guideline. NICE, London, UK.

Nelson-Piercy, C., 2015. Handbook of obstetric medicine, fifth ed. Informa Healthcare, New York, NY.

Royal College of Obstetricians and Gynaecologists (RCOG), 2007. The acute management of thrombosis and embolism during pregnancy and the puerperium. RCOG green-top guideline no. 37b. RCOG, London, UK.

Royal College of Obstetricians and Gynaecologists (RCOG), 2011. Obstetric cholestasis. RCOG green-top guideline no. 43. RCOG, London, UK.

Royal College of Obstetricians and Gynaecologists (RCOG), 2009. Reducing the risk of thrombosis and embolism during pregnancy and the puerperium. RCOG green-top guideline no. 37a. RCOG, London, UK.

Williamson, C., 2011. Obstetric cholestasis. In Oxford desk reference obstetrics & gynaecology. Oxford University Press, Oxford, UK.

ABDOMINAL PAIN IN PREGNANCY

The important differential diagnosis when assessing abdominal pain in pregnancy is whether the cause is obstetric or non-obstetric. Table 23.1 shows the systems that might be involved.

Do not forget to take a history, which includes the non-obstetric causes of abdominal pain. Some of them are more common than the obstetric causes, such as a urinary tract infection.

History

With diverse differential diagnoses, the history is very important to identify the cause of the pain. Table 23.2 gives a summary of the points elicited from the history and examination that help to make the diagnosis.

Current obstetric history

This should include the current gestation and the parity. The antenatal history may be relevant. For example, if the patient has a history of pregnancy-induced hypertension (see Chapter 21), then she is at risk of preeclampsia and placental abruption (see Chapter 20). She may already have been admitted earlier in the pregnancy with suspected preterm labour (see Chapter 25) or with a urinary tract infection. Check that these two conditions were treated adequately.

Presenting symptoms

As with any history of pain, its characteristics are important. The acronym SOCRATES can be used for assessing pain:

Site – generalized or specific
Onset – sudden or gradual
Character – continuous or intermittent, stabbing or burning
Radiation – to the pelvis, back or thighs
Associations – gastrointestinal or genitourinary
Time course – duration
Exacerbating/relieving factors
Severity

Obstetric history

A history of pre-eclampsia or preterm labour in a previous pregnancy puts the patient at increased risk of these conditions in her current pregnancy.

Gynaecological/medical/surgical history

Ultrasound scans earlier in the current pregnancy may have diagnosed an ovarian cyst or uterine fibroids. There may be a history of peptic ulcer disease or gallstones. If the patient has previously had an appendicectomy or a cholecystectomy, these differential diagnoses can be excluded.

Examination

General examination

As with any clinical examination, the general condition of the pregnant patient should be assessed, including:

- temperature
- pulse
- blood pressure
- respiratory rate
- cardiovascular system
- respiratory system

Abdominal palpation

The abdomen should be inspected for any previous operation scars. In the presence of a gravid uterus, abdominal palpation to establish the cause of the symptoms may not be straightforward because the site of the tenderness might not be typical. The uterus should be palpated to determine:

- lie, presentation and engagement of the fetus (see Chapter 1)
- presence of uterine contractions
- generalized or specific areas of uterine tenderness
- presence of uterine fibroids

Table 23.1 Differential diagnoses of abdominal pain in pregnancy

System involved	Pathology
Obstetric	Labour Placental abruption Symphysis pubis dysfunction Ligament pain Preeclampsia/HELLP syndrome Acute fatty liver of pregnancy
Gynaecological	Ovarian cyst rupture/torsion/haemorrhage Uterine fibroid degeneration
Gastrointestinal	Constipation Appendicitis Gallstones/cholecystitis Pancreatitis Peptic ulcer disease
Genitourinary	Cystitis Pyelonephritis Renal stones/renal colic

HELLP, Haemolysis, elevated liver enzymes, low platelets.

Table 23.2 Making a diagnosis from the history and examination

Differential diagnosis	Clinical features
Labour (see Chapter 26)	Intermittent pain, usually regular in frequency, associated with uterine tightening. The presenting part of the fetus is usually engaged. Vaginal examination shows cervical change.
Placental abruption (see Chapter 20)	Mild or severe pain, more commonly associated with vaginal bleeding. The uterus is usually tender on palpation and can be irritable or tense. There might be symptoms and signs of preeclampsia.
Symphysis pubis dysfunction	Pain is usually low and central in the abdomen just above the symphysis pubis, which is tender on palpation. Symptoms are worse with movement.
Ligament pain	Commonly described as sharp pain, which is bilateral and often associated with movement.
Preeclampsia/HELLP (see Chapter 21)	Epigastric or right upper quadrant pain, associated with nausea and vomiting, headache and visual disturbances. On examination there is hypertension and proteinuria.
Acute fatty liver of pregnancy	Epigastric pain or right upper quadrant pain, associated with nausea, vomiting, anorexia and malaise.
Ovarian cyst (see Chapter 11)	Unilateral pain, which is intermittent and might be associated with vomiting.
Uterine fibroids (see Chapter 5)	Pain is localized and constant. Fibroid may be noted on palpation and is tender.
Constipation	Usually suggested by the history, can cause lower abdominal discomfort and bloating.
Appendicitis	Pain associated with nausea and vomiting. Tenderness with guarding and rebound might be localized to the right iliac fossa depending on gestation. Patient may be pyrexial and have raised inflammatory markers.
Gallstones/cholecystitis	Right upper quadrant or epigastric pain which might radiate to the back or to the shoulder tip. Tenderness in the right hypochondrium, pyrexia present with cholecystitis.
Pancreatitis	Epigastric pain radiating to the back, associated with nausea and vomiting. Occurs more commonly in the third trimester.
Peptic ulcer	Epigastric pain associated with food. There might be heartburn, nausea and even haematemesis.
Cystitis	Usually suggested by history of dysuria, with pain and tenderness in the lower abdomen or suprapubically.
Renal stones/renal colic/ pyelonephritis	Loin pain that might radiate to the abdomen and groin, possibly associated with vomiting and rigors. Pyrexia is present with pyelonephritis.

HELLP, Haemolysis, elevated liver enzymes, low platelets.

COMMON PITFALLS

When examining a nonpregnant patient who has an ovarian cyst torsion is likely to elicit tenderness and guarding in the iliac fossa. Depending on the gestation, this might not be so specific in a pregnant patient because the gravid uterus interferes with the usual anatomical markings. Similarly, tenderness at McBurney's point, which is typical of appendicitis, may be difficult to elicit in a patient who is late in the second or in the third trimester of pregnancy for a similar reason.

HINTS AND TIPS

When examining an obstetric patient, remember that she might feel faint if she lies flat on her back for too long, secondary to pressure on the large vessels reducing venous return to the heart and causing supine hypotension. She should be examined with left lateral tilt.

Vaginal examination

A speculum examination is appropriate to exclude bleeding, for example, in the presence of a placental abruption (see Chapter 20). A digital examination may be indicated if the history and abdominal palpation suggest that the patient is in labour, to determine if there is cervical change.

Investigations

Box 23.1 gives a summary of the investigations that should be considered and Fig. 23.1 provides an algorithm for the investigation of abdominal pain.

Full blood count/clotting studies/group and save serum

The full blood count can show a reduced haemoglobin if the patient is bleeding, for example. in the case of a placental abruption. The platelet count is usually low in association with pre-eclampsia or HELLP syndrome (*h*aemolysis, *el*evated liver enzymes, *l*ow *p*latelets; see Chapter 21).

This may be associated with abnormal clotting studies. A group-and-save sample of serum is essential if there is ongoing bleeding, in case cross-matched blood is required for transfusion. With the non-obstetric causes of pain, the white blood cell count and C-reactive protein will be raised if there is infection, for example, with pyelonephritis or cholecystitis.

Urea/electrolytes/glucose/liver function tests

In pre-eclampsia or HELLP syndrome, urea, creatinine and the liver transaminases can be raised. Serum uric acid is also high in pre-eclampsia and in acute fatty liver disease. The latter is associated with hypoglycaemia.

Urinalysis/midstream urine sample

In pre-eclampsia, there is proteinuria on dipstick urinalysis. A single sample protein-to-creatinine ratio or 24-hour urine collection will quantify the amount of protein to determine the severity of the disease. Proteinuria may also be present with a urinary tract infection and may be associated with microscopic haematuria, particularly in the presence of renal stones. If leucocytes or nitrites are present on a urine dipstick test, a sample should be sent for microscopy, culture and sensitivity to identify the causative organism of a urinary tract infection. Empirical antibiotic treatment can be started until sensitivity results are back.

Cardiotocograph

Before 26 weeks' gestation, the fetal heart should be auscultated with a Pinard or a Sonicaid. A cardiotocograph is performed after 26 weeks' gestation (see Chapter 27) and is important to determine fetal well-being, particularly in the case of placental abruption. The recording will also detect uterine activity including the presence and frequency of uterine contractions.

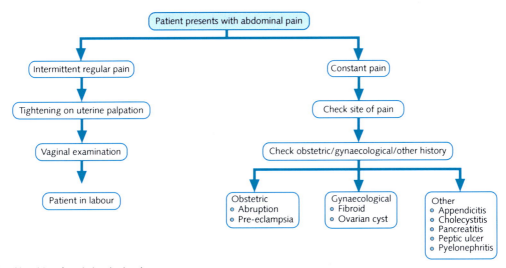

Fig. 23.1 Algorithm for abdominal pain.

Ultrasound scan (uterus/ovaries/kidneys/liver/gall bladder)

Although generally a clinical diagnosis, an ultrasound scan may show a retroplacental haematoma in the case of severe placental abruption. If preterm delivery is necessary, for example, in acute fatty liver disease, fetal well-being and growth should be assessed, and the fetal weight estimated to inform the paediatricians. For the other systems, ultrasound examination can assist diagnosis and management. An ovarian cyst might be seen if haemorrhage, rupture or torsion of the cyst is suspected. Renal stones or gallstones can be visualized.

Management

This depends on the cause of the pain and the gestation of the pregnancy. With regard to the obstetric causes, caesarean section or induction of labour might need to be considered. For example, in severe pre-eclampsia, the benefits of delivery to the mother's health can outweigh the risks to the fetus of preterm birth. Placental abruption might be severe enough to compromise the fetus, and then delivery should be expedited.

However, most conditions can be managed conservatively. This includes analgesia in the presence of renal stones, or antibiotics for pyelonephritis. Multidisciplinary management with other specialties is important, for example, with gastroenterology in a patient suspected of having gallstones or a peptic ulcer. Depending on the clinical findings, an operation is necessary for an acute appendicitis or for ovarian torsion.

> **HINTS AND TIPS**
>
> Multidisciplinary team management of patients with suspected medical or surgical complications in pregnancy is essential (e.g. renal stones or cholecystitis). In the case of preterm labour, management must be in conjunction with the paediatricians. Do not forget to liaise with the anaesthetists for analgesia if delivery is indicated or for assistance with fluid replacement and airway management.

LARGE FOR DATES OR SMALL FOR DATES

Differential diagnosis

The growth of a pregnancy is estimated by measuring the symphysis–fundal height (SFH) after 24 weeks' gestation (see Chapter 1). This takes into account the size of the fetus, the liquor volume and the maternal structures, including the uterus. National guidelines recommend that every woman should have a dating scan between 11 and 14 weeks of pregnancy to establish the estimated date of delivery. Before deciding whether the SFH is abnormal or not, the dates of the last menstrual period and the scan reports should be checked to confirm the gestation of the pregnancy, and also whether it is a singleton pregnancy.

The differential diagnoses of the large-for-dates (LFD) or small-for-dates (SFD) uterus can be considered in two categories:

1. fetal or placental
2. maternal

A fetus found to be SFD can be categorized according to its growth pattern diagnosed with serial ultrasound scans:

- Small for gestational age (SGA): the fetus is small for the expected size at a certain gestation, but continues to grow at a normal rate as the pregnancy progresses.
- Intrauterine growth restriction (IUGR): the fetus is small or normal sized for the expected size at a certain gestation, but the growth rate slows down as the pregnancy progresses.

> **HINTS AND TIPS**
>
> The symphysis–fundal height (SFH) measurement should be ±3 cm equal to the number of weeks of pregnancy after 24 weeks (i.e. at 32 weeks a normal SFH will be between 29 and 35 cm). Discrepancy of more than 3 cm is large for date, less than 3 cm is small for dates.

History

Obstetric history

With respect to the LFD uterus, a patient who had gestational diabetes in a previous pregnancy is at risk of developing the same condition again (see Chapter 22). This disorder puts the pregnancy at risk of fetal macrosomia and polyhydramnios (increased liquor volume).

A previous history of a baby that was SGA or IUGR, whether in relation to pre-eclampsia or not, increases the risk of a future pregnancy being similarly affected.

Gynaecological history

A diagnosis of uterine fibroids or an ovarian cyst, either prior to pregnancy or in early pregnancy, can cause the SFH to palpate as LFD.

Medical history

Pre-existing diabetes increases the chance of fetal macrosomia and polyhydramnios. The abdomen will palpate LFD, as in gestational diabetes. Fetal infection with cytomegalovirus or rubella may produce polyhydramnios, so the woman should be asked about recent flu-like illness or rash.

Current maternal disease increases the risk of IUGR, and therefore an SFD uterus (see Chapter 22):

- renal disease including renal transplantation
- hypertension
- congenital heart disease
- severe anaemia
- sickle-cell disease
- systemic lupus erythematosus
- cystic fibrosis
- human immunodeficiency virus (HIV) infection

Family history

In relation to an LFD uterus, a family history of diabetes will put the patient at increased risk of developing gestational diabetes in her current pregnancy.

There is also evidence that a family history of pre-eclampsia is relevant. This disorder can be associated with IUGR (see Chapter 21).

Social history

The ethnic group of the patient can be relevant in an SFD patient. The growth charts used in most units were derived from Caucasian populations, in whom the average birthweight is greater than, for example, an Asian population. Hence some units have developed customized growth charts for each particular patient group.

Smoking in pregnancy is a major cause of a fetus being SGA, so that the abdomen palpates as SFD. It affects growth in the third trimester. Alcohol and illegal drug use are also causes of being SGA, and so all these factors must be checked in the antenatal history.

Examination

Chapter 1 discusses examination of the pregnant patient and the uterus. General examination should include checking blood pressure, and urinalysis for proteinuria or glycosuria. Body mass index (BMI) should be routinely calculated at the booking visit. If it is below the normal range, the fetus is at risk of measuring SFD in the third trimester. Conversely, a raised BMI may make it difficult to assess fetal size accurately, as well as increasing the risk of gestational diabetes. In both situations, it is appropriate to arrange serial growth scans. The following should be noted on abdominal palpation in relation to LFD or SFD:

- SFH
- number of fetuses
- fetal lie
- liquor volume
- presence of uterine fibroids
- presence of adnexal masses

> **COMMON PITFALLS**
>
> Patients with a raised body mass index (BMI) can have undiagnosed small-for-gestational-age or intrauterine growth restriction babies as their symphysis–fundal height measurements are not accurate due to their body habitus. Serial growth scans should be arranged for women with a BMI > 35 kg/m^2.

Investigations

Figs 23.2 and 23.3 provide algorithms for the investigation of the LFD and SFD uterus.

Blood tests

In the case of an LFD uterus where fetal macrosomia is diagnosed, a glucose tolerance test should be arranged to establish whether gestational diabetes has developed (see Chapter 22). If polyhydramnios is found in the absence of diabetes, fetal infection may be the cause, so maternal antibodies [immunoglobulin M (IgM) and IgG] to rubella and cytomegalovirus should be investigated.

A patient who is SFD and is also hypertensive should be investigated for pre-eclampsia (see Chapter 21). The blood investigations include a full blood count, liver and renal function tests.

> **HINTS AND TIPS**
>
> If there is no evidence of uteroplacental insufficiency, the other causes of the fetus being small for dates should be excluded. Ultrasound scan should examine for fetal abnormalities and check for signs of in-utero infection. Prior screening for chromosomal abnormalities should be reviewed.

Ultrasound of the fetus

Plotting ultrasound measurements of head circumference, abdominal circumference and femur length on a growth chart is the main method of monitoring fetal growth, either LFD or SFD. In the case of SFD, serial measurements, at least 2 weeks apart, should be taken to distinguish between SGA and IUGR. The latter is often secondary to uteroplacental insufficiency. With IUGR, the fetus preferentially diverts blood to the vital organs. There is less blood to the kidneys, and therefore reduced production of liquor (oligohydramnios), as well as less storage of glycogen in the fetal liver. The latter results in a tailing off of the abdominal circumference measurement.

Fig. 23.2 Algorithm for a large-for-dates (LFD) uterus.

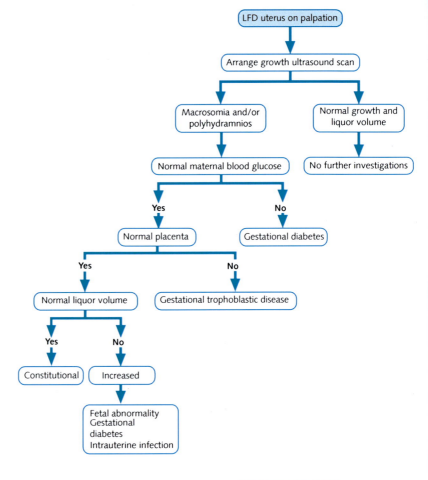

Fig. 23.3 Algorithm for a small-for-dates (SFD) uterus.

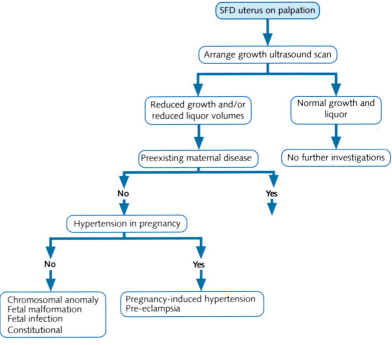

Ultrasound of the placenta and liquor volume

Trophoblastic disease is usually excluded at the 12-week dating scan by checking the structure of the placenta (see Chapter 18). This condition very rarely presents later in pregnancy with a uterus that palpates LFD.

A scan can also be used to measure the liquor volume objectively. The amniotic fluid index is the sum of the fluid pockets in the four quadrants of the abdomen. The amount varies with gestation, but the normal range is 5–25 cm. Liquor volume is also measured in terms of the deepest vertical pocket. During scan, the deepest pocket of fluid that is free of umbilical cord or fetal parts is measured vertically. A measurement of <2 cm indicates oligohydramnios, 2–8 cm is normal and >8 cm indicates polyhydramnios. Box 23.2 shows the causes of increased or decreased liquor.

Doppler studies

In conjunction with growth scans and measurement of the liquor volume, Doppler waveforms of the blood flow in the uteroplacental and fetal circulations can be used to assess the fetus. Increased placental vascular resistance, for example, in pre-eclampsia, changes the pattern of the flow in the umbilical artery. There is normally flow towards the placenta during fetal diastole. However, as the placental resistance increases, diastolic flow becomes absent and then reversed. Other vessels can also be examined within the fetus, including the middle cerebral artery and the ductus venosus, to look for patterns of flow redistribution or, in severe cases, heart failure which can occur if the placental blood flow is insufficient.

Maternal ultrasound

Ultrasound scan is useful to diagnose uterine fibroids or the presence of ovarian cysts which make the maternal abdomen palpate as large for dates.

Cardiotocography

The cardiotocography (CTG) can be used to assess the IUGR fetus. When not in labour, the tracing might be abnormal if the uteroplacental insufficiency is severe. The presence of the following should be excluded:

- reduced variability
- bradycardia
- tachycardia
- decelerations

REDUCED FETAL MOVEMENTS

A woman first feels fetal movements between 18 and 20 weeks' gestation and it is recognized as a sign of fetal wellbeing. Fetal movements quickly develop a regular pattern and any reduction or change in this pattern may be an important clinical sign that may indicate the fetus is not thriving in utero. Women should be taught to recognize their baby's own pattern of movements and present to hospital if they have noticed a reduction or absent movements.

History

Normal fetal movements imply that the fetus' central nervous system and musculoskeletal systems are functioning. In the history, identify if this is the first episode of reduced fetal movement, and quantify the duration and nature of reduced fetal movements. Risk factors for stillbirth and growth restriction need to be identified, these include:

- hypertension
- IUGR
- diabetes
- smoking
- previous stillbirth
- primiparous
- multiple episodes of reduced fetal movements
- congenital malformation
- maternal obesity

A drug and social history should be taken as some sedating drugs such as alcohol, benzodiazepines, methadone

BOX 23.2 CAUSES OF INCREASED OR DECREASED LIQUOR VOLUME	
Increased liquor volume	**Decreased liquor volume**
Diabetes	Ruptured membranes
Fetal abnormality	Fetal abnormality
Multiple pregnancy	Aneuploidy
Fetal infection	Fetal infection
	Intrauterine growth restriction
	Maternal drugs (e.g., atenolol)

or opioids can cross the placenta and cause reduced fetal movements.

A review of the anomaly ultrasound and placenta location should be undertaken as those women with an anterior placenta may have a reduced perception of fetal movements. Fetuses with major congenital malformations may move less due to abnormalities within their muscular, skeletal or central nervous systems.

RED FLAG

Fetal movements plateau around 32 weeks and then continue in this pattern. There is no reduction in movements in the third trimester.

Examination

Palpation of the abdomen may reveal that the fetal spine is anterior – this can give women a reduced perception of movements. The SFH should be measured, as a lower-than-expected measurement could indicate an IUGR

baby, whereas an increased measurement may represent polyhydramnios both of which can be causes of reduced fetal movements. The fetal heart should be auscultated, as this will reassure an anxious mother.

Investigations

A CTG should be performed. A normal CTG (see Chapter 27) over a 20-minute period will indicate that the fetus is healthy with an intact autonomic nervous system.

An ultrasound scan for growth and liquor volume assessment should be performed if there are persistent reduced movements even with a normal CTG, or if there is an abnormal SFH measurement.

Management

If all the investigations are normal after one episode of reduced fetal movements, the woman can be reassured and discharged. She should be advised to contact her hospital if she experiences any further episodes of reduced fetal movements. Induction of labour may be considered in cases of persistent reduced movements at term with no cause identified.

Chapter Summary

- Taking a thorough history from a patient presenting with abdominal pain in the second and third trimesters of pregnancy can identify treatable causes.
- You should perform an abdominal, speculum and vaginal examination for patients presenting with abdominal pain in the second and third trimesters of pregnancy.
- Undertake the appropriate investigations to establish a diagnosis.
- Perform an ultrasound to assess fetal growth in patients who present measuring large or small for dates and investigate further if the ultrasound scan is abnormal.
- When a woman presents with reduced fetal movements, she should be fully assessed and induction of labour should be considered if the pregnancy is at full-term gestation.

FURTHER READING

National Institute for Health and Care Excellence (NICE), 2008. Guidelines – CG63 diabetes in pregnancy: full guideline. NICE, London, UK. Available at: www.nice.org.uk.

Royal College of Obstetricians and Gynaecologists (RCOG), February 2011. Reduced fetal movements: RCOG green-top guideline no. 57. RCOG, London, UK. Available at: www.rcog.org.uk.

Royal College of Obstetricians and Gynaecologists (RCOG), 2013. Small for gestational age fetus, investigation and management: RCOG green-top guideline no. 31. RCOG, London, UK. Available at: www.rcog.org.uk.

A multiple pregnancy is one in which two or more fetuses are present (i.e. it is not a singleton pregnancy). Such pregnancies are important to the obstetrician because they represent a high-risk pregnancy. The risk of all pregnancy complications is greater than in a singleton pregnancy; in particular, preterm labour (see Chapter 25) and intrauterine growth restriction (IUGR). Perinatal mortality for a multiple pregnancy is about six times greater than that of a singleton.

> ### RED FLAG
>
> A multiple pregnancy is a high-risk pregnancy. Perinatal mortality rate is increased six times compared with a single fetus, mainly due to the risk of preterm delivery.

INCIDENCE

The most common type of multiple pregnancy is a twin pregnancy, with an incidence of 1 in 80 pregnancies. The incidence of spontaneous triplets is 1 in 80^2 or 1 in 6400. The incidence of any multiple pregnancy increases with:

- increasing maternal age
- increasing parity
- ethnic variation – dizygous pregnancies are more common in Africa compared with Far East
- improved nutrition
- assisted conception

The latter accounts for a significant rise in the numbers of multiple pregnancies over the last two decades, especially in Western countries.

DIAGNOSIS

Nowadays, multiple pregnancies are normally diagnosed by routine dating ultrasound scan at 11–14 weeks' gestation. Clinical situations in which the diagnosis should be suspected include a patient who presents with hyperemesis gravidarum, or if clinical examination reveals either a large-for-dates uterus or multiple fetal parts in later pregnancy.

AETIOLOGY OF TWINS

Zygosity and chorionicity

The majority of twins (75%) are dizygotic, that is, they arise from the fertilization of two ova by two sperm. Each fetus has its own chorion, amnion and placenta – dichorionic diamniotic placentation. The placentae can appear fused if implantation occurs close together. These twins can be of the same or different sexes and will have different genetic constitutions (i.e. they have no more similarities than any siblings; Fig. 24.1).

Monozygotic twins (25%) arise following the fertilization of a single ovum by a single sperm, which then completely divides, so that each twin has the same genetic make-up. Cell division may occur at different stages of embryonic development, giving rise to different structural arrangements of the membranes (Fig. 24.1). A third of monozygotic twins establish at the eight-cell stage, so that two separate blastocysts form and implant. These twins will thus have dichorionic diamniotic placentation. About two-thirds of monozygotic twins have monochorionic diamniotic placentation: that is, a single blastocyst implants, developing a single chorion; the inner cell mass divides into two so that each embryo has its own amnion. The least common type of monozygotic twins occurs by later splitting of the inner cell mass, before the appearance of the primitive streak, to produce a single amniotic cavity – monochorionic monoamniotic twins. Splitting even later than this results in conjoined twins. The incidence of monozygotic twins is constant around the world, at about 4 per 1000 births.

The clinically important issue is the **chorionicity** of the pregnancy. This relates to the placentation. If the placentae are separate, with separate amnions and chorions (**dichorionic diamniotic twins**), the blood supply to each fetus during the pregnancy is independent.

Conversely, if there are blood vessel anastomoses between the placentae (**monochorionic diamniotic** twins or **monochorionic monoamniotic** twins), then there is a risk of uneven distribution of blood. This may result in discordant growth, with one twin showing signs of growth restriction and the other getting larger (see the 'Twin-to-twin transfusion syndrome' section). Thus diagnosing **chorionicity** determines the level of surveillance necessary in that particular pregnancy.

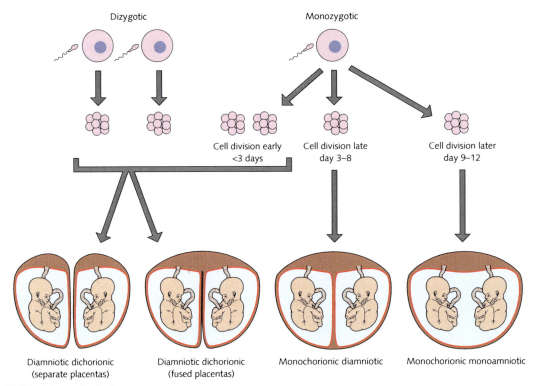

Fig. 24.1 Aetiology of twinning.

Diagnosis of chorionicity

Antenatally

Ultrasound assessment of the membrane dividing the amniotic sacs diagnoses the chorionicity; ideally this is done by 14 weeks' gestation. Fig. 24.2 shows the thicker membrane (chorion and amnion), known as the 'lambda sign' at the point where it meets the placenta, which is seen in a dichorionic pregnancy. By contrast, the thinner T sign (amnion only) is seen in a monochorionic pregnancy. If there is no dividing membrane between the fetuses, they are monochorionic monoamniotic twins.

Fetal sex can also be assessed by ultrasound. If they are discordant, then the pregnancy must be dichorionic (as the fetuses must come from two separate ova and sperm). Localization of the placental sites may also be helpful. If the placentae can be seen as being completely separate, then similarly, the pregnancy must be dichorionic.

Postnatally

At this stage, chorionicity can be determined by:

- macroscopic and microscopic examination of membranes

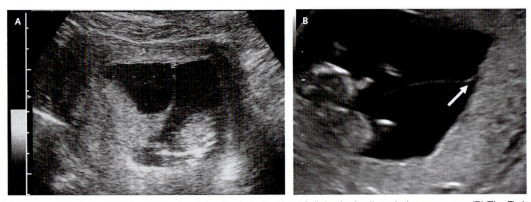

Fig. 24.2 Diagnosis of chorionicity. (A) The lambda sign is indicative of dichorionic diamniotic pregnancy. (B) The T sign is indicative of monochorionic diamniotic pregnancy. (B, from D'Addario V, Rossi C: Diagnosis of chorionicity: the role of ultrasound, *Diagn Prenat* 25:58–64, 2014. Elsevier.)

- analysis of red blood cell markers
- DNA probes

COMPLICATIONS

A multiple pregnancy must be treated as a high-risk pregnancy. The majority of pregnancy-related complications are more common in multiple pregnancies (e.g. gestational diabetes or pre-eclampsia). There are also certain problems that are specific to multiple pregnancies.

> **RED FLAG**
>
> The mother with a multiple pregnancy is at risk of any complication associated with a singleton pregnancy but all the risks are increased.

Fetal malformations

The frequency of fetal malformations is thought to be almost double in a twin pregnancy compared with a singleton pregnancy, especially for monochorionic twins (4% cf. 2%). In terms of screening for chromosomal anomalies, parents can be offered nuchal translucency and combined blood test screening. They must be counselled about the possibility of a screen positive result in one baby, but a negative one in the other. With an invasive procedure, there is a greater risk of pregnancy loss than in a singleton pregnancy. Separate sampling must be performed with dichorionic twins.

ETHICS

There is the potential dilemma of finding an abnormality in only one fetus at the anomaly ultrasound scan. Selective fetocide can result in the miscarriage of both babies (i.e. the apparently normal fetus as well as the abnormal one). The procedure may not be acceptable to some couples on moral or religious grounds.

Antenatal assessment of fetal wellbeing and growth

In a multiple pregnancy, antenatal care should be more frequent, managed by a hospital consultant in a unit with facilities for regular ultrasound scans to check fetal growth and neonatal care facilities in case of preterm labour and delivery.

Serial ultrasounds are usually performed every 4 weeks from 24 weeks in a dichorionic pregnancy, and every 2 weeks from 16 weeks in a monochorionic pregnancy, to exclude IUGR. In a monochorionic pregnancy, the scans also monitor the development of twin-to-twin transfusion syndrome (see below).

Preterm labour

Spontaneous preterm labour occurs in 30% of twin pregnancies. There is some evidence to suggest that cervical length screening by transvaginal ultrasound may be a useful screening tool. In higher-order multiple pregnancies, some physicians opt to put in an elective cervical suture at the start of the second trimester, which may reduce the risk of preterm labour.

If preterm labour is diagnosed, tocolytics should be considered to allow in-utero transfer to a hospital with neonatal intensive care facilities and to allow time for steroids administered to the mother to improve lung maturation (see Chapter 25).

Pregnancy-induced hypertension and pre-eclampsia

Hypertension is about three times more common in multiple pregnancies than in singleton pregnancies because of the larger size of the placental bed (see Chapter 21). Hypertension and pre-eclampsia often develop earlier and can be more severe than in a singleton pregnancy. National guidelines recommend consideration for aspirin 75 mg daily from 12 weeks' gestation to reduce the risk of preeclampsia.

Antepartum haemorrhage

The incidence of placental abruption and placenta praevia is increased in multiple pregnancies (see Chapter 20).

Twin-to-twin transfusion syndrome

This occurs in 15% of monochorionic twin pregnancies – blood is shunted across placental interfetal vascular anastomoses, such that the donor becomes anaemic and growth restricted, with oligohydramnios, and the recipient becomes fluid overloaded with polyhydramnios. This syndrome usually occurs in the second trimester, and therefore scanning every 2 weeks is advised from 16 weeks. The condition results in fetal death in up to 80% of cases if left untreated and a 10% risk of handicap in the surviving twin. Depending on the stage of the disease at diagnosis, up to 26 weeks, laser treatment to the placental anastomoses is generally the advised option to reduce discordant blood flow between the fetuses (known as 'fetoscopic laser ablation of the placenta'). Amniodrainage may be appropriate at later gestations.

With monochorionic placentation, fetal death of a twin in-utero puts the surviving twin at risk of neurological damage (15%–26%) and the mother at risk of developing disseminated intravascular coagulation as thromboplastins are released into the circulation. Magnetic resonance imaging of the surviving twin has been used in some centres to assess the neurological morbidity. The pregnancy can be managed conservatively until the surviving twin reaches a gestation with improved likelihood of survival.

HINTS AND TIPS

The psychological sequelae of a multiple pregnancy for the mother and her family, including existing children, should be remembered.

INTRAPARTUM MANAGEMENT OF A TWIN PREGNANCY

Box 24.1 summarizes the management of a vaginal delivery in a twin pregnancy.

Delivery of twin pregnancy

Delivery of multiple pregnancies should be managed in a unit with neonatal intensive care facilities. For a twin pregnancy, the mode of delivery depends on the presentation of the first twin; twin one is cephalic in more than 80% of pregnancies. If presentation of twin one is anything other than cephalic, caesarean section is advised. In the case of higher-order multiple pregnancies, delivery is almost always by caesarean section.

BOX 24.1   THE INTRAPARTUM MANAGEMENT OF TWIN PREGNANCY

- Neonatal unit intensive care facilities.
- Allow vaginal delivery if normal pregnancy and twin 1 has cephalic presentation.
- Intravenous (IV) access/full blood count/group and save.
- Regional anaesthesia.
- Continuous cardiotocography monitoring with or without fetal scalp electrode to twin 1.
- IV syntocinon infusion to start after delivery of twin 1 to maintain contractions.
- IV syntocinon infusion for third stage to reduce risk of postpartum haemorrhage.
- Neonatal team presents for delivery.
- Stabilize the lie of twin 2.

For a vaginal delivery, the onset of labour can be spontaneous or induced; induction is advised by 36–37 weeks for a monochorionic twin pregnancy and by 37–38 weeks for a dichorionic pregnancy. The woman needs intravenous access and a sample of serum saved in the blood transfusion laboratory because of the risk of postpartum haemorrhage (see below). An epidural block is often recommended to allow for possible manipulation of the second twin in the second stage of labour.

Both fetal heart rates should be monitored continuously, either per abdomen or with a fetal scalp electrode on the first twin. If there is an abnormality in the heart rate pattern of twin one, fetal blood sampling might be appropriate (see Chapter 27). Concerns with twin two should lead to immediate delivery by caesarean section. The reasons for augmentation of labour and for instrumental delivery are similar to those in a singleton pregnancy (see Chapter 28).

Once the first twin is delivered, the lie and presentation of the second twin must be determined by abdominal palpation and ultrasound. External cephalic version can be used to establish a longitudinal lie. Intravenous syntocinon may be necessary to maintain uterine contractions and the delivery of the second twin occurs either as a cephalic presentation or by internal podalic version and breech extraction. Again, the reasons for instrumental delivery or caesarean section are similar to those of a singleton pregnancy.

Complications

Postpartum haemorrhage
Postpartum haemorrhage (see Chapter 31) is more likely with a multiple pregnancy than a singleton because of the larger placental site. Uterine atony due to the increased volume of the uterine contents – two fetuses, placentae, etc. – is a contributing factor. Active management of the third stage of labour is, therefore, appropriate, including routine use of a postpartum syntocinon infusion.

Locked twins
This is a very rare complication of vaginal deliveries when the first twin is breech. As the delivery proceeds, the aftercoming head of the first twin is prevented from entering the pelvis by the head of the cephalic second twin. If this is diagnosed in the first stage of labour, a caesarean section should be performed; during the second stage, general anaesthesia is necessary to allow manipulation.

HIGHER-ORDER MULTIPLE PREGNANCIES

In comparison to twin pregnancies, higher-order multiples are associated with a higher perinatal mortality rate and an increased incidence of the aforementioned antenatal complications. Fertility treatments have increased the numbers of high-order pregnancies and, in the case of in-vitro fertilization, guidelines in the UK now advise that a maximum of two embryos should be replaced in a woman under the age of 40 years (see Chapter 16). Pregnancies of higher-order multiples may be formed by separate embryos. Alternatively, one of the embryos may split to form a monochorionic pair of twins.

Selective fetocide (multifetal pregnancy reduction)

With triplets or more, it is appropriate to counsel the parents about selective fetal reduction, with the aim of reducing the risks of late miscarriage and preterm labour by keeping only one or two babies. Selective fetocide is a technique in which intracardiac potassium chloride is given to one or more fetuses under ultrasound guidance. The chorionicity of the pregnancy must be known to select the appropriate fetus. The procedure cannot be performed on a monochorionic twin because it shares placental circulation with its co-twin and, therefore, the drugs would affect both fetuses. It is usually performed at 12–14 weeks' gestation, after results of screening for Down syndrome have been obtained if the parents wish this test. Despite the procedure-related risk of miscarriage of about 6%, the incidence of complications is low.

ETHICS

Care must be taken to establish a couple's religious and moral views regarding abortion, when counselling about selective fetal reduction in high-order multiple pregnancies. It must be balanced against the chances of taking home babies who have not been compromised by premature birth.

● Chapter Summary

- Monozygotic twins arise following fertilization of a single ovum by a single sperm which then divides, so that each twin has the same genetic material (identical twins).
- Dizygotic twins arise following fertilization of two ova by two sperm.
- Chorionicity relates to placentation and is ideally diagnosed on the dating ultrasound scan performed before 14 weeks' gestation.
- Twin pregnancies are high risk and consultant-led antenatal care is required and screening for pregnancy-related conditions such as gestational diabetes and pre-eclampsia should be undertaken.

FURTHER READING

National Institute for Health and Care Excellence (NICE), 2011. Guideline multiple pregnancy CG129. NICE, London, UK. Available at: www.nice.org.uk.

Nicolaides, K.H., Sebire, N.J., Snijders, J.M., 2004. The 11–14 week scan. Fetal Medicine Foundation, London, UK. Available at: www.fetalmedicine.com/fmf.

Royal College of Obstetricians and Gynaecologists (RCOG), 2016. Monochorionic twin pregnancy, management. RCOG green-top guideline no. 51. RCOG, London, UK. Available at: www.rcog.org.uk.

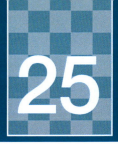
PRETERM LABOUR

Preterm labour is defined as labour occurring after 24 weeks and before 37 weeks' gestation, therefore diagnosis depends upon the accurate calculation of the estimated date of delivery at the first ultrasound scan between 11 and 14 weeks. It is important to establish whether labour is preterm for several reasons:

1. Preterm labour has more risk of complications than labour at term, for example, abnormal lie.
2. Prematurity has potentially significant risk of morbidity to the baby – the paediatric team must be consulted.
3. Up to 34 + 0 weeks' gestation attempts should be made to stop the labour to administer corticosteroids to the mother, which will boost fetal lung surfactant production and, therefore, reduce neonatal respiratory distress.

RED FLAG

With improving standards of neonatal care, it is easy to forget that prematurity is the single largest cause of neonatal mortality and long-term handicap in otherwise normal babies – preterm babies have a significantly increased mortality rate compared with term babies.

INCIDENCE

The incidence of preterm labour is currently around 8% in England and Wales, but this varies in different populations and the incidence is increasing. Risk factors for premature labour are presented in Box 25.1.

The main causes of preterm delivery are given in Box 25.2.

Infection is thought to play a part in at least 20% of cases (Box 25.3 lists common pathogens implicated in preterm labour).

Iatrogenic preterm delivery, accounting for one-third of preterm deliveries, occurs when obstetricians decide that delivery is necessary in the interests of fetal or maternal health, due, for example, to severe preeclampsia, or when scans have shown severe intrauterine growth restriction of the fetus.

BOX 25.1 RISK FACTORS FOR PRETERM LABOUR

- Previous preterm labour.
- Smoking.
- Low socioeconomic group.
- Body mass index <19 kg/m^2.
- Lack of social support.
- Afro-Caribbean ethnicity.
- Extreme of reproductive age (<20 or >35 years).
- Domestic violence.
- Bacterial vaginosis.
- Chronic medical conditions.
- Multiple pregnancy.
- Previous cone biopsy or large loop excision of the transformation zone procedure.

The most significant association is a history of a previous preterm labour.

BOX 25.2 CAUSES OF PRETERM LABOUR

- Infection (e.g. chorioamnionitis, maternal pyelonephritis).
- Uteroplacental ischaemia (e.g. abruption).
- Uterine overdistension (e.g. polyhydramnios, multiple pregnancy).
- Cervical incompetence.
- Fetal abnormality.
- Iatrogenic (e.g. delivery for severe intrauterine growth restriction caused by pre-eclampsia).

BOX 25.3 PATHOGENS IMPLICATED IN PRETERM LABOUR

- Sexually transmitted: Chlamydia, Trichomonas, Syphilis, Gonorrhoea.
- Enteric organisms: Escherichia coli, Streptococcus faecalis.
- Bacterial vaginosis: Gardnerella, Mycoplasma and anaerobes.
- Group B streptococcus (if a very heavy growth).

HISTORY

Preterm labour may be rapid in onset and progress, and is almost always unexpected. Therefore history taking must be done as comprehensively as possible, taking into account the fact that some women will arrive in an advanced state of labour.

The history should include the timing of onset of the abdominal pain (see Chapter 23). Intermittent, but regular abdominal pain suggests uterine contractions. Frequency and intensity over time should be assessed. Preterm labour may be associated with clear watery vaginal discharge, suggesting possible rupture of the membranes, or bleeding, as with an antepartum haemorrhage (see Chapter 20). A history of normal fetal movements should be checked. With regard to possible infection, urinary and gastrointestinal symptoms should be elicited, as well as systemic symptoms such as fever. A past medical history and a social history should be taken to identify the risk factors shown in Box 25.1.

EXAMINATION

Examination must include baseline observations – pulse, blood pressure, respiratory rate and temperature – to look for possible infection. Abdominal palpation will assess:

- abdominal tenderness – site, guarding, rebound
- uterine tenderness – site
- uterine tone – soft or irritable (e.g. abruption)
- uterine contractions – frequency and strength
- fetal lie, presentation and engagement

Sterile speculum examination should be performed on a woman with abdominal pain and/or discharge. A vaginal swab should be taken if there is a clear watery loss suggesting ruptured membranes or if an abnormal vaginal discharge is present. If there is no obvious pooling of liquor but the patient provides a good history of ruptured membranes, then a test for the presence of amniotic fluid can be performed (e.g. AmniSure test). A fetal fibronectin test is appropriate between 24 + 0 and 33 + 6 weeks – the vaginal swab should be taken at this time (see below). A digital examination is necessary to check the dilatation of the cervix. A closed cervix in the presence of palpable uterine contractions is termed 'threatened preterm labour'.

INVESTIGATIONS

As abnormal lie and presentation are far more common in preterm pregnancy, an ultrasound scan should be performed (see Chapter 29). Up to 25 + 6 weeks' gestation, presence of the fetal heart beat should be confirmed with a Sonicaid. After this gestation, a cardiotocograph should

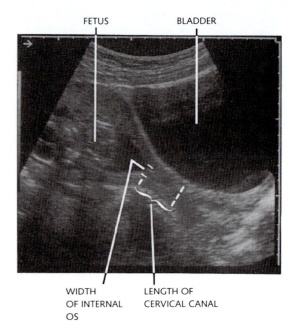

Fig. 25.1 Transvaginal scan of cervical canal. From Chudleigh T: Obstetric ultrasound: how, why and when (3rd ed.), London, 2004, Churchill Livingstone. Elsevier, with permission.

be performed, which will assess fetal wellbeing as well as indicating uterine activity.

Evidence of fetal fibronectin in the mother's cervical secretions can be checked using a specific kit and a vaginal swab; absence of fetal fibronectin, i.e. a negative test, suggests that delivery is less likely and this may assist with management decisions such as the need for fetal steroids and tocolysis. Transvaginal scans may be used to examine the length of the cervix because cervical shortening is a predictor of preterm delivery (Fig. 25.1). Urinalysis must be performed to look for nitrites, which suggest a urinary tract infection.

MANAGEMENT

Box 25.4 summarizes the management plan for a woman who appears to be in preterm labour.

Liaison with the neonatal team and administration of steroids are vital. Some hospitals do not have facilities for treating babies born under certain gestations and in these cases transfer to the nearest appropriate unit is made, preferably prior to delivery known as an 'in-utero transfer'. If the mother is very unwell or if delivery is imminent, transfer of the baby can be arranged after delivery known as an 'ex-utero transfer'. Ideally, the neonatologist will have an opportunity to counsel the woman and her partner about expectations when the baby is born and some of the problems that premature babies encounter. A tour of the neonatal intensive care unit could be arranged.

BOX 25.4 MANAGEMENT CHECKLIST FOR A PATIENT PRESENTING IN THREATENED PRETERM LABOUR

- Assess for signs of a precipitant of preterm labour (e.g. sepsis, polyhydramnios, abruption, severe preeclampsia, obstetric cholestasis).
- Investigate with blood tests as appropriate, perform urin analysis and send midstream sample of urine.
- Determine frequency and regularity of contractions.
- Ascertain fetal presentation.
- Monitor fetal heart with Sonicaid or cardiotocography if appropriate gestation.
- Perform a sterile speculum examination to examine the cervix and assess if membranes have ruptured. Take a high vaginal swab. Vaginal examination may be required to ascertain cervical dilatation.
- Give corticosteroids.
- Give antibiotics if the membranes have ruptured or obvious signs of sepsis are present.
- Consider tocolysis.
- Contact neonatal team and arrange transfer if necessary and appropriate.
- Discuss mode of delivery.

COMMUNICATION

Parents need to be warned of problems encountered by children surviving extreme premature delivery, which include cerebral palsy, chronic lung disease, visual and hearing deficits and learning difficulties.

Tocolysis and steroids

Administration of drugs to reduce the uterine activity should be considered depending on:

- cervical dilatation
- need to administer steroids and allow time for them to be effective
- need for in-utero transfer

The different drugs used to try to stop contractions are shown in Table 25.1. They have been shown to delay the number of women who deliver within 48 hours, but there is no clear evidence that they improve perinatal morbidity and

HINTS AND TIPS

Corticosteroids (betamethasone or dexamethasone) are given to the woman as two intramuscular injections 12–24 hours apart. They have been shown to significantly reduce neonatal respiratory distress by stimulating fetal surfactant production and are recommended for any woman in threatened preterm labour between 24 + 0 and 33 + 6 weeks' gestation. This can be extended up to 35 + 6 weeks if there are other risk factors such as intrauterine growth restriction (see Chapter 23). Consideration should be given up to 38 + 6 weeks for women being delivered by elective caesarean section. Repeated courses of steroid administration are currently not recommended.

Table 25.1 Drugs used to treat preterm labour

Drug	Route of administration	Comments/ side-effects
Calcium-channel blockers (e.g. nifedipine)	Oral	Block calcium channels in the myometrium to reduce contractions. Not licensed in UK for this use. Side-effects include headache, flushing and tremor.
Oxytocin receptor antagonists (e.g. Atosiban)	Intravenous	Well tolerated but expensive. 8% experience headache

mortality overall. They allow time for corticosteroids and, if necessary, transfer to another hospital able to offer neonatal care, as above. With all drugs, the side-effects on mother and fetus must be balanced against the benefit of prolonging the pregnancy. Tocolysis should not be used in the following circumstances:

- maternal illness that would be helped by delivery (e.g. pre-eclampsia)
- evidence of fetal distress
- in the presence of chorioamnionitis
- when there has been significant vaginal bleeding, particularly if abruption is suspected
- once the membranes have ruptured

Magnesium sulphate

In cases of established labour or planned preterm delivery where the gestation is below 30 weeks, a magnesium sulphate infusion should be commenced. This drug causes cerebral vasodilation and therefore acts as neuroprotection for the fetus. It has been proven to reduce rates of cerebral palsy in preterm infants. At gestations between 30 and 33 + 6 weeks an infusion can be considered.

Antibiotic therapy

If the membranes are intact in preterm labour, the mother is screened for infection (vaginal and cervical swabs, midstream urine sample, blood cultures if pyrexial) and only given antibiotics if there are signs or confirmatory tests for sepsis. Antibiotics (erythromycin) are given prophylactically if the membranes have ruptured before term (around one-third of cases) to protect the fetus from ascending vaginal infection.

Mode of delivery

In most cases of preterm labour, it is possible to plan for a normal vaginal birth. There is no firm evidence to show that caesarean section is safer for the baby than vaginal delivery, especially when the presentation is cephalic. However, the caesarean section rate is higher than for term pregnancies because of a higher incidence of low-lying placenta, fetal distress and abnormal lie in prematurity. Caesarean section might have higher morbidity for the mother, particularly at very early gestations because the lower segment is less well formed, increasing the necessity of having to use a classical uterine incision.

> **RED FLAG**
>
> The following procedures are contraindicated in preterm labour:
> - application of fetal scalp electrode
> - fetal blood sampling
> - ventouse delivery

PRETERM PRELABOUR RUPTURE OF MEMBRANES

Preterm prelabour rupture of membranes (PPROM) occurs in only 2% of pregnancies, but is associated with 40% of preterm deliveries. The principal issue is the risk of sepsis, both maternal and fetal. Maternal sepsis with ascending uterine infection can rapidly become overwhelming if not monitored and may cause severe morbidity and mortality, as well as affecting future fertility. Sepsis in the infant is one of the three leading causes of mortality in the preterm infant, along with prematurity and pulmonary hypoplasia.

History and examination

History and examination should be performed as described above. Abdominal palpation and ultrasound scan should be done to check fetal lie and presentation. There is a risk of cord prolapse with an abnormal lie or with a high presenting part and ruptured membranes, particularly in a preterm infant.

Ruptured membranes are confirmed by the visualization of a pool of liquor in the posterior fornix on sterile speculum examination. If there is no obvious pooling of liquor but the patient provides a good history of ruptured membranes, then a test for the presence of amniotic fluid can be performed (e.g. AmniSure test). A digital examination should only be performed if there are obvious signs of labour, as it may introduce infection higher up into the genital tract. A high vaginal swab should be taken.

Management

Management involves monitoring for symptoms and signs of clinical chorioamnionitis. These include:

- feeling unwell such as fever or shivering
- abdominal pain
- change in colour of vaginal loss from clear to green or brown
- foul smelling vaginal loss
- raised maternal temperature, pulse or respiratory rate
- tender uterus on palpation

Investigations include a cardiotocograph to exclude a fetal tachycardia. Maternal blood tests can suggest infection including a raised C-reactive protein and white blood cell count. However, chorioamnionitis should not be discounted if these tests are normal in the presence of obvious clinical signs.

Expectant management (i.e. with no symptoms or signs of infection) involves:

- administration of erythromycin (250 mg) four times a day for 10 days to reduce chorioamnionitis
- administration of corticosteroids to improve fetal lung maturity

Some women will start to labour within 72 hours, but for those who do not, the general principle is to aim to deliver from 34 + 0 weeks gestation onwards. This will be either by induction of labour with a cephalic presentation or by caesarean section with an abnormal lie. Tocolytics are not used in PPROM.

Management of future pregnancies

Any woman who has laboured prematurely in a previous pregnancy is at risk of doing so again in her next pregnancy. In many cases there is currently no specific prevention strategy except for serial monitoring of the cervical length by transvaginal ultrasound scan. The woman should be advised of the increased risk of repeat preterm labour and the need to attend early if she develops abdominal pain.

In some cases, such as repeated second-trimester miscarriage, or with repeated delivery at extreme prematurity, cervical incompetence is diagnosed. This can be treated by insertion of a cervical suture, either electively in early pregnancy (usually around 12–14 weeks after the high risk of early miscarriage and once results of Down syndrome screening tests have been obtained), or, if the cervix is monitored regularly in pregnancy with transvaginal scanning, when scans show that the cervix is shortening. There is some evidence to advise prophylactic vaginal progesterone in some women with a history of preterm labour. The prescription of prophylactic oral tocolytics to women is not helpful.

Cervical cerclage

The more common type of cervical suture is the MacDonald suture, which is inserted vaginally as high in the cervix as possible (Fig. 25.2). Other options are the Shirodkar suture, which is inserted vaginally, but involves the dissection of the bladder off the cervix, or a suture can be inserted into the cervix at laparotomy, which will therefore be placed higher and is known as an 'abdominal cerclage'. However, insertion of any suture can introduce infection and result in rupture of the membranes during the procedure or within a couple of weeks. This may lead to miscarriage or preterm labour depending on the gestation.

Indications for cervical cerclage

Insertion of a cervical cerclage can be as a prophylactic measure or an emergency procedure.

A prophylactic cerclage can be considered in women who have had a previous preterm birth or midtrimester loss (between 16 and 34 weeks' gestation) and who have a shorted cervix on ultrasound scan.

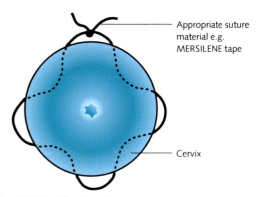

Appropriate suture material e.g. MERSILENE tape

Cervix

Fig. 25.2 The MacDonald suture.

An emergency cerclage, also known as a 'rescue' cerclage, can be considered in women between 16 + 0 and 27 + 6 weeks' gestation if they present in preterm labour with a dilated cervix and intact membranes.

RED FLAG

Contraindications to cervical cerclage include:
- signs of infection
- vaginal bleeding
- uterine contractions
- ruptured membranes

Chapter Summary

- Preterm labour is defined as labour occurring after 24 weeks' and before 37 weeks' gestation.
- Prematurity is the single largest cause of neonatal mortality and long-term handicap in otherwise normal babies.
- A course of corticosteroids should be administered to women in suspected preterm labour as this has been shown to significantly reduce neonatal respiratory distress.
- A magnesium sulphate infusion is neuroprotective for fetuses below 30 weeks and can be considered up to 33 + 6 weeks' gestation.
- Antibiotic treatment should be commenced once the membranes have ruptured in threatened preterm labour.
- The neonatal team should be informed at the earliest opportunity as they need to counsel the parents and prepare for the preterm delivery.

FURTHER READING

National Institute for Health and Care Excellence (NICE), 2015. NG25 Preterm labour and birth. NICE, London, UK 2015.

Update Software Ltd. Available at: www.update-software.com/cochrane

Royal College of Obstetricians and Gynaecologists (RCOG), 2010. Antenatal corticosteroids to reduce neonatal morbidity. RCOG green-top guideline no. 7. RCOG, London, UK.

Royal College of Obstetricians and Gynaecologists (RCOG), 2010. Preterm prelabour rupture of membranes. RCOG green-top guideline no. 44. RCOG, London, UK.

Royal College of Obstetricians and Gynaecologists (RCOG), 2011. Cervical cerclage. RCOG green-top guideline no. 60. RCOG, London, UK.

Royal College of Obstetricians and Gynaecologists (RCOG), 2011. Preterm labour, tocolytic drugs. RCOG green-top guideline no. 1b. RCOG, London, UK.

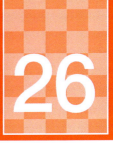
INTRODUCTION

Labour is divided into three stages:

- First stage: from the onset of established labour until the cervix is fully dilated.
- Second stage: from full dilatation until the fetus is born.
- Third stage: from the birth of the fetus until delivery of the placenta and membranes.

ONSET OF LABOUR

Prior to the onset of labour, painless irregular uterine tightenings, known as 'Braxton Hicks' contractions, become increasingly frequent. As the presenting part becomes engaged, the uterine fundus descends, reducing upper abdominal discomfort, and pressure in the pelvis increases. The signs and symptoms that define the actual onset of established labour are:

- painful regular contractions.
- cervical dilatation of ≥4 cm and effacement [see Fig. 1.10.

These factors diagnose labour, with or without a 'show' (passage of a mucoid plug from the cervix, often blood stained)] or ruptured membranes. Irregular contractions prior to cervical dilatation and effacement are part of the latent phase of labour, which may be very variable in duration.

The exact cause of the onset of labour is not known. To some degree it is thought to be mechanical, as preterm labour is seen more commonly in circumstances in which the uterus is overstretched, such as multiple pregnancies and polyhydramnios. Inflammatory markers such as cytokines and prostaglandins also play a role. The latter are thought to be present in the decidua and membranes in late pregnancy and are released if the cervix is digitally stretched at term to separate the membranes and help to initiate labour (a cervical sweep).

NORMAL PROGRESS IN LABOUR

Once the diagnosis of established labour has been made, progress is assessed by monitoring:

- uterine contractions
- dilatation of the cervix
- descent of the presenting part

The rate of cervical dilatation is expected to be approximately 0.5–1 cm/h in a nulliparous woman and 1–2 cm/h in a multiparous woman. A partogram is commonly used to chart the observations made in labour (Fig. 26.1) and to highlight slow progress, particularly a delay in cervical dilatation or failure of the presenting part to descend (see Chapter 29).

Progress is determined by three factors:

- passages
- passenger
- power

Passages

Bony pelvis

The pelvis is made up of four bones:

- two innominate bones
- sacrum
- coccyx

The passage that these bones make can be divided into inlet and outlet, with the cavity between them (Fig. 26.2). The pelvic inlet is bounded by the pubic crest, the iliopectineal line and the sacral promontory. It is oval in shape, with its wider diameter being transverse. The cavity of the pelvis is round. The pelvic outlet is bounded by the lower border of the pubic symphysis, the ischial spines and the tip of the sacrum. Again, the shape is oval, but the wider diameter is anteroposterior.

When a woman stands upright, the pelvis tilts forwards. The inlet makes an angle of about 55° with the horizontal; this angle varies between individuals and different ethnic groups. The presenting part of the fetus must negotiate the axis of the birth canal with the change of direction occurring by rotation at the level of the pelvic floor muscles (see the 'Soft tissues' section).

Soft tissues

The soft passages consist of:

- uterus (upper and lower segments)
- cervix
- pelvic floor
- vagina
- perineum

The upper uterine segment is responsible for the propulsive contractions that deliver the fetus. The lower segment is the part of the uterus that lies behind the uterovesical fold of the peritoneum and above the cervix. It develops gradually during the third trimester, and then more rapidly during labour. It incorporates the cervix as the cervix effaces, to allow the presenting part to descend.

Fig. 26.1 A partogram showing progress and observations in labour. *PP*, presenting part; *IV*, intravenous; *SRM*, spontaneous rupture of membranes; *LOA*, position of the fetal head - left occipito-anterior; *DOA*, direct occipito-anterior; *SVD*, spontaneous vaginal delivery; *C*, clear liquor; *P*, pink liquor.

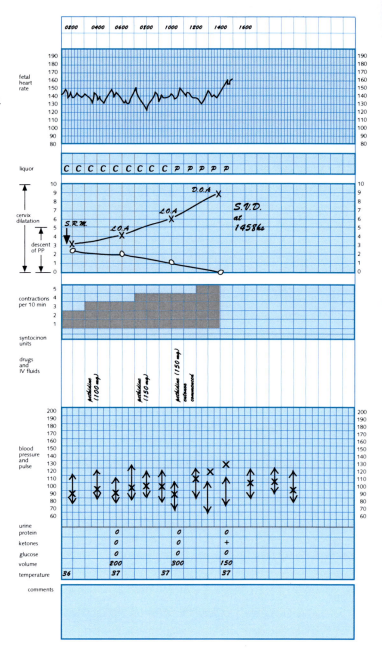

The pelvic floor consists of the levator ani group of muscles, including pubococcygeus and iliococcygeus arising from the bony pelvis to form a muscular diaphragm along with the internal obturator muscle and piriformis muscle. As the presenting part of the fetus is pushed out of the uterus it passes into the vagina, which has become hypertrophied during pregnancy. It reaches the pelvic floor, which acts like a gutter to direct it forwards and allow rotation. The perineum is distal to this and stretches as the head passes below the pubic arch and delivers.

Passenger

The fetal skull consists of the face and the cranium. The cranium is made up of two parietal bones, two frontal bones and the occipital bone (see Figs 26.3 and 1.11), held together by a membrane that allows movement. Up until early childhood, these bones are not fused and so can overlap to allow the head to pass through the pelvis during labour; this overlapping of the bones is known as 'moulding'.

Fig. 26.3 shows the anatomy of the fetal skull, including the sutures between the bones, and the spaces known

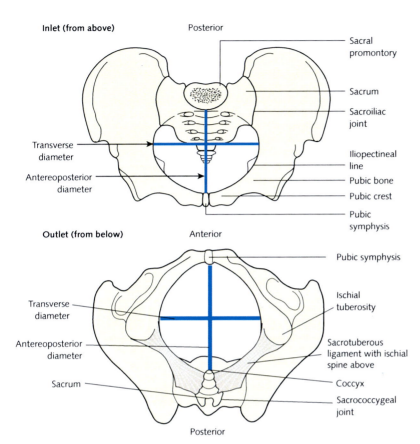

Fig. 26.2 The boundaries of the pelvic inlet and the pelvic outlet.

Inlet (from above)

Posterior

Sacral promontory
Sacrum
Sacroiliac joint
Iliopectineal line
Pubic bone
Pubic crest
Pubic symphysis

Transverse diameter
Antereoposterior diameter

Outlet (from below)

Anterior

Pubic symphysis
Ischial tuberosity
Sacrotuberous ligament with ischial spine above
Coccyx
Sacrococcygeal joint

Transverse diameter
Antereoposterior diameter
Sacrum

Posterior

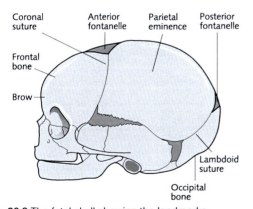

Coronal suture
Anterior fontanelle
Parietal eminence
Posterior fontanelle
Frontal bone
Brow
Lambdoid suture
Occipital bone

Fig. 26.3 The fetal skull showing the landmarks.

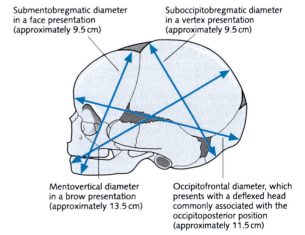

Submentobregmatic diameter in a face presentation (approximately 9.5 cm)

Suboccipitobregmatic diameter in a vertex presentation (approximately 9.5 cm)

Mentovertical diameter in a brow presentation (approximately 13.5 cm)

Occipitofrontal diameter, which presents with a deflexed head commonly associated with the occipitoposterior position (approximately 11.5 cm)

Fig. 26.4 Diameters of the fetal skull.

as 'fontanelles'. These are important landmarks that can be felt on vaginal examination in established labour and enable the position of the fetus to be assessed (see Fig. 1.12). The position is described in terms of the occiput in a cephalic presentation, and the sacrum in a breech presentation.

The degree of flexion and the position of the fetal skull determine the ease with which the fetus passes through the birth canal. Fig. 26.4 shows the diameters of the fetal skull. The diameter that presents during labour depends on the degree of flexion of the head. The head usually becomes more flexed with the increasing strength of the uterine contractions. Thus the smallest diameters for delivery are the suboccipitobregmatic diameter, which represents a flexed vertex presentation, and the submentobregmatic diameter, which corresponds to a face presentation. The widest diameter is mentovertical, a brow presentation, which usually precludes vaginal delivery.

Power

The myometrial component of the uterus acts as the power to deliver the fetus. It consists of three layers:

- thin outer longitudinal layer
- thin inner circular layer
- thick middle spiral layer

From early pregnancy, the uterus contracts painlessly and irregularly (Braxton Hicks contractions). These contractions increase after the 36th week until the onset of labour. In labour, a contraction starts from the junction of the fallopian tube and the uterus on each side, spreading down and across the uterus with its greatest intensity in the upper uterine segment. Like any other muscle, the myometrium contracts and relaxes, but it also has the ability to retract so that the fibres become progressively shorter. This effect is seen in the lower segment: progressive retraction causes the lower segment to stretch and thin out, resulting in effacement and dilatation of the cervix (see Fig. 1.10).

During labour, the contractions are monitored for:

- strength
- frequency
- duration

The resting tone of the uterus is about 6–12 mmHg; to be effective in labour this increases to an intensity of 40–60 mmHg. There are usually three or four co-ordinated strong contractions every 10 minutes, each lasting approximately 60 seconds, to progress in labour.

In the second stage of labour, additional power comes from voluntary contraction of the diaphragm and the abdominal muscles as the mother pushes to assist delivery.

HINTS AND TIPS

The mechanism of delivery can be more easily remembered in four stages, thinking about how the head and shoulders must negotiate the transverse and anteroposterior diameters of the maternal pelvis inlet and outlet:

- flexion of the head
- internal rotation
- extension
- external rotation (restitution)

DELIVERY OF THE FETUS

Active contractions of the uterus of increasing strength, frequency and duration cause passive movement of the fetus down the birth canal. At the beginning of labour, the fetus usually engages in the occipitotransverse or occipitoanterior

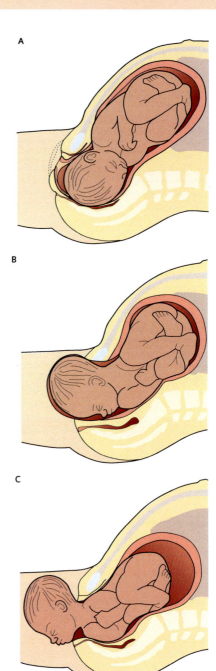

Fig. 26.5 (A) Early labour. There has been flexion of the fetal head. The cervix is effacing and has begun to dilate. (B) The second stage of labour. The head has undergone internal rotation to bring the occiput into the anterior position. The cervix is fully dilated. (C) Delivery of the head. Extension of the fetal neck occurs as the head passes under the pubic symphysis for its delivery.

position (i.e. in a position appropriate to the wider transverse diameter of the pelvic inlet). As labour progresses (Fig. 26.5A), the head becomes fully flexed so that the suboccipitobregmatic diameter is presenting.

As descent occurs through the pelvic cavity, internal rotation brings the occiput into the anterior position as it reaches the pelvic floor. This means that the head is now in the appropriate position to negotiate the wider diameter of the pelvic outlet, which is anteroposterior. In the second stage of labour, the occiput descends below the symphysis pubis (Fig. 26.5B) and delivers by extension. Increasing extension around the pubic bone delivers the face (Fig. 26.5C).

Delivery of the head brings the widest diameter of the shoulders (the bisacromial diameter) through the transverse diameter of the pelvic inlet into the pelvic cavity. External rotation or restitution occurs where the head rotates to a transverse position in relation to the shoulders (Fig. 26.6). This progresses with continuing descent and

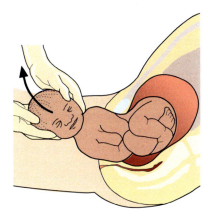

Fig. 26.7 Delivery of the shoulders. The anterior shoulder passes below the pubic symphysis, aided by axial traction of the head by the midwife or doctor. The posterior shoulder delivers as the head is gently guided upwards.

rotation of the shoulders to bring the bisacromial diameter into the anteroposterior diameter of the pelvic outlet. Further contractions and maternal effort enable the anterior shoulder to pass under the pubis, usually assisted by gentle downward traction on the head. Lateral flexion of the fetus delivers the posterior shoulder and the rest of the body follows (Fig. 26.7).

HINTS AND TIPS

Descent of the presenting part is assessed by both abdominal palpation (amount of head felt above the pelvic brim expressed in fifths = engagement) and vaginal examination (descent in relation to level of ischial spines = station).

MANAGEMENT OF LABOUR

The first stage of labour

When a patient presents in the first stage of labour, routine assessment of the mother and fetus is performed.

Maternal monitoring

Regular examination of the mother should include:
- pulse, blood pressure, respiratory rate, temperature
- urinalysis
- analgesia requirements
- abdominal palpation: symphysis fundal height, lie, presentation, engagement
- contractions: strength, frequency, duration

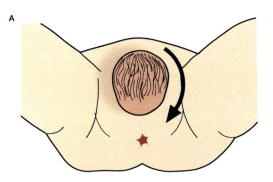

A

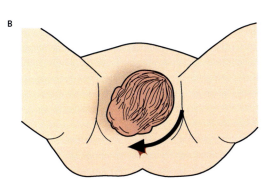

B

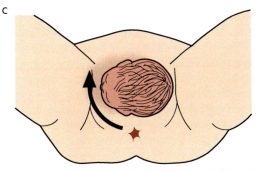

C

Fig. 26.6 External rotation (restitution). The head distends the perineum as it delivers in the occipitoanterior position and the external rotation occurs to allow delivery of the shoulders.

- vaginal examination: degree of cervical effacement, cervical dilatation, station of presenting part in relation to ischial spines, position of presenting part, presence of caput or moulding (see Chapter 29)

As well as regular observations, the patient is encouraged to mobilize if possible and is allowed to eat, depending on her risk of needing an operative procedure. There is delayed gastric emptying during pregnancy and labour. If an emergency general anaesthetic is needed, there is an increased risk of inhalation of regurgitated acidic stomach contents, causing Mendelson syndrome. Therefore, some women may be advised to remain nil by mouth and take an antacid therapy.

If the membranes are ruptured, then the colour of the liquor must be documented, usually clear, blood-stained or having meconium present.

The need for analgesia during labour varies markedly between different women, different ethnic groups and depending on their antenatal preparation. Non-pharmacological techniques include the use of psychoprophylaxis, hypnosis, massage and transcutaneous electrical nerve stimulation. The pharmacological methods are summarized in Table 26.1.

Fetal monitoring

Intermittent or continuous fetal heart rate monitoring is appropriate, depending on the clinical picture antenatally and in labour. In a low-risk pregnancy, intermittent monitoring with a Sonicaid or with a Pinard stethoscope is sufficient, every 15 minutes during and after a contraction for 60 seconds in the first stage of labour, and every 5 minutes in the second stage.

If there are any risk factors during the pregnancy that have been present antenatally or are identified in labour, then continuous electronic monitoring with cardiotocography (CTG) should be performed. See Box 27.1 for indications for continuous monitoring.

Table 26.1 Pharmacological methods of analgesia in labour

	Technique	Indication	Effectiveness	Duration of effect	Side-effects
Oxygen/ nitrous oxide (entonox)	Inhalation of 50:50 mixture with onset of contraction	First stage	<50% Takes 20–30 seconds for peak effect	Time of inhalation only	Does not relieve pain
Pethidine	Intramuscular injection 100–150 mg	First stage	<50% Takes 15–20 minutes for peak effect	Approximately 3 hours	Nausea and vomiting – give with an antiemetic Respiratory depression in the neonate (this is easily reversed with intramuscular naloxone)
Pudendal block	Infiltration of right and left pudendal nerves (S2, S3 and S4) with 0.5% lidocaine	Second stage for operative delivery	Within 5 minutes	45–90 minutes	–
Perineal infiltration	Infiltration of perineum with 0.5% lidocaine at posterior fourchette	Second stage prior to episiotomy Third stage for suturing of perineal lacerations	Within 5 minutes	45–90 minutes	–
Epidural anaesthesia	Injection of 0.25% or 0.5% bupivacaine via a catheter into the epidural space (L3–4)	First or second stage Caesarean section	Complete pain relief in approximately 95% of women within 20–30 minutes	Bolus injection every 3–4 hours or continuous infusion or patient-controlled administration	Transient hypotension – give intravenous fluid load Dural tap Risk of haemorrhage if abnormal maternal clotting Increased length of second stage because of reduced pelvic floor tone and loss of bearing-down reflex
Spinal anaesthesia	Injection of 0.5% bupivacaine into the subarachnoid space	Any operative delivery; manual removal of the placenta	Immediate effect	Single injection lasting 3–4 hours	Respiratory depression

In some patients, abdominal monitoring of the heart rate can be difficult, for example, if the patient is obese, and so a fetal scalp electrode can be applied directly to the head once the cervix dilates and the membranes are ruptured. If monitoring suggests that the fetal heart rate pattern is pathological, it may be appropriate to measure the fetal pH by taking a blood sample from the fetal scalp known as a 'fetal blood sample' (see Chapter 27).

The second stage of labour

Once the cervix is fully dilated, the patient is encouraged to use voluntary effort to push with the contractions. If she has an epidural anaesthetic in-situ, she might be less aware of an urge to push, and so a further hour can be allowed for the presenting part to descend with the contractions alone. Without an epidural, the mother may adopt various positions for delivery of the fetus. As the head descends, the perineum distends and the anus dilates. Finally, the head crowns: the biparietal diameter has passed through the pelvis and there is no recession between contractions. The attendant can apply pressure on the perineum for support during delivery of the head and give consideration of an episiotomy. Once delivered, the neck is felt to exclude the presence of the umbilical cord which should be looped over the fetal head to prevent excessive tension in the cord as the body delivers.

After external rotation, lateral flexion of the head towards the anus (also known as 'axial traction') dislodges the anterior shoulder from behind the pubic symphysis with the next contraction. Lifting the head gently in the opposite direction delivers the posterior shoulder (Fig. 26.7). Holding the shoulders, the rest of the body is delivered either onto the bed or onto the mother's abdomen. Finally, the umbilical cord is secured with clamps and cut.

The third stage of labour

Management of the third stage of labour can be:
- physiological
- active

Women who have had an uncomplicated pregnancy and labour may choose to have a physiological third stage. This means that they do not receive any oxytocic drugs, the attendant waits for the umbilical cord to stop pulsating before it is cut and delivery of the placenta occurs passively. In situations where there is an increased risk of postpartum haemorrhage (PPH) or depending on parental choice, active management is advised.

Active management of the third stage has been shown to reduce the incidence of PPH (see Chapter 31). Management involves:
- using an oxytocic drug
- clamping and cutting the cord
- controlled cord traction

In most units, syntocinon (5 units of oxytocin) or syntometrine (5 units of oxytocin with 0.5 mg ergometrine) is

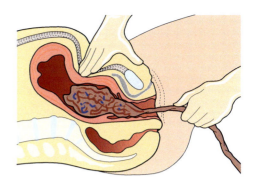

Fig. 26.8 Controlled cord traction to deliver the placenta.

given intramuscularly with delivery of the anterior shoulder; it takes about 2–3 minutes to act. As the placenta detaches from the uterine wall, the cut cord will appear to lengthen. There is usually some bleeding and the fundus becomes hard. Brandt-Andrews method of controlled cord traction is commonly used to deliver the placenta once it has separated to reduce the incidence of uterine inversion (Fig. 26.8). The placenta and membranes must be checked to ensure they are complete.

Finally, the vagina, labia and perineum are examined for tears that may require suturing (see Chapter 28). The uterine fundus is palpated to check that it is well contracted, approximately at the level of the umbilicus. The estimated blood loss should be recorded.

LACTATION

There are two main hormonal influences on breast tissue during pregnancy:
- oestrogen increases the number and the size of the ducts
- progesterone increases the number of alveoli

Colostrum, which is rich in antibodies, is secreted in late pregnancy and production increases after delivery. The level of oestrogen falls in the first 48 hours after delivery so that prolactin can act on the alveoli and initiate lactation.

Suckling stimulates two maternal reflexes:
1. The anterior part of the pituitary gland releases prolactin into the bloodstream, which induces the alveoli to secrete milk.
2. The posterior part of the pituitary gland releases oxytocin into the bloodstream, which causes contraction of the myoepithelial cells surrounding the alveoli so that the milk is ejected.

In most units, breastfeeding is positively encouraged due to the beneficial effects on both mother and baby. Breastfeeding reduces the baby's risk of:
- infections
- diarrhoea and vomiting

- sudden infant death syndrome
- childhood leukaemia
- type 2 diabetes
- obesity
- cardiovascular disease in adulthood

Breastfeeding lowers the mother's risk of:

- breast cancer
- ovarian cancer
- osteoporosis (weak bones)
- cardiovascular disease
- obesity

INDUCTION OF LABOUR

Definition

Induction of labour is the artificial initiation of uterine contractions prior to spontaneous onset resulting in delivery of the baby.

Indications

The rate of induction varies widely between different units. Table 26.2 shows possible reasons for induction of labour. In the UK, the most common indication is prolonged pregnancy, which is when a pregnancy continues beyond 41 weeks' gestation.

Methods

Prior to induction of labour, the favourability of the cervix should be assessed. This is usually done by using the Bishop score (see Fig. 1.2); a higher score suggests a more favourable cervix.

HINTS AND TIPS

With regard to the Bishop score to assess the cervix:

- unfavourable cervix = hard, long, closed, not effaced (low Bishop score)
- favourable cervix = soft, beginning to dilate and efface (high Bishop score)

Table 26.2 Indications for the induction of labour

Maternal	Severe pre-eclampsia
	Recurrent antepartum haemorrhage
	Pre-existing disease (e.g. diabetes)
	Social
Fetal	Prolonged pregnancy
	Intrauterine growth restriction
	Rhesus disease

Prostaglandins

Local application of a prostaglandin, usually prostaglandin E2, given as a vaginal gel, tablet or pessary, has been shown to ripen the cervix as part of the induction process and reduce the incidence of operative delivery when compared with the use of oxytocin alone. Used locally instead of systemically, the gastrointestinal side-effects are minimized. National Institute for Health and Care Excellence (NICE) guidelines have been produced to advise on the dose of prostaglandin given, to reduce the risk of uterine hyperstimulation.

HINTS AND TIPS

Tachysystole versus hyperstimulation

Tachysystole – more than five contractions in a 10-minute period associated with a normal fetal heart trace and the absence of fetal distress.

Hyperstimulation – more than five contractions in a 10-minute period associated with an abnormal fetal heart rate pattern indicating the presence of fetal distress.

Amniotomy

Artificial rupture of the membranes is thought to cause local release of endogenous prostaglandins. It is done using an amnihook and may be part of the induction process or performed to accelerate slow progress in labour. It can also be done with an abnormal CTG to exclude meconium staining of the liquor, or to allow application of a fetal scalp electrode. Table 26.3 shows the complications associated with amniotomy.

Oxytocin

An intravenous infusion of synthetic oxytocin (syntocinon) is commonly used to induce labour, and to stimulate contractions after amniotomy or spontaneous rupture of membranes. The dose must be carefully titrated according to the strength and frequency of the uterine contractions, and continuous fetal monitoring is necessary. Table 26.3 shows the complications associated with oxytocin.

Table 26.3 Complications associated with the use of amniotomy and oxytocin

Treatment	Complication
Amniotomy	Cord prolapse
	Infection
	Bleeding from a vasa praevia
	Placental separation
	Failure to induce efficient contractions
	Amniotic fluid embolism
Oxytocin	Abnormal fetal heart rate pattern
	Hyperstimulation of the uterus
	Rupture of the uterus
	Fluid overload

Chapter Summary

- Labour is defined as the onset of regular painful contractions associated with cervical change (dilatation and effacement).
- Progress in labour is determined by three factors: passage, passenger and power.
- Delivery of the fetus involves flexion of the head, internal rotation, extension and external rotation (restitution).
- Analgesia in labour is dependent on patient choice and includes entonox, intramuscular opioids, local anaesthetic and regional anaesthetic.
- Induction of labour is the artificial initiation of uterine contractions to deliver the fetus. This can be with the use of prostaglandin agents and/or artificial rupture of the membranes followed by the use of syntocinon.

FURTHER READING

National Institute for Health and Care Excellence (NICE), 2014. National evidence-based clinical guidelines. Intrapartum care of healthy women and babies. CG190. NICE, London, UK. Available at: www.nice.org.uk.

National Institute for Health and Care Excellence (NICE), 2008. National evidence-based clinical guidelines. Induction of labour. NICE, London, UK. Available at: www.nice.org.uk.

Royal College of Obstetricians and Gynaecologists (RCOG), 2007. Working party report. Safer Childbirth: Minimum Standards for the Organisation and Delivery of Care in Labour. RCOG, London, UK. Available at: www.rcog.org.uk.

Fetal monitoring in labour 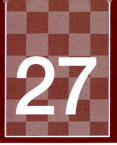 27

FETAL MONITORING IN LABOUR

There are two ways to monitor the fetal heart rate (FHR) in labour, intermittently or continuously. Intermittent auscultation involves the use of a Pinard stethoscope or Sonicaid and is discussed below.

The cardiotocograph (CTG) is a form of continuous electronic FHR monitoring used to evaluate fetal well-being antenatally and during labour. As well as the FHR, the uterine activity is recorded. It has been used increasingly in the UK since the 1970s, with the aim of detecting fetal hypoxia before it causes perinatal morbidity or mortality, in particular cerebral palsy. However, the expected reduction in hypoxia-induced intrapartum perinatal mortality has not occurred and the role of CTG monitoring has been questioned as the rate of caesarean section increases. The need to constantly educate staff about the appropriate use of the CTG and its interpretation by fetal physiology and pattern recognition, and to audit standards in relation to patient care is essential. There is currently debate about guidelines produced by National Institute for Health and Care Excellence (NICE) and International Federation of Gynaecology and Obstetrics (FIGO). In the UK, there are more units using the NICE guidelines at present and so these are presented here.

Monitoring in an uncomplicated pregnancy in labour

Intermittent auscultation of the FHR with a Pinard stethoscope or a Sonicaid may be appropriate for a healthy woman in labour who has had an uncomplicated pregnancy. This involves documenting the heart rate for a minimum of 60 seconds at least:

- every 15 minutes including after a contraction in the first stage of labour
- every 5 minutes including after a contraction in the second stage of labour

Continuous monitoring is recommended if intermittent auscultation is abnormal or any risk factors develop during the course of the labour, such as meconium-stained liquor.

Who should have continuous cardiotocograph monitoring?

Table 27.1 shows the maternal and fetal indications for recommending continuous monitoring.

Table 27.1 Indications for recommending continuous fetal monitoring

Categories	Indication for continuous monitoring
Maternal	Previous caesarean section Preeclampsia Diabetes Antepartum haemorrhage Other maternal medical disease
Fetal	Intrauterine growth restriction Prematurity Oligohydramnios Abnormal Doppler artery studies Multiple pregnancy Breech presentation
Intrapartum	Meconium-stained liquor Vaginal bleeding in labour Use of oxytocin for augmentation Epidural analgesia Maternal pyrexia Post-term pregnancy Prolonged rupture of membranes >24 hours Induced labour

FEATURES OF THE CARDIOTOCOGRAPH

There are four features of the CTG, which should all be assessed individually and then taken together with the clinical picture to determine the appropriate management of the patient. For example, an antepartum haemorrhage or the presence of meconium-stained liquor should prompt more timely intervention:

> **HINTS AND TIPS**
>
> Use the following tool to assess the cardiotocograph DR C BRAVADO:
>
> D define
> R risk
> C contractions
> B baseline
> R rate
> A accelerations
> V variability
> A and
> D decelerations
> O overall assessment

Table 27.2 Categorization of the features of the fetal heart rate according to National Institute for Health and Care Excellence (NICE) guidelines

Feature	Baseline [beats per minute (bpm)]	Variability (bpm)	Decelerations	Accelerations
Reassuring	110–160	5–25	None present	Present
Nonreassuring	100–109 161–180	<5 for 50 minutes		None present
Abnormal	<100 >180	≤5 for ≥90 minutes	Atypical variable decelerations Late decelerations Single deceleration >3 minutes	None present

- **Baseline FHR**: this is the mean level of FHR over a period of 5–10 minutes. It is expressed as beats per minute (bpm) and is determined by the fetal sympathetic and parasympathetic nervous systems. The normal range is 110–160 bpm. In the preterm fetus, the baseline tends to be at the higher end of the normal range.
- **Baseline variability**: minor fluctuations occur in the baseline FHR at three to five cycles/min. It is measured by estimating the difference in bpm between the highest peak and the lowest trough of change in a 1-minute segment of the trace. Normal baseline variability is 5–25 bpm.
- **Accelerations**: these are increases in the FHR of 15 bpm or more above the baseline rate, lasting 15 seconds or more. These are a feature of a normal CTG.
- **Decelerations**: these are falls in the FHR of more than 15 bpm below the baseline, lasting 15 seconds or more. Different types of decelerations can be seen, depending on their timing with the uterine contractions:
  1. Early decelerations: the FHR slows at the same time as the onset of the contraction and returns to the baseline at the end of the contraction in an identical pattern with every contraction. These are usually benign.
  2. Variable decelerations: the timing of the slowing of the FHR in relation to the uterine contraction varies within the time frame of the contraction. The deceleration is of rapid onset and recovery, with a particular shape on the recording, known as 'shouldering'. It represents a normal physiological response by the fetus to the stress of a contraction in association with compression of the umbilical cord. However, other features might make this type of deceleration more suspicious, such as loss of the normal baseline variability or loss of the shouldering.
  3. Late decelerations: the FHR begins to fall during the contraction, with its trough more than 20 seconds after the peak of the contraction and returning to baseline after the contraction.

The CTG has been categorized by NICE guidelines, as shown in Table 27.2:

- normal: all four features are reassuring (Fig. 27.1)
- suspicious: one feature is nonreassuring, the others are reassuring
- pathological: two or more features are nonreassuring, one is abnormal (Fig. 27.2)

HINTS AND TIPS

When presenting a cardiotocograph, note:

- patient's name
- date and time
- maternal pulse
- baseline fetal heart rate
- baseline variability
- presence or absence of accelerations
- presence or absence of decelerations

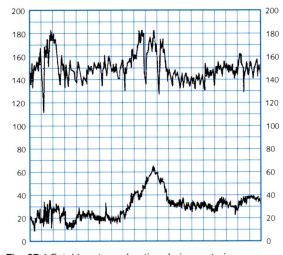

Fig. 27.1 Fetal heart acceleration during a uterine contraction with normal baseline variability.

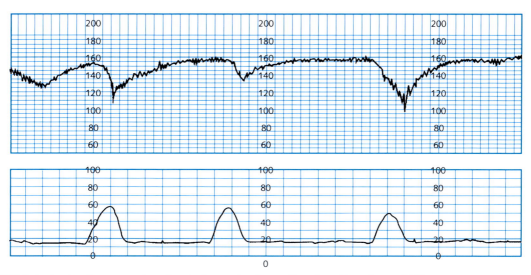

Fig. 27.2 Late decelerations occurring after uterine contractions with reduced baseline variability.

PHYSIOLOGY

The principle of monitoring during labour is to detect fetal hypoxia and, therefore, prevent fetal acidaemia and cell damage.

Acute fetal hypoxia

In a previously well fetus, this can occur secondary to:

- uterine hyperstimulation
- placental abruption
- umbilical cord compression
- sudden maternal hypotension (e.g. insertion of regional anaesthesia)

These conditions can result in a increase in the FHR baseline, with decelerations, produced by a baroreceptor-mediated response, as the fetal blood pressure is affected. If the FHR baseline falls, and this is prolonged to more than 3 minutes (i.e. a fetal bradycardia), the ongoing fetal hypoxia may result in myocardial ischaemia.

Chronic fetal hypoxia

If there has been chronic uteroplacental insufficiency during the pregnancy, for example, secondary to preeclampsia, then the fetus is at increased risk of hypoxia during labour. Reduced intervillous perfusion during uterine contractions or maternal hypotension can exacerbate underlying reduced placental perfusion. This can result in FHR decelerations persisting after the uterine contraction has stopped (late decelerations), and an increase in the fetal cardiac output with an increase in the baseline heart rate. This may be followed by reduced heart rate variability as the fetal chemoreceptors respond to ongoing fetal hypoxia. Prolonged hypoxia eventually produces cerebral and myocardial damage.

CLINICAL NOTES

Remember to look at the changes in the cardiotocograph over time. For example, after 8 hours in labour in a term baby, the baseline rate may be 155 bpm (i.e. within the normal range). But if it was 120 bpm at the start of labour, then this rise is significant and pathology such as fetal infection should be excluded.

MONITORING UTERINE CONTRACTIONS

As well as monitoring the FHR, the CTG also monitors the frequency of the uterine contractions. This is important, for example, if the patient is having intravenous oxytocin to stimulate the contractions. Contractions more than five in 10 minutes will reduce the time of return to resting tone between contractions and this may lead to fetal hypoxia if occurring over a prolonged period.

The actual strength and the length of each contraction should be checked by palpation of the uterus, because the size of the peaks shown on the tracing may be related to positioning of the monitor on the maternal abdomen or thickness of the maternal abdominal wall.

HISTORY OF THE PATIENT WHO PRESENTS WITH AN ABNORMAL CARDIOTOCOGRAPH IN LABOUR

The need to act on an abnormal CTG in labour is influenced by maternal, fetal and intrapartum factors.

Table 27.1 gives the indications for continuous CTG monitoring as well as showing the relevant points in the patient's antenatal history that should make the staff more concerned if the CTG is suspicious. The intrapartum factors are particularly important. In the presence of meconium-stained liquor, for example, the CTG should be acted upon promptly as hypoxia may cause the fetus to gasp and inhale the meconium.

EXAMINATION OF THE PATIENT WHO PRESENTS WITH AN ABNORMAL CARDIOTOCOGRAPH IN LABOUR

Baseline maternal observations

Temperature
A raised maternal temperature might explain fetal tachycardia, for example, if there are ruptured membranes for >24 hours increasing the risk of fetal and maternal infection.

Pulse
This might be raised in conjunction with maternal pyrexia. In the presence of fetal bradycardia, maternal pulse should be checked to ensure the monitoring is recording FHR and not the mother's heart rate. This can be excluded by checking with an ultrasound scan. To aid differentiation between FHR and maternal heart rate, a fetal scalp electrode (FSE) can be applied, provided the cervix is at least 1–2-cm dilated and the membranes are ruptured.

Blood pressure
Administering epidural anaesthesia can be associated with maternal hypotension. This results in reduced blood flow to the uterus and can cause fetal bradycardia. Therefore intravenous fluids are administered and blood pressure regularly checked when the medication is given.

Abdominal palpation

- Uterine size.
- Engagement of presenting part.
- Scar tenderness in a patient with a previous caesarean section.
- Uterine tone.

The size of the maternal abdomen should be assessed to check if it is large or small for dates (see Chapter 23). The engagement of the presenting part is important to assess progress in labour (see Chapter 26). In a patient who has previously had a caesarean section, the presence of scar tenderness should be elicited; scar rupture is commonly associated with an abnormal CTG and vaginal bleeding. Another cause of vaginal bleeding with an abnormal CTG is placental abruption (see Chapter 20). If this is suspected, the uterus will typically feel hard and tender.

The uterine contractions should be palpated, especially if the patient's labour is being stimulated by intravenous oxytocic agents. Hyperstimulation can cause an abnormal FHR. There should be resting tone between contractions.

Vaginal examination

As well as assessing the dilatation of the cervix to determine the progress in labour and the ability to perform a fetal blood sample, the presence of the fetal cord must be excluded. A cord prolapse, as it is known, is associated with a fetal bradycardia as the blood vessels in the cord spasm. This is an emergency situation requiring immediate delivery by caesarean section if the cervix is not fully dilated.

A vaginal examination may also be indicated to apply an FSE to aid distinguishing between maternal heart rate and FHR.

INVESTIGATING THE ABNORMAL CARDIOTOCOGRAPH

If the CTG is categorized as suspicious, the patient can be managed conservatively (Fig. 27.3), for example, by changing maternal position to relieve pressure on the umbilical cord or reducing the dose of syntocinon.

If the CTG is pathological, fetal blood sampling (FBS) should be considered if there are the appropriate facilities. The procedure involves taking a sample of capillary blood from the fetal scalp with the mother in the left lateral position, ruptured membranes and the cervix dilated at least 2–3 cm. A sample of blood from the fetal scalp gives the fetal pH (i.e. a measure of acidosis). The result might indicate that delivery is necessary (pH ≤ 7.20) or that the test should be repeated within 30 minutes (pH 7.21–7.24) or 60 minutes (pH ≥ 7.25). If FBS is not possible, delivery should be expedited by caesarean section.

RED FLAG

Contraindications to fetal blood sampling:
- maternal infection (human immunodeficiency virus/hepatitis B/herpes simplex)
- fetal bleeding disorder (haemophilia/thrombocytopaenia)
- prematurity (<34 weeks)

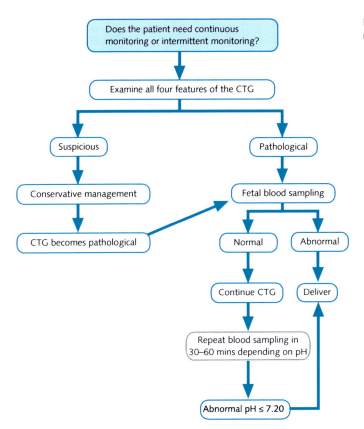

Fig. 27.3 Algorithm for cardiotocograph (CTG) monitoring.

Does the patient need continuous monitoring or intermittent monitoring?

Examine all four features of the CTG

Suspicious

Pathological

Conservative management

Fetal blood sampling

CTG becomes pathological

Normal

Abnormal

Continue CTG

Deliver

Repeat blood sampling in 30–60 mins depending on pH

Abnormal pH ≤ 7.20

● Chapter Summary

- Fetal monitoring in labour can be intermittent or continuous depending on the risk factors associated with the pregnancy.
- The four features of a CTG are baseline rate, variability, acceleration and decelerations.
- The principle of monitoring during labour is to detect fetal hypoxia and, therefore, prevent fetal acidaemia and cell damage.
- A fetal blood sample can be obtained and analysed if the CTG is pathological to establish fetal wellbeing.

FURTHER READING

Gibb, D., Arulkumaran, S., 2017. Fetal monitoring in practice, fourth ed. Churchill Livingstone, London, UK.

International Federation of Gynaecology and Obstetrics (FIGO), 2015. Consensus guidelines on intrapartum fetal monitoring.

FIGO, London, UK. Available at: www.ijgo.org/article/S0020-7292(15)00395-1/fulltext.

National Institute for Health and Care Excellence (NICE), 2014. Intrapartum care for healthy women and babies. CG190. NICE, London, UK. Available at: www.nice.org.uk.

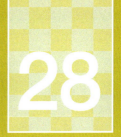
INTRODUCTION

For all interventions in obstetrics, the following general principles apply:

- Make sure all documentation includes the time and date, a legible signature and printed name.
- Clearly record the indication for the intervention, the abdominal and vaginal examination findings as appropriate and the operative findings including any complications.
- Obtain informed consent from the patient, either verbal or written, depending on the procedure.

Table 28.1 Complications of instrumental delivery

Type of complication	Description
Maternal	Genital tract trauma (cervical/vaginal/vulval) with risk of haemorrhage and/or infection
Fetal	Ventouse delivery is likely to cause a chignon (scalp oedema) or, less commonly, a cephalohaematoma (subperiosteal bleed) Forceps can cause bruising if not appropriately applied, or rarely facial nerve palsy or depression skull fracture

VENTOUSE DELIVERY

Since the 1950s, when the vacuum extractor was invented in Sweden, it has increasingly been seen as the instrument of choice for assisted vaginal delivery. Metal cups (Fig. 28.1C) were used initially, either anterior cups or posterior cups. Subsequently, silicone rubber ones (Fig. 28.1A) were developed and more recently, the disposable handheld KIWI cup (Fig. 28.1B). The metal cups are more likely to be associated with trauma to the vagina or the fetal scalp, but may be more appropriate for delivery in certain situations, such as the presence of excessive caput on the fetal head. Along with the KIWI cups, they are useful in the presence of a fetal malposition. Both the metal and silicone cups are available in different diameters depending on the gestation of the fetus. It is not an appropriate instrument at less than 34 weeks' gestation and should be used with caution between 34 and 36 weeks' gestation. Table 28.1 presents the complications of instrumental delivery.

Indications for use of the ventouse cup are:

- Maternal – delay in the second stage of labour due to maternal exhaustion.
- Fetal – abnormal cardiotocograph (CTG) or slow progress in the second stage of labour due to fetal malposition.

Technique for ventouse

The criteria shown in Box 28.1 must be fulfilled.

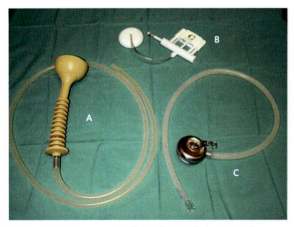

Fig. 28.1 Ventouse cups. (From Simms R, Hayman R: Instrumental vaginal delivery. *Obstet Gynaecol Reprod Med* 23:270–78, 2013. Elsevier Ltd.)

BOX 28.1 CRITERIA FOR INSTRUMENTAL VAGINAL DELIVERY

1. Adequate analgesia: perineal infiltration/pudendal block/epidural anaesthesia (see Chapter 26)
2. Abdominal examination: estimation of fetal size, head either 1/5 or 0/5 palpable
3. Vaginal examination: cervix fully dilated, head either at or below the ischial spines, known fetal position, note presence of caput or moulding
4. Adequate maternal effort and regular contractions necessary for ventouse delivery
5. Empty bladder for forceps delivery

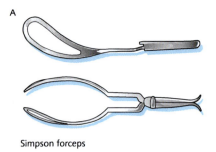

Simpson forceps

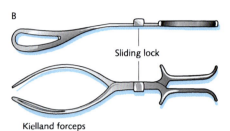

Sliding lock

Kielland forceps

Fig. 28.2 Types of forceps.

All types of cup rely on the same technique. The cup is applied in the midline over or just anterior to the occiput, avoiding the surrounding vaginal mucosa. The suction pressure in the cup is raised to $-0.8\,\text{kg/cm}^2$ or equivalent, either by connection to a separate machine or with the handheld mechanism found within the KIWI cup.

Traction with the maternal contractions and with maternal effort should be along the pelvic curve, that is, initially in a downwards direction and then changing the angle upwards as the head crowns. This action basically mimics the passage of the fetal head during a normal delivery, but uses the vacuum pump to increase traction and flexion.

The operator should judge whether an episiotomy is needed and the procedure should be complete within approximately 15 minutes of cup application. The cardiotocograph should monitor the fetal heart rate throughout and, in most units, it is standard practice for a paediatrician to be present. Complications are listed in Table 28.1.

Table 28.2 Indications for forceps rather than ventouse delivery

Type of indication	Description
Maternal	Medical conditions complicating labour (e.g. cardiovascular disease) Unconscious mother (i.e. conditions where the mother is unable to assist with pushing)
Fetal	Gestation less than 34 weeks Face presentation Known or suspected fetal bleeding disorder After-coming head of a breech At caesarean section

FORCEPS DELIVERY

Over the last three to four centuries, forceps have been used for delivery. There are two main types of forceps (Fig. 28.2):

- non-rotational or traction forceps (Simpson, Anderson, Neville Barnes or Wrigley)
- rotational forceps (Kielland)

Indications for forceps

These are shown in Table 28.2. They differ slightly from those for the ventouse, mainly because the ventouse requires maternal effort and adequate contractions. Non-rotational forceps are suitable only for certain positions of the fetal head – direct occipito-anterior or direct occipito-posterior. By contrast, the mode of action of the ventouse cup allows rotation to take place during traction and so it is suitable for a malposition (see Chapter 29).

With a decline in the use of rotational forceps in some units due to fetal and maternal complications such as extended vaginal wall tears, it is essential to define the fetal position before attempting delivery, so that the appropriate instrument is chosen and the correct technique used.

Technique for forceps

As for the ventouse, the necessary criteria must be fulfilled (see Box 28.1). The blades of non-rotational forceps are applied to the head, avoiding trauma to the vaginal walls. The direction of traction is similar to that of the ventouse, with episiotomy performed when the head crowns to give more space (Fig. 28.3).

Use of the rotational forceps involves a slightly different technique: the knobs on the blades must always point towards the occiput; asynclitism can be corrected using the sliding mechanism of the handles and then rotation achieved prior to traction in the manner described above.

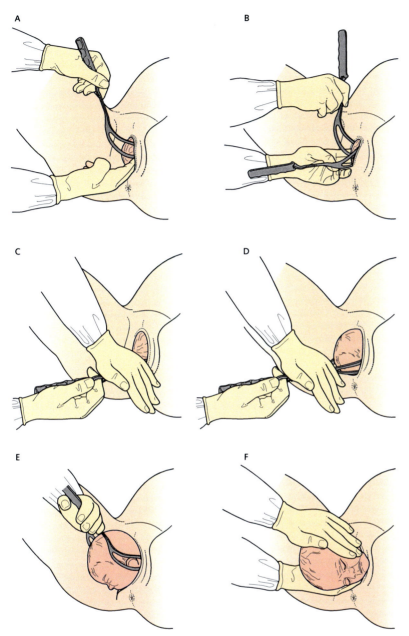

A B

C D

E F

Fig. 28.3 Forceps delivery: change the application of blades.

EPISIOTOMY

The purpose of an episiotomy is to increase the diameter of the vulval outlet by making an incision in the perineal body. Since the 1980s, the routine episiotomy rate has been reduced dramatically because studies have demonstrated its association with increased blood loss, as well as long-term morbidity such as pain and dyspareunia. However, there are still indications for its use (Table 28.3).

Two techniques are used for episiotomy (Fig. 28.4). Both should be performed with adequate analgesia, either an

Table 28.3 Indications for episiotomy

Type of indication	Description
Maternal	Female circumcision [Consider if previous perineal reconstructive surgery]
Fetal	Instrumental delivery
	Breech delivery
	Shoulder dystocia
	Abnormal cardiotocograph

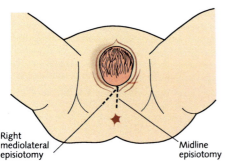

Right mediolateral episiotomy   Midline episiotomy

Fig. 28.4 Types of incision for episiotomy.

epidural, pudendal or perineal infiltration with local anaesthetic, and should start in the midline at the posterior fourchette:

1. Mediolateral: widely used in the UK, this type of incision is more likely to protect the anal sphincter if the incision extends during delivery.
2. Midline: this technique is widely used in the USA and, although it is easier to repair and likely to result in less postpartum pain, it is more likely to involve the anal sphincter if it extends.

Repair of an episiotomy should be performed by an experienced operator. There should be adequate light and appropriate analgesia. A three-layer technique is normally practised, with absorbable sutures (Fig. 28.5):

*   First layer – vaginal skin: identify the apex of the incision and suture in a continuous layer to the hymen to oppose the cut edges of the posterior fourchette.
*   Second layer – perineal body: deep sutures to realign the muscles of the perineal body.

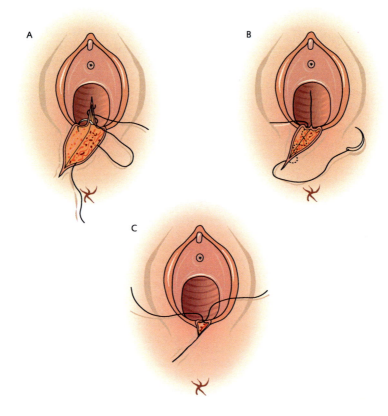

Fig. 28.5 Repair of an episiotomy. (A) Suturing the vaginal wall. (B) Suturing the perineal muscles. (C) Subcuticular sutures to the perineal skin. Tying the strands together – the knot disappears beneath the vaginal mucosa.

- Third layer – perineal skin: continuous subcuticular or interrupted sutures to close the skin.

An examination of the vagina should be performed to ensure that the apex of the episiotomy is secure. Rectal examination should ensure the rectal mucosa has not been broached by any deep sutures because this can result in fistula formation.

RED FLAG

At the end of the procedure all needles and swabs should be accounted for as a retained swab or instrument is classified by NHS Improvement as a 'Never event'.

PERINEAL REPAIR

Approximately 70% of mothers who deliver vaginally will sustain some degree of perineal trauma. This can be classified as:

- first degree: involves skin only
- second degree: involves skin and perineal muscle
- third degree: includes partial or complete rupture of the anal sphincter (see Table 28.4)
- fourth degree: as for third degree, but also involves the anal mucosa

The principles for repair are the same as for episiotomy. Some first-degree tears can be allowed to heal by primary or secondary intention if they are not actively bleeding. It is very important to recognize and repair appropriately any damage to the anal sphincter or mucosa; failure to do so can result in long-term morbidity, such as urgency of stool, or incontinence of flatus or faeces (this occurs in approximately 5% of women).

COMMUNICATION

Approximately 3% of patients sustain a third- or fourth-degree tear. These patients need to be debriefed postnatally regarding the extent of their tear. They should be advised to take antibiotics, analgesia and laxatives during their recovery. They may also require referral for physiotherapy depending on local policy. The discussion should involve mode of delivery and risks in a future pregnancy alongside a patient information leaflet.

Table 28.4 Classification of third-degree tears

Grade 3a tear	Less than 50% of external anal sphincter (EAS) thickness torn
Grade 3b tear	More than 50% of EAS thickness torn
Grade 3c tear	Both EAS and internal anal sphincter (IAS) torn
Fourth-degree tear	Injury to the perineum involving the anal sphincter complex (EAS and IAS) and anorectal mucosa

CAESAREAN SECTION

Caesarean section was first described by the ancient Egyptians. It was used increasingly throughout the 20th century such that rates of 25% are now common in units in the UK. The lower segment procedure [lower segment caesarean section (LSCS)] was introduced in the 1920s and has largely replaced the 'classical' midline uterine incision. Although the latter is sometimes indicated for preterm delivery with a poorly formed lower segment or for a preterm abnormal lie, it is associated with higher rates of haemorrhage and rupture in future labours (up to 5% for midline operation, <1% for lower segment procedure).

Indications for lower segment caesarean section

These are shown in Table 28.5.

Table 28.5 Indications for lower segment caesarean section

Type of indication	Description
Maternal	Two previous lower segment caesarean section Placenta praevia Maternal disease (e.g. fulminating preeclampsia) Maternal request with no obstetric indication Active primary genital herpes simplex virus Human immunodeficiency virus disease depending on viral load
Fetal	Breech presentation Twin pregnancy if the presentation of first twin is not cephalic Abnormal cardiotocograph or abnormal fetal blood sample in first stage Cord prolapse Delay in first stage of labour (e.g. due to malpresentation or malposition)

Technique for lower segment caesarean section

An elective LSCS is usually performed at 39 or more weeks' gestation. Delivery at this gestation reduces the respiratory morbidity in the infant – transient tachypnoea of the newborn. With regional analgesia more commonly used than general analgesia, a low transverse skin incision is made. The rectus sheath is cut and the rectus muscles divided. The uterovesical peritoneum is incised to allow the bladder to be reflected inferiorly. The lower uterine segment is incised transversely and the fetus is delivered manually.

Intravenous oxytocin is given by the anaesthetist and the placenta and membranes are removed. The angles of the uterine incision are secured to ensure haemostasis and then the uterus is closed with an absorbable suture, usually in two layers. The rectus sheath is closed to avoid incisional hernias and, finally, the skin is closed with either an absorbable or nonabsorbable suture.

> **ETHICS**
>
> You cannot proceed to caesarean section without consent from the mother even if there is acute fetal distress. This can be verbal or written consent.

Complications of lower segment caesarean section

Although LSCS has become an increasingly safe procedure, particularly with the introduction of regional anaesthesia, there is still significant morbidity associated with it:

- Haemorrhage – all patients should have a group-and-save sample sent; cross-match blood for certain patients (e.g. those with placenta praevia).
- Infection – reduced by routine use of prophylactic antibiotics.

- Thromboembolic disease – prophylaxis in all patients for up to 6 weeks depending on other risk factors.
- Visceral injury – damage to bladder or bowel, particularly with a history of previous abdominal surgery, most commonly a previous LSCS.
- Gastric aspiration – particularly with general anaesthetic (Mendelson syndrome), this is reduced by routine use of antacids.
- Future pregnancy – may be suitable for vaginal birth after caesarean (VBAC; see the following section) or may be advised repeat LSCS. This carries an increasing risk of complications (e.g. placenta praevia).

Vaginal birth after caesarean

In patients who have had a pregnancy complicated by caesarean section, options for future deliveries should be discussed. For the majority of women who have had one previous LSCS, vaginal delivery can be offered if they go into spontaneous labour (VBAC). The main serious fetal and maternal risk is scar rupture, which occurs in 0.5% of pregnancies. In the case of a classical caesarean, the possibility of scar rupture in labour is high (up to 5%) and thus repeat LSCS would be recommended.

Patients who agree to VBAC need to be counselled regarding care in labour, as well as possible recourse to repeat LSCS:

- intravenous cannula
- full blood count and group-and-save sample available in laboratory
- continuous CTG monitoring
- monitor vaginal loss to exclude bleeding
- monitor abdominal pain: scar rupture can present with continuous pain, as opposed to intermittent contractions

With appropriate monitoring, vaginal delivery rates of approximately 70% can be expected.

● **Chapter Summary**

- The aim of operative vaginal delivery is to replicate a vaginal delivery to expedite the delivery and reduce neonatal and maternal morbidity.
- Perineal trauma should be assessed by appropriately trained staff who can correctly identify a third-degree tear after delivery and arrange immediate repair to reduce maternal morbidity.
- A caesarean section is major abdominal surgery and is associated with an increased risk of bleeding, infection, thromboembolic disease and visceral injury.
- A vaginal birth after caesarean section is associated with a 0.5% risk of scar rupture and women should be counselled adequately.

FURTHER READING

National Institute for Health and Care Excellence (NICE), 2011. CG 132. Caesarean section. NICE, London, UK.

Royal College of Obstetricians and Gynaecologists (RCOG), 2011. Operative vaginal delivery. RCOG green-top guidelines no. 26. RCOG, London, UK. Available at: www.rcog.org.uk.

Royal College of Obstetricians and Gynaecologists (RCOG), 2015. Birth after previous caesarean birth. RCOG green-top guidelines no. 45. RCOG, London, UK. Available at: www.rcog.org.uk.

Royal College of Obstetricians and Gynaecologists (RCOG), 2015. Third and fourth degree perineal tears: management. RCOG green-top guidelines no. 29. RCOG, London, UK. Available at: www.rcog.org.uk.

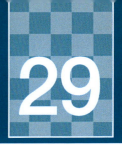
MALPRESENTATION

Any presentation other than a vertex presentation is a malpresentation. The vertex is the area between the parietal eminences and the anterior and posterior fontanelles. The most common malpresentation is the breech presentation, whilst others include shoulder, brow and face presentations.

Malpresentation can occur by chance, but it can also be caused by fetal or maternal conditions that prevent the vertex from presenting to the pelvis (Table 29.1). In all cases, management of malpresentation must begin by exclusion of important conditions such as fetal abnormality, pelvic masses and placenta praevia.

Breech presentation

Apart from the general causes of malpresentation, breech presentation is particularly associated with prematurity. The incidence of breech presentation increases with decreasing gestation:

- term: 3%
- 32 weeks: 15%
- 28 weeks: 25%

Classification of breech presentation

There are three types of breech presentation:

- extended or frank breech (approximately 50%)
- flexed or complete breech (approximately 25%)
- footling breech (approximately 25%)

Table 29.1 Causes of malpresentation	
Maternal	Contraction of the pelvis
	Pelvic tumour
	(e.g. fibroid)
	Mullerian abnormality
	Multiparity
Fetoplacental	Prematurity
	Placenta praevia
	Polyhydramnios
	Multiple pregnancy
	Fetal anomaly
	• hydrocephalus
	• extension of the fetal head by neck tumours
	• anencephaly
	• decreased fetal tone

With an extended breech, the hips are flexed and the knees extended with the feet situated adjacent to the fetal head. Flexed and footling breeches are flexed at both the hips and knees, but in the latter the feet present to the maternal pelvis not the breech (Fig. 29.1).

Diagnosis

The head can be felt as a hard lump at the uterine fundus by the examiner and the patient. Auscultation of the fetal heart at a higher level than is usual with a cephalic presentation might suggest a breech presentation, although this is not a reliable sign. Vaginal examination in labour can confirm the diagnosis, If there is any doubt, ultrasound examination is indicated, which will also determine the type of breech presentation.

Complications

There is increased perinatal mortality and morbidity associated with vaginal breech delivery when compared with cephalic presentation of comparable birthweight at term. This is usually associated with difficulty in delivering the aftercoming head. The fetal trunk is softer than the head and can pass through the pelvis easily. Compared with a cephalic delivery, there is relatively little time for moulding to occur, which may result in entrapment of the aftercoming head. If the fetal arms become extended behind the head during delivery (known as 'nuchal arms'), this may also reduce the available space for the head. Rapid compression and decompression of the head during delivery can produce intracranial injury. Unfortunately, no method of antenatal assessment, clinical, radiological or ultrasonic, will guarantee easy delivery of the aftercoming head.

Cord prolapse may occur if the cervix is poorly applied to the presenting part and is most likely to occur with a footling breech and a preterm breech. Birth trauma is associated with difficulty in delivery of the aftercoming head or soft-tissue injury due to excessive traction to the fetus. The causes of morbidity and mortality associated with birth trauma following vaginal breech delivery include:

- intracranial haemorrhage/tentorial tear
- spinal cord injury
- soft-tissue injury
- liver rupture
- adrenal haemorrhage
- nerve palsies (e.g. brachial plexus or facial nerve)
- fractures of the clavicle or humerus

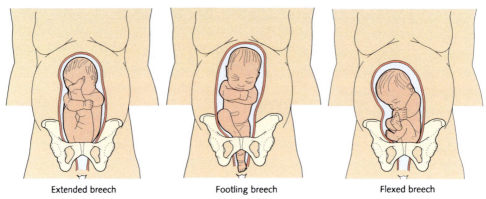

| Extended breech | Footling breech | Flexed breech |

Fig. 29.1 Classification of breech presentation.

MANAGEMENT

There are three management options for a breech presentation:

- external cephalic version (ECV)
- elective caesarean section
- planned vaginal breech delivery

All women with a term breech presentation should be offered ECV, preferably at around 37 weeks gestation. If this is not successful or they decline, then the options are caesarean section or vaginal delivery. Following the publication of a large, randomized, prospective trial, the gold-standard management of a breech presentation at term is delivery by caesarean section. This trial indicated a significantly lower incidence of complications in term breech babies born by caesarean section than by the vaginal route.

External cephalic version

An attempt is made to turn the fetus to a cephalic presentation by manual manipulation through the maternal anterior abdominal wall. This is usually performed at around 37 weeks' gestation, to allow time for spontaneous version, and to minimize the number of successful versions turning back to breech. Contraindications to ECV include:

- pelvic mass
- antepartum haemorrhage
- placenta praevia
- multiple pregnancy
- ruptured membranes

ECV can be performed with the aid of tocolytics, to reduce uterine activity, or under spinal anaesthesia, to reduce discomfort felt by the patient, and under ultrasound control. It should be performed on the labour ward because of the small risk of fetal distress requiring immediate caesarean section (1:300). The fetus can be rolled forwards or backwards and version is successful in about half the cases. Extended breeches are more difficult to turn because the legs 'splint' the fetus. Rhesus-negative women should be given anti-D immunoglobulin following attempted version because of the possibility of feto-maternal transfusion.

Antenatal assessment for vaginal breech delivery

For those women who choose to undergo a trial of vaginal breech delivery prior assessment should include fetal size. It is important to exclude a macrosomic fetus by ultrasound-estimated fetal weight (EFW). A fetus with an

EFW of greater than 4 kg may be best delivered by caesarean section. However, ultrasound EFW at term is associated with an error of 10%–20%.

Management of labour with a breech presentation

Delivery should be in an obstetric unit with an attendant neonatologist, as vaginal breech delivery should be regarded as high risk. Management of the first stage of labour should be as for a vertex presentation, although some obstetricians do not advocate the use of syntocinon for slow progress – preferring to perform a caesarean section instead. Continuous fetal heart rate monitoring is recommended. Exclusion of cord prolapse is mandatory when the membranes rupture or if the fetal heart rate pattern becomes abnormal. Epidural anaesthesia is recommended because of the increased level of manipulation during delivery. Approximately half of planned vaginal breech deliveries will be successful because of the lower threshold to perform caesarean section.

During the second stage, the breech should be allowed to descend onto the pelvic floor before active pushing is commenced. If descent does not occur, this could indicate disproportion or an unexpectedly large fetus, and caesarean section is indicated. Delivery in the lithotomy position allows access for the attendant to perform any necessary manipulation to the fetus. Lovset manoeuvre, as the body delivers, keeps the fetal spine anterior and aims to reduce the incidence of nuchal arms. Mauriceau–Smellie–Veit manoeuvre improves flexion of the head to allow easier delivery. Routine episiotomy is recommended to further increase access and prevent delay due to the soft tissues.

Transverse lie and unstable lie

A transverse lie occurs when the long axis of the fetus lies transverse or oblique to the long axis of the uterus, usually with the shoulder presenting (Fig. 29.2). When the fetal lie is different at each palpation, the lie is said to be 'unstable'. The incidence of transverse lie diagnosed in labour with a single fetus is approximately 1 in 500 women, but many more will have been identified and managed appropriately antenatally. On abdominal palpation, the fetal head is lateral in the maternal abdomen, and the symphysis-fundal height (SFH) is lower than expected by gestation. Vaginal examination, which should be avoided until placenta praevia has been excluded, will reveal an empty pelvis.

The causes of transverse lie include the general causes of malpresentation shown in Table 29.1, but there is particular association with:

- multiparity, where the tone of the uterus and anterior abdominal wall is poor
- premature labour (see Chapter 25)
- the second twin (see Chapter 24)

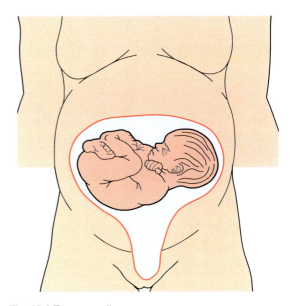

Fig. 29.2 Transverse lie.

The most serious complication of a transverse lie is cord prolapse, and this is associated with spontaneous rupture of membranes, either antenatally or in labour.

Management

Antenatal

Exclusion of causes of malpresentation is important. Elective caesarean section at term is indicated in the presence of placenta praevia or a pelvic mass. In their absence, ECV can be attempted. If reversion to a malpresentation occurs, or an unstable lie is diagnosed, then admission to hospital from 37 weeks gestation is indicated when immediate delivery is possible if the membranes spontaneously rupture. At term, an unstable lie can be managed expectantly because spontaneous version to a cephalic presentation often occurs due to the increase in uterine activity. Transverse lie can be corrected by ECV followed by immediate induction of labour. If the lie remains unstable, then caesarean section is indicated.

Intrapartum

If a transverse lie is diagnosed in early labour, ECV may be attempted only if the membranes are intact. If successful, artificial rupture of membranes (ARM) with the head in the pelvis can stabilize the lie by inducing uterine contractions. If version is not successful or the membranes have ruptured, caesarean section is indicated. ECV of a second twin in transverse lie may be appropriate if the fetal monitoring is normal, as described in Chapter 24, with ARM once the presenting part is in the pelvis.

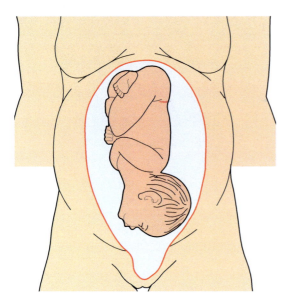

Fig. 29.3 Face presentation.

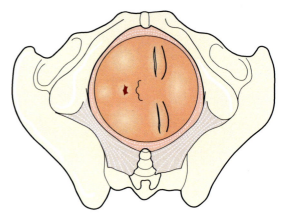

Fig. 29.4 Vaginal examination findings in face presentation.

Face presentation

The incidence of face presentation in labour is 1 in 300 labours and occurs when the head is fully extended (Fig. 29.3). Causes include:

- normal fetus with an extended neck
- congenital tumour of neck
- anencephaly

Diagnosis is usually made during vaginal examination in labour when the supraorbital ridges, the bridge of the nose and the alveolar margins in the mouth are palpable (Fig. 29.4). During labour, the face becomes oedematous and may be mistaken for a breech presentation.

Mechanism of labour

The chin (mentum) is the denominator and the submentobregmatic diameter is 9.5 cm (Fig. 26.4), i.e. the same as the suboccipitobregmatic diameter when the head is fully flexed, so vaginal delivery is possible. Flexion of the head to allow vaginal delivery is possible only in the mentoanterior position, which occurs in 75% of cases.

> **HINTS AND TIPS**
>
> Face presentation will deliver vaginally if it is mentoanterior but not if it is mentoposterior.

Management of a face presentation in labour is essentially the same as for a vertex presentation. Vaginal examination should be performed when the membranes rupture to exclude a cord prolapse. Mentoposterior positions rotate spontaneously to mentoanterior in 50% of cases, usually in the second stage of labour, and in those that do not, a caesarean section is indicated. Caesarean section should also be performed when the fetal heart rate pattern is abnormal, because a fetal blood sample for pH measurement should not be taken from the face. Traction forceps can be applied to a mentoanterior position to correct delay in the second stage.

> **COMMUNICATION**
>
> Patients with a face presentation need to be counselled that during labour the face becomes swollen and the baby can look very bruised when delivered and that this is not permanent and will settle.
>
> Care must be taken during vaginal examination because the fetal eyes can be damaged by trauma or antiseptic lotions.

Brow presentation

The incidence of brow presentation in labour is approximately 1 in 500 and the causes are the same as for a face presentation. Vaginal examination reveals a high presenting part, a palpable forehead with orbital ridges in front and the anterior fontanelle behind.

Mechanism of labour

The membranes tend to rupture early in labour and there is an increased risk of cord prolapse. With a brow presentation, the mentovertical diameter of 13.5 cm presents (Fig. 26.4). An average-sized fetus will not engage with a normal-sized pelvis and obstructed labour results. When the fetal head is small in relation to the maternal pelvis, descent might occur, allowing flexion of the head as it reaches the pelvic floor. In the absence of disproportion, labour should be allowed to continue. Further extension might occur to a face presentation or flexion to a vertex position.

Table 29.2 Differential diagnoses for failure to progress in labour

Bony passages	Abnormal shaped pelvis Cephalopelvic disproportion
Soft passages	Uterine/cervical fibroids Cervical stenosis Circumcision
Passenger	Fetal size Fetal abnormality Fetal malpresentation Fetal malposition
Power	Lack of coordinated regular strong uterine contractions

FAILURE TO PROGRESS IN LABOUR

As described in Chapter 26, labour and delivery require the interaction of three components – the passages, the passenger and power – as part of a dynamic process:

- passages: the shape and size of the hard bony pelvis and soft tissues
- passenger: the size, presentation and position of the fetus
- power: this is both involuntary (strength and frequency of uterine contractions) and voluntary (diaphragm and abdominal muscles)

Any of these factors can be involved in the failure of labour to progress normally, as summarized in Table 29.2 Once the diagnosis of labour has been made, a primiparous patient is expected to progress at approximately 0.5–1 cm/h and a multiparous patient at 1–2 cm/h.

Failure to progress related to the bony pelvis

Abnormal bony shape
Antenatal X-ray pelvimetry and routine pelvic assessment by vaginal examination are no longer performed. However, certain points in a patient's history and examination can give clues to the likelihood of failure to progress in labour due to an abnormal pelvis (Table 29.3). Although still rare, one of the common problems is a previous pelvic fracture.

Table 29.3 Causes of abnormalities of the bony pelvis

Congenital	Acquired
Osteogenesis imperfecta Ectopia vesicae Dislocation of the hip	Kyphosis of the thoracic or lumbar spine Scoliosis of the spine Spondylolisthesis Pelvic fractures Rickets/osteomalacia Poliomyelitis in childhood

Cephalopelvic disproportion
With true cephalopelvic disproportion (CPD), the size of the pelvis is not in proportion to the fetus. It should be suspected antenatally if the head does not engage at term, particularly in a woman of short stature. Usually, a trial of labour is still appropriate, but in some cases an elective caesarean section is planned. During labour, CPD is diagnosed if the head remains unengaged on abdominal palpation. This is confirmed by assessing station on vaginal examination and by the presence of caput (swelling under the fetal scalp caused by reduction in venous return) and moulding. However, these signs are more commonly found simply with malposition rather than with true CPD.

Failure to progress related to the soft tissues of the pelvis

Uterus
A uterine malformation, such as the presence of a midline septum (a müllerian or developmental abnormality), might prevent the fetus from lying longitudinally, so that a malpresentation is responsible for failure to progress. This can also be rarely caused by uterine fibroids, which may increase the SFH measurement during pregnancy and obstruct labour. The presence of a cervical fibroid might even necessitate caesarean section.

Cervix
Failure of the cervix to dilate during labour despite adequate uterine contractions is rarely secondary to cervical scarring causing stenosis. This could be the result of cervical amputation or cone biopsy.

Vagina
Congenital anomalies of the vagina rarely cause problems with respect to labour and delivery, except in patients who have had reconstructive surgery. Other types of surgery, such as a colposuspension for urinary stress incontinence or repair of a vesicovaginal fistula, generally indicate the need for an elective caesarean section at term, but more to prevent recurrent symptoms rather than because of possible slow progress in labour.

Vulva
Previous perineal tears or episiotomy should not present difficulties during delivery. More problematic is a female circumcision [female genital mutilation (FGM)], which may necessitate an anterior episiotomy to prevent more severe tears and the risk of fistula formation. Ideally, this patient should have been assessed antenatally to make the appropriate plan of care including surgery for reversal of FGM before 20 weeks' gestation.

Ovary

Ovarian cysts in pregnancy are usually incidental findings at routine ultrasound. They can present with abdominal pain during pregnancy, secondary to torsion or haemorrhage (see Chapter 11). They do not cause slow progress in labour because they rise up out of the pelvis as the uterus increases in size.

Failure to progress related to the passenger

Fetal size

The possibility of a large fetus might be suggested by the patient's past medical history, for example, type 1 diabetes, or from the antenatal history, with development of gestational diabetes or hydrops fetalis from rhesus isoimmunization or parvovirus infection (see Chapter 23). In a multiparous patient, it is useful to check the weights of previous deliveries as an assessment of ability to deliver the current infant.

Abdominal palpation is not always accurate as a method of diagnosing a large fetus, although this should be done to assess engagement of the presenting part in labour. Ultrasound is more accurate, provided that gestational age has been correctly estimated early in pregnancy.

During labour, on vaginal examination, the cervix may be felt to be increasingly oedematous. Signs of caput or moulding may be noted on the fetal head. Caput is the boggy swelling on the fetal head as subcutaneous oedema of the scalp develops. Moulding is described in Chapter 26, when the fetal skull bones overlap.

Fetal abnormality

Routine ultrasound scanning is likely to diagnose abnormalities such as a congenital goitre or a lymphangioma. These extend the neck, so that the normal process of flexion cannot take place. This may result in a face or brow presentation (see earlier). Abdominal enlargement caused by the presence of ascites, multicystic kidneys or an umbilical hernia may make delivery difficult. Abnormalities of the fetal skull such as anencephaly should be suspected in labour if the head does not engage and the sutures feel widely spaced on vaginal examination. This condition is a type of spina bifida, again routinely diagnosed on ultrasound scan.

Fetal malposition

The fetal head normally engages with an occipitotransverse position. With descent, the head rotates to an occipitoanterior position as described in Chapter 26. Any position other than occipitoanterior can be associated with failure to progress in labour, namely:

- occipitoposterior (OP) position
- occipitotransverse position

Approximately 20% of vertex presentations in early labour are occipitoposterior. Diagnosis is determined by abdominal palpation:

- maternal lower abdomen that is flattened or concave
- fetal back cannot be palpated anteriorly
- fetal limbs that can be palpated anteriorly

On vaginal examination, the positions of the sutures and fontanelles are determined (see Chapter 26). If the anterior fontanelle is palpable vaginally, then the head is deflexed. If only the posterior fontanelle can be felt, then the head is flexed. This degree of flexion allows the smallest diameter of the head to present. It will, therefore, be more likely to rotate at the pelvic floor and proceed to normal vaginal delivery. The majority of OP positions will rotate during labour in the presence of adequate contractions. The minority will not rotate, but will deliver vaginally in the OP position (face to pubes) if the pelvis is large enough, whilst some will need rotation either manually or with an instrument (see Chapter 28).

Fetal malpresentation

Malpresentation of the fetus is defined as a non-vertex presentation (see above). This can be:

- breech
- shoulder
- face
- brow

Failure to progress related to the power

Uterine palpation monitors frequency, duration and strength of the contractions. The cardiotocograph checks the frequency and duration. However, the recording of the strength can be altered by position of the monitor on the abdomen and maternal obesity and so this must be assessed on palpation. Inefficient uterine action can be diagnosed if labour is prolonged and the contractions are:

- uncoordinated
- fewer than 3–4 in 10 minutes
- lasting less than 60 seconds

After thorough abdominal and vaginal examinations, and with normal fetal monitoring, careful use of oxytocic drugs, usually intravenous syntocinon infusion, can improve the contractions. Caution must be taken to avoid too frequent contractions because this can reduce the oxygen exchange in the placental bed and lead to fetal hypoxia. Continuous electronic monitoring is advisable.

Particular care is essential in a multiparous patient because the diagnosis of inefficient uterine action is much less common than in a primiparous patient. A fetal malposition, malpresentation or increased fetal size should be considered as the cause of the slow progress; inappropriate use of oxytocic drugs is associated with uterine rupture in this group.

MANAGEMENT OF FAILURE TO PROGRESS

This depends on the cause. Contractions may be improved with:

- artificial rupture of membranes (ARM)
- use of intravenous syntocinon

ARM is thought to release local prostaglandins and can increase the rate of labour progression. The strength and frequency of the uterine contractions can also be improved by administration of an infusion of intravenous syntocinon (synthetic oxytocin). However, caution must be exercised in a multiparous patient. In general, labour proceeds more rapidly in a second pregnancy. Therefore if progress is slow, fetal size and position must be considered so that excessive contractions do not put the patient at risk of uterine rupture with syntocinon. Regular strong contractions will help to correct a fetal malposition by rotating the head against the pelvic floor muscles, as well as improving descent. Malpresentation may be managed as described above.

The presence of good contractions over several hours but without significant progression in terms of cervical dilatation and descent of the presenting part should alert the physician to consider delivery by caesarean section.

Failure to progress in the second stage of labour should be assessed in the manner already described and instrumental delivery considered (see Chapter 27). If the head is almost crowning, then an episiotomy might be all that is necessary to expedite vaginal delivery.

SHOULDER DYSTOCIA

Shoulder dystocia is a problem of the pelvic inlet preventing delivery of the shoulders once the head is out. This occurs because the shoulders fail to pass through the pelvic inlet; it is not a problem with the outlet or the perineum. The essential point is not to use excessive traction on the fetal head to facilitate delivery of the shoulders because this risks damage to the brachial plexus nerve roots in the neck. Increasing hypoxia occurs while the fetus is lodged in the vagina, with pressure on the umbilical cord. The more common injury to the fetus is Erbs palsy caused by damage

to nerve roots C4, C5 and C6, which can have serious long-term neurological sequelae. Manoeuvres to aid delivery include:

- Lie the patient flat.
- McRoberts position — the hips are flexed in knee–chest position to widen the anteroposterior diameter of the pelvis.
- Suprapubic pressure to dislodge the anterior shoulder.
- Internal rotation techniques to try and rotate the anterior shoulder from under the pubic symphysis.
- Deliver the posterior arm.

This situation is an emergency and should therefore be practised as a regular drill by all the staff on the maternity unit. A senior neonatologist should be called to attend urgently to assess the baby at delivery.

HINTS AND TIPS

A useful pneumonic for management of a shoulder dystocia – HELPERR

call for *help*
*e*valuate for episiotomy
*l*egs into McRoberts
su*p*rapubic *p*ressure
*e*nter manoeuvres (internal rotation)
*r*emove posterior arm
*r*oll onto all fours

COMMUNICATION

Because of the high rate of litigation associated with shoulder dystocia due to the long-term sequelae of an Erbs palsy, good documentation is important. Shoulder dystocia proformas should be used with careful documentation of the timing of each manoeuvre and who performed it. There must be clear documentation as to which shoulder was anterior during the delivery.

Chapter Summary

- The most common malpresentation is a breech presentation, for which an external cephalic version, vaginal breech delivery or caesarean section is offered depending on the history and the patient's wishes.
- Other malpresentations include transverse lie, oblique lie, face presentation and brow presentation.
- Failure to progress in labour can be due to an abnormality of the passage, passenger or powers.
- Management of failure to progress in labour due to inadequate contractions can be treated with ARM followed by the use of a syntocinon infusion.
- Shoulder dystocia occurs when the anterior shoulder of the baby fails to pass under the symphysis pubis; however, there are various manoeuvres to aid delivery.

FURTHER READING

Hannah, M.E., Hannah, W.J., Hewson, S.A., et al., 2000. Planned caesarean section versus planned vaginal birth for breech presentation at term: a randomized multicentre trial. Term Breech Trial Collaborative Group. Lancet 356, 1375–1383. https://doi.org/10.1016/S0140-6736(00)02840-3.

National Institute for Health and Care Excellence (NICE), 2007. Intrapartum care. NICE, London, UK. Available at: www.nice.org.uk.

Royal College of Obstetricians and Gynaecologists (RCOG), 2017. External Cephalic Version and Reducing the Incidence of Term Breech Presentation. RCOG green-top guidelines no.20a. RCOG, London, UK. Available at: www.rcog.org.uk.

Royal College of Obstetricians and Gynaecologists (RCOG), 2017. Breech presentation, management. RCOG green-top guidelines no. 20b. RCOG, London, UK. Available at: www.rcog.org.uk.

Royal College of Obstetricians and Gynaecologists (RCOG), 2009. Female genital mutilation, management. RCOG green-top guidelines no. 53. RCOG, London, UK. Available at: www.rcog.org.uk.

Royal College of Obstetricians and Gynaecologists (RCOG), 2012. Shoulder dystocia. RCOG green-top guidelines no. 42. RCOG, London, UK. Available at: www.rcog.org.uk.

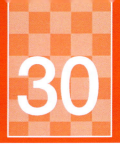

Stillbirth 30

INTRODUCTION

Despite advances in prenatal and antenatal care, stillbirth is still a common occurrence and has a massive impact on the families affected. Investigations into the cause of stillbirth by means of maternal investigations and a postmortem are aimed at reducing the risk of this devastating situation recurring in a future pregnancy and potentially identifying causes, which may help reduce the overall incidence (Table 30.1).

DEFINITIONS

- Stillbirth: A baby that is born with no signs of life at or after 24 completed weeks of pregnancy.
- Intrauterine death: A fetus in-utero greater than 24 completed weeks of pregnancy found to have no cardiac activity.

Table 30.1 Causes of stillbirth

Type of condition	Causes of stillbirth
Maternal condition	Diabetes (pre-existing and gestational) Pre-eclampsia Sepsis Obstetric cholestasis Acute fatty liver Thrombophilias (e.g. protein C and protein S resistance, factor V Leiden mutation, antithrombin III deficiency)
Fetal condition	Infection: *Toxoplasma*, *Listeria*, syphilis, parvovirus Chromosomal abnormality Structural abnormality Rhesus disease leading to severe anaemia Twin-to-twin transfusion syndrome (affects monochorionic twins only) Intra-uterine growth restriction Alloimmune thrombocytopaenia
Placental condition	Postmaturity Abruption Placenta praevia: significant bleed Cord prolapse

INCIDENCE

As mentioned above stillbirth is common, with a rate of 3.87 per 1000 total births. In 2015 there were 3032 stillbirths in the UK, with Wales having the highest rate. More than 50% of stillbirths were found to be unexplained.

DIAGNOSIS

Most commonly a diagnosis of an intrauterine death is made when the patient presents with a history of reduced fetal movements. Occasionally it will be made during a routine antenatal visit when the clinician is unable to auscultate the fetal heart. It can also present with symptoms of the event that caused the baby to die, for example, antepartum haemorrhage and abdominal pain associated with a placental abruption (see Chapter 20).

When a patient presents with reduced fetal movements and one is unable to auscultate the fetal heart using a cardiotocography machine or handheld Doppler, this should prompt rapid referral to a trained clinician to perform an ultrasound scan. If there is no fetal heart activity, then the diagnosis of an intrauterine death can be made. Ideally, this should be verified by a second appropriately trained individual.

TELLING THE PARENTS

Conveying the diagnosis of an intrauterine death to the parents can be one of the most challenging things a clinician ever has to do. It is imperative that the parents are told straight away in a sensitive and empathetic manner using clear unambiguous terms. Occasionally, if a mother presents on her own, one should offer to call her partner or a relative to come and join her.

COMMUNICATION

Breaking bad news is an important skill for all clinicians. Think about the environment in which you are going to do this and ensure the patient has appropriate support. Also try to give the patient the time she needs, so if possible, hand over bleeps to colleagues as these could be a distraction.

HISTORY

Taking a history from a patient diagnosed with an intrauterine death is aimed at:

- assessing maternal wellbeing
- identifying potential causes

Using the handheld obstetric notes to review their past obstetric and medical history or by direct questioning of the patient, the following points should be identified:

- Maternal rhesus group – mothers that are rhesus negative should be investigated to rule out the possibility of rhesus disease as cause of the stillbirth (see Chapter 19: Antenatal booking and prenatal diagnosis).
- Trisomy screening – trisomy screening is usually offered to patients in the first trimester, and the results should be checked. In patients found to be high risk, a chromosomal abnormality may be the cause.
- Ultrasound – the anomaly ultrasound scan and any subsequent growth scans should be reviewed, as any abnormality (either structural or growth related) may indicate a potential cause.
- Antepartum haemorrhage – recurrent bleeds or, indeed, a large bleed may indicate a placental abruption or vasa praevia (a situation where unprotected placental vessels course through the membranes and if ruptured can lead to rapid loss of fetal blood and fetal death). See Chapter 20.
- Ruptured membranes – any history of vaginal fluid loss may indicate a breach in the fetal membranes exposing the fetus to ascending infection (chorioamnionitis).
- Itching – itching mainly affecting the palms and soles may indicate obstetric cholestasis, which is associated with an increased risk of stillbirth (see Chapter 22).
- Signs of maternal illness – fever, rash or vomiting may indicate an intercurrent illness as the cause of the fetal demise. Listeria, toxoplasmosis and parvovirus are all possible infections that can lead to intrauterine death.

EXAMINATION

A thorough general examination is important to identify any potential signs of maternal illness. Even in the absence of a preceding maternal illness, an intrauterine death can lead to maternal sepsis and/or coagulopathy. Examination should include:

- maternal pulse
- blood pressure
- respiratory rate
- temperature
- looking for rashes (may indicate maternal infection) or
- excoriations (may indicate obstetric cholestasis)

The uterus should also be palpated to assess its size, tone and contour. A uterus that is larger than one would expect for the gestation may indicate polyhydramnios, which can be secondary to maternal diabetes (see Chapter 22). A uterus that is smaller than expected may indicate intrauterine growth restriction. A tender firm uterus may indicate a placental abruption, whereas a tender but soft uterus may indicate chorioamnionitis.

INVESTIGATIONS

Investigations in the setting of an intrauterine death are aimed at:

1. assessing the current state of maternal wellbeing
2. identifying a potential cause of the stillbirth
3. possibly identifying any prognostic factors for future pregnancy

It is important that parents are told that in around 50% of all cases, no cause will be found. However, investigation is still essential – if a cause is found, this may be vital in preventing recurrence.

Haematology and biochemistry

- Full blood count – Assess maternal haemoglobin levels in the context of a haemorrhage, maternal white cells if infection is suspected and platelets if a coagulopathy is suspected.
- C-reactive protein – Useful in infection, although non-specific as to the site.
- Urea and electrolytes – Assess renal function in pre-eclampsia, haemorrhage and sepsis, also useful as a baseline.
- Liver function tests – Assess in pre-eclampsia, obstetric cholestasis, haemorrhage and sepsis, also useful as a baseline.
- Coagulation screen – Assess the possibility of coagulopathy.
- Kleihauer – Essential for ALL women (not just those who are rhesus negative) to estimate a fetomaternal haemorrhage AND allows dose calculation of anti-D in rhesus-negative patients.
- Maternal thrombophilia screen with or without antibody screen – Indicated if intrauterine growth restriction or hydrops is identified, respectively.
- Random blood sugar and HbA1c – May indicate gestational diabetes or indeed previously undiagnosed type 1 or type 2 diabetes.
- Maternal thyroid function – May indicate occult thyroid disease.
- Parental karyotyping – Indicated if fetal karyotype indicates an unbalanced translocation or if fetal karyotyping is not possible and features indicate a chromosomal cause.

Microbiology

- Urinalysis and midstream urine – Assess the possibility of urinary tract infection; proteinuria may indicate pre-eclampsia and ketonuria in a diabetic patient would prompt assessment to rule out ketoacidosis.
- Blood cultures, vaginal swabs, cervical swabs – Should be performed if sepsis is suspected as they will allow accurate identification of a pathogen and appropriate antibiotic therapy.
- Placental and fetal swabs should be taken to rule out chorioamnionitis.
- Maternal infection serology – Parvovirus B19, toxoplasmosis, rubella, cytomegalovirus, syphilis (TORCH screen).

Pathology

A postmortem examination should be offered to all parents when an intrauterine death has been diagnosed. It is carried out by a specialist perinatal pathologist. A full postmortem involves examination of the placenta and fetal karyotype, as well as the fetus. A limited postmortem allows the parents to specify the organs or body compartments they wish to be examined. This can be of relevance when a specific organ abnormality was suspected antenatally, for example, on the anomaly scan. An external postmortem examination can be performed using imaging modalities, but this is likely to give only limited information. It is important to inform parents that agreeing to a postmortem may affect the timing of funeral arrangements.

ETHICS

Some individuals may have religious or cultural beliefs against a postmortem and these should be respected. An external postmortem examination with imaging or placental examination only may be acceptable. Informed consent involves explaining that such tests will give less information.

MANAGEMENT

Once an intrauterine death has been confirmed and the parents have been informed, it is important to allow them the time to absorb the information, as well as starting to grieve.

Subsequently, a plan of care needs to be made detailing the method of delivery.

In most cases a vaginal delivery will be the most suitable way to deliver the fetus, having less impact on mode of delivery for a subsequent pregnancy. An antiprogesterone (mifepristone) is given orally and then after 36–48 hours, a course of prostaglandins (e.g. misoprostol) is administered, either orally or vaginally. For gestations nearer term, an oxytocin infusion may be used as an alternative to the prostaglandin.

Rarely, labour is contraindicated (e.g. multiple previous caesarean sections or extensive uterine surgery), and a caesarean section may be required.

COMMUNICATION

Following delivery, the parents are encouraged to hold the baby (if they wish to do so) and mementoes such as pictures and foot/hand prints are taken. Religious ceremonies can also take place if the parents wish.

AFTER DELIVERY

Most units have a specialist midwife who acts as a direct contact for the patient and ensures appropriate follow-up counselling and investigations take place. They will report all stillbirths to MBRRACE-UK who are responsible for the confidential enquiries. In the UK, support should include details about the Stillbirth & Neonatal Death charity (SANDS), which offers support to parents. The immediate period following a stillbirth is a very vulnerable time for the mother and she is at significant risk of postnatal depression (see Chapter 31). Mothers should be offered cabergoline to suppress lactation if they wish to do so.

It is very important to arrange a follow-up appointment with the consultant in charge of their care to ensure all investigations that were performed are reviewed and a plan made for future pregnancies. If no particular cause for the stillbirth was identified, then the couple can be offered consultant-led antenatal care with regular growth scans in the next pregnancy and induction of labour at an appropriate gestation can be considered. As always, cases need to be handled with great sensitivity and care.

Chapter Summary

- A stillbirth occurs when a baby is born with no signs of life at or after 24 completed weeks of pregnancy.
- An intrauterine death occurs when a fetus in-utero greater than 24 completed weeks of pregnancy is found to have no cardiac activity.
- More than 50% of stillbirths have no cause identified.
- Diagnosis of an intrauterine death is by detecting no fetal heart activity on ultrasound scan. A second clinician should confirm this.
- Investigations to identify a cause for the stillbirth should be undertaken and include haematology, biochemistry, microbiology and a postmortem.
- Vaginal delivery is the most suitable mode of delivery in majority of cases unless there are other risk factors.
- A follow-up appointment should be offered to these couples to discuss results from investigations performed, plans for future pregnancies and concerns or questions that the couple may have.

FURTHER READING

MBRRACE-UK Perinatal Mortality Surveillance for Births in 2016. Available at: www.npeu.ox.ac.uk/mbrrace-uk.

Royal College of Obstetricians and Gynaecologists (RCOG), 2011. Late intrauterine fetal death and stillbirth. RCOG green-top guideline no. 55. Available at: www.rcog.org.uk.

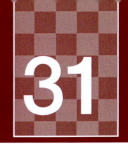
POSTPARTUM HAEMORRHAGE

Definition

Postpartum haemorrhage (PPH) is bleeding from the genital tract of more than 500 mL after delivery of the infant. It is classified as either primary or secondary:

Primary PPH: bleeding more than 500 mL within 24 hours of delivery.

Secondary PPH: bleeding more than 500 mL that starts 24 hours after delivery and occurs within 6 weeks.

In practice, blood loss of more than 1000 mL is more clinically relevant. Most units classify bleeding of more than 1500 mL as major obstetric haemorrhage.

Incidence

The incidence of primary PPH in the developed world is about 5% of deliveries, in contrast to developing countries where it can occur in up to 28% of deliveries and remains the major cause of maternal mortality. The incidence of secondary PPH is lower than that of primary PPH.

Differential diagnoses

Table 31.1 presents the differential diagnoses that should be considered for primary and secondary PPH. About 90% of cases of primary PPH are caused by uterine atony, and about 7% are due to genital tract trauma.

PRIMARY POSTPARTUM HAEMORRHAGE

History

Uterine atony

Risk factors in the patient's history that suggest an increase in the risk of a primary PPH secondary to uterine atony include:

- multiple pregnancy
- grand multiparity
- fetal macrosomia
- polyhydramnios
- fibroid uterus
- prolonged labour
- previous PPH
- antepartum haemorrhage

Table 31.1 Differential diagnoses of postpartum haemorrhage

Type of postpartum haemorrhage	Differential diagnosis
Primary	Uterine atony
	Genital tract trauma (cervix, vagina, perineum)
	Retained placenta/placenta accreta
	Coagulation disorders
	Uterine inversion
	Uterine rupture
Secondary	Retained products
	Endometritis

In a multiple pregnancy, the placental site is larger than with a singleton (see Chapter 24). There is overdistension of the uterus, which is also seen in cases of macrosomia and polyhydramnios (see Chapter 23).

RED FLAG

When the patient presents with primary postpartum haemorrhage, always ask the midwife to check that the placenta and membranes are complete, to exclude retained products of conception.

Mode of delivery

The mode of delivery may increase risk of PPH. Genital tract trauma can occur with a normal vaginal delivery, either from an episiotomy (see Chapter 28) or from a vaginal, cervical or perineal tear. Trauma is more common with an instrumental delivery, especially forceps, in particular Kielland forceps. Therefore the genital tract, including a rectal examination, should always be checked for signs of trauma once the placenta has been delivered.

Average blood loss at caesarean section is 500 mL. Placenta praevia (see Chapter 20) or a prolonged labour may increase this. In the latter, the presenting part may become impacted in the pelvis, making delivery more difficult. This can cause the incision on the uterus to tear, which may increase blood loss.

Rarely, PPH is secondary to uterine inversion that occurs after delivery of the placenta. With bleeding, the patient complains of abdominal pain, which can be severe, associated with a feeling of prolapse. Rupture of the uterus is also an uncommon cause of PPH. It is seen in association with labour in a patient who has previously had a caesarean section.

Other causes

Coagulation disorders can be acute or chronic. The chronic conditions such as inherited vascular disorders are usually known about antenatally. Disseminated intravascular coagulation can present acutely, secondary to placental abruption or severe preeclampsia.

HINTS AND TIPS

When thinking about the causes of primary postpartum haemorrhage, think of the 4 Ts:

- tissue (ie. retained placenta)
- trauma (ie. tears)
- tone (ie. atonic uterus)
- thrombin (ie. coagulation disorders)

The blood loss must be estimated as accurately as possible to manage the patient appropriately. Examination must include the ABC (airways, breathing, circulation) of basic resuscitation (see Chapter 32), as well as pallor, pulse and blood pressure. Abdominal palpation should assess whether the uterus is contracted or not. The fundal height should be at or below the umbilicus. If it is above, there might be retained products of conception or the uterus could be filling with clots.

RED FLAG

Always remember airways, breathing, circulation and basic examination when the patient presents with postpartum haemorrhage.

Uterine inversion should be considered if the fundus is indented or cannot be palpated. Vaginal examination will assess the degree of inversion, either up to the cervical os or complete inversion of the uterus and vagina.

If the placenta and membranes have been delivered, they must be carefully examined to see that the cotyledons appear complete and that there is no suggestion of a succenturiate lobe.

If the uterus is well contracted and the placenta is out and complete, then the bleeding might be from trauma to the

---

BOX 31.1   EXAMINATION OF THE PATIENT WHO PRESENTS WITH PRIMARY POSTPARTUM HAEMORRHAGE

- Airways, breathing, circulation.
- Quantify amount of blood loss.
- Pulse.
- Blood pressure.
- Monitor urine output.
- Assess uterine contraction.
- Assess fundal height.
- Confirm placenta and membranes are complete.
- Assess for genital tract trauma.

---

genital tract. The patient should be examined in sufficient light and with adequate analgesia (either local or regional) to exclude lacerations to the cervix, vagina and perineum. The examination is summarized in Box 31.1.

Investigations

Having established intravenous access, blood should be sent for haemoglobin, platelets, clotting screen including fibrin degradation products and serum save. Depending on the estimated blood loss, cross-matching blood might be necessary. Urea and electrolytes should be tested if the urine output is poor.

Management

Treatment must start with basic resuscitation (ABC) depending on the patient's condition and the extent of the bleeding. It is important to make an accurate estimation of the blood loss, for example, by weighing pads; it is frequently underestimated. Intravenous access must be established. Blood is sent for haemoglobin, platelets, clotting and cross-matching, as above. In cases of massive obstetric haemorrhage, generally classified as ≥1500 mL,

---

COMMUNICATION

Good interdisciplinary communication is essential in obstetrics:
- haematologists in cases of massive postpartum haemorrhage
- microbiologists in cases of sepsis of uncertain origin that does not respond to regular treatment
- psychiatrists in cases of postnatal mental illness

All these disorders are associated with significant maternal morbidity and mortality.

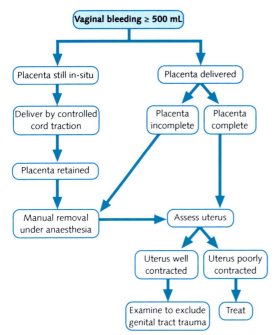

Fig. 31.1 Algorithm for the management of primary postpartum haemorrhage.

a multidisciplinary approach to management is very important, involving liaison between the obstetrician, the anaesthetist and the haematologist. The cause of the bleeding must be identified so that appropriate management can be instigated. Fig. 31.1 provides an algorithm for the management of primary PPH.

Uterine atony

With uterine atony, the uterus is palpated and a contraction rubbed up by massaging the uterus abdominally. Bimanual compression may also be tried. Further oxytocic drugs are given, commonly intravenous syntocinon, initially as a single dose, then proceeding to an intravenous infusion. Intravenous ergometrine can be given if maternal blood pressure has been normal in pregnancy. Prostaglandins may be beneficial, either carboprost can be injected intramuscularly or intramyometrially (also known as 'Hemabate') or misoprostol can be given rectally.

An intrauterine balloon can be inserted either vaginally or via the abdomen if inserted during a caesarean section. The balloon is filled with water so that pressure is applied to the uterine cavity wall and bleeding is reduced.

In severe cases, surgery is necessary and even life-saving. This includes bilateral uterine artery ligation or bilateral internal iliac artery ligation. A B-Lynch compression suture can be performed to avoid hysterectomy and this preserves future fertility. Depending on local facilities, then interventional radiology procedures can be considered. However, prompt recourse to hysterectomy is essential to reduce maternal morbidity and mortality. This management is summarized in Box 31.2.

BOX 31.2   TREATMENT OF PRIMARY POSTPARTUM HAEMORRHAGE SECONDARY TO UTERINE ATONY

- Airways, breathing, circulation.
- Large-bore intravenous (IV) access X2.
- Send full blood count, cross-match, clotting and urea and electrolytes.
- Rub-up uterine contractions by massaging the uterine fundus.
- Give IV oxytocin and ergometrine.
- Start oxytocin infusion.
- Give per rectum/intramuscular/intramyometrial prostaglandin.
- Consider surgical options or uterine artery embolization.

Genital tract trauma

Bleeding while the uterus is firmly contracted is strong evidence of genital tract trauma. In the case of trauma, this should be repaired as soon as possible with appropriate analgesia (see Chapter 28 for perineal repair). There should be good light and an aseptic technique should be applied to minimize infection. Suturing may be necessary in theatre, for example, cervical lacerations bleed profusely and may need to be repaired under general anaesthesia.

Retained or incomplete placenta

If the placenta is still in-situ, delivery should be attempted by controlled cord traction. Once delivered, the placenta must be examined to ensure the cotyledons and the membranes are complete. If the placenta is still retained, manual removal is necessary under regional analgesia in the situation of a PPH. This is usually performed with antibiotic cover and with further doses of oxytocics.

Examination of the patient under anaesthetic allows exploration of the uterus if the placenta is thought to be incomplete. It also enables suturing of genital tract trauma such as cervical or vaginal lacerations once uterine atony is excluded as the cause of the PPH.

Placenta accreta

With routine active management of the third stage of labour, the placenta is usually delivered within minutes of the infant delivery. If the patient is not bleeding, up to an hour can be left before undertaking manual removal of the placenta under anaesthesia. Rarely, the placenta is found to be morbidly adherent to the uterine wall, known as a 'placenta accreta'. Invasion of the myometrium by the placenta is known as 'placenta increta' and if it invades through the myometrium, it is known as 'placenta percreta'. These conditions are associated with paucity of underlying decidua in situations such as:

- previous placenta praevia
- uterine scar such as previous caesarean section
- multiparity

If the patient is not bleeding, it may be appropriate to leave the placenta in-situ. Conservative management includes observation and antibiotics, as well as considering the use of the folate antagonist methotrexate. However, more commonly, the patient has significant bleeding and surgery is necessary, including hysterectomy.

> **RED FLAG**
>
> The potential morbidity and mortality associated with postpartum haemorrhage are so significant that earlier rather than delayed recourse to hysterectomy is essential.

Uterine inversion

The placenta and membranes should be delivered by controlled cord traction to prevent this rare complication of labour. It can be either complete, when the uterine fundus passes through the cervix, or incomplete, when the fundus is still above the cervix. It can occur spontaneously, for example, in association with a fundal placental site or a unicornuate uterus, or it may be the result of mismanagement of the third stage.

The more serious presentation is of severe lower abdominal pain followed by collapse (due to neurogenic shock) and haemorrhage. The pain is secondary to tension on the infundibulopelvic ligaments. Treatment involves resuscitation of the patient, replacement of the uterus, either manually or hydrostatically, and oxytocin infusion.

Uterine rupture

This is seen very rarely in the UK, except in association with a previous caesarean section. It is associated with high rates of maternal and fetal morbidity and mortality. The incidence has fallen dramatically with the introduction of the lower segment procedure (<1%), as opposed to the classical vertical incision of the uterus (up to 5%). Spontaneous rupture is much less common. It is seen in a patient of high parity, associated with the use of syntocinon to augment labour.

Uterine rupture can present with an abnormal cardiotocograph in labour (see Chapter 27), or with continuous abdominal pain and vaginal bleeding. Diagnosis is made at laparotomy and the treatment is surgical – either repair of the rupture or hysterectomy.

Complications of primary postpartum haemorrhage

Sheehan syndrome

Severe PPH can lead to avascular necrosis of the pituitary gland, resulting in hypopituitarism. This can present as secondary amenorrhoea or failure of lactation.

Prevention of primary postpartum haemorrhage

In the first instance, prevention of primary PPH involves treatment of anaemia during pregnancy and identifying patients who might be at risk. These women might be obvious antenatally, such as the patient with a known inherited coagulation factor deficiency or one who has had a previous PPH. Equally, PPH might be anticipated during labour, for example, the patient who has a prolonged labour ending with a difficult instrumental delivery of a large baby.

Active management of the third stage of labour is routine in most obstetric units, with the patient's consent. It involves:

- use of an oxytocic drug
- controlled cord traction to deliver the placenta (Brandt–Andrews method)
- clamping and cutting the umbilical cord

Prophylactic use of oxytocics in particular is known to reduce the incidence of PPH by 30%–40%. Intramuscular Syntometrine is commonly used in the UK (5 units of syntocinon and 0.5 mg ergometrine). If the patient has hypertension, syntocinon is given alone.

SECONDARY POSTPARTUM HAEMORRHAGE

History

Table 31.1 shows the differential diagnoses that need to be considered when someone presents with a secondary PPH. In the presence of retained products of conception, either placenta or membranes, the common presenting complaint is prolonged heavy vaginal bleeding or persistent offensive discharge.

In the presence of infection, the patient may also present with fever and lower abdominal pain.

Examination

Basic observations should include pulse, blood pressure, respiratory rate and temperature. Tachycardia and pyrexia may be present with endometritis. The height of the uterine fundus should be checked because the uterus will usually

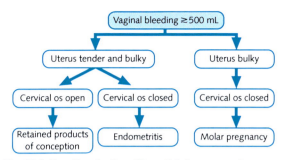

Fig. 31.2 Algorithm for the differential diagnoses of secondary postpartum haemorrhage.

remain poorly contracted if there are retained products of conception. Tenderness should be excluded to rule out endometritis.

Speculum examination excludes vaginal discharge if there is suspicion of infection. Bimanual palpation examines the size of the uterus, because it might be bulky with retained products. Tenderness is present with endometritis. If the cervical os is open, there might be retained products of conception. Fig. 31.2 provides an algorithm for the differential diagnoses of secondary PPH, depending on the examination findings.

Investigations

A full blood count should be taken to estimate haemoglobin. A raised white blood cell count is an indication of infection. Again, cross-matching blood for transfusion might be necessary, depending on the clinical situation and the haemoglobin result. A high vaginal swab should be taken to exclude endometritis.

An ultrasound scan should be arranged to check that the uterus is empty and exclude retained products. Care should be taken to interpret the findings in conjunction with the clinical picture because blood clot might have a similar scan appearance.

Evacuation of the uterus will yield tissue for histological analysis to confirm the diagnosis.

Management

The management of a secondary PPH starts with basic resuscitation using an ABC approach. The definitive management depends on the cause. As described in the 'Investigations' section earlier, retained products of conception will need evacuation under general anaesthesia (ERPC evacuation of retained products of conception). This may need antibiotic cover. Suspected infection or endometritis without retained products needs broad-spectrum antibiotics, including anaerobic cover. Depending on the assessment of the woman, these may need to be given intravenously, or could be simply oral.

POSTNATAL INFECTION

Definition

Also known as 'puerperal infection', this is defined as a maternal temperature of 38°C maintained for 4–6 hours in the first 14 days after delivery. The causative agent is commonly Group A streptococcus.

Incidence

Infection remains a major cause of maternal mortality (see Chapter 32). The Sepsis Six pathway has been developed internationally to provide a quick reference guide to the urgent measures that will reduce morbidity and mortality from severe infection if undertaken promptly. With improved hygiene and the use of antibiotics, the incidence of postnatal infection has fallen over the last 50 years.

RED FLAG

Sepsis Six pathway for the immediate management of suspected sepsis:

- administer oxygen – maintain saturations >94%
- take blood cultures, consider urine microscopy, culture and sensitivity, vaginal swab, sputum, etc. as indicated
- give broad-spectrum antibiotics
- give intravenous fluids
- check serial lactate, call critical care if >4
- measure urine output, start fluid balance chart with or without urinary catheter

---

Sites of infection

- Uterus.
- Abdominal incision.
- Perineum.
- Chest.
- Urinary tract.
- Breast.

History

The site of infection is usually obvious from the patient's history. Dysuria and urine frequency would suggest a urinary tract infection. If there is also loin pain, then there might be an ascending infection to the kidneys causing pyelonephritis. If the patient has a productive cough and complains of feeling breathless, then she may have a chest infection. This is typically a postoperative complication, seen after caesarean section.

A uterine infection is also more common after an operative intervention, such as a caesarean section or a manual removal of placenta. It typically presents with lower abdominal pain, sometimes with unpleasant-smelling vaginal discharge. Retained products of conception must be excluded. It is now routine practice to give prophylactic antibiotics at the time of a caesarean section to decrease the incidence of wound and uterine infection.

Infection in the perineum can also present with vaginal discharge, as well as localized discomfort. There is usually a history of a vaginal tear or an episiotomy. Acute mastitis, or infection of the breast, typically presents at the end of the first week after birth, as organisms that colonize the baby affect the breast. Infection presents with pain and/or erythema of one or both breasts associated with fever.

Examination

Examine the patient from head to toe, as suggested in Fig. 31.3. Pyrexia, tachypnoea, hypotension and tachycardia will be present with infection.

Investigations

White blood cell count and C-reactive protein level may be raised. Blood cultures are indicated if the patient's temperature is ≥38°C.

Other investigations depend on the system that is involved:

- high vaginal swab for uterine infection
- perineal swab
- wound swab for caesarean section patient
- midstream urine sample
- sputum sample

Management

The antibiotic of choice will depend on local protocol, but usually involves a broad-spectrum antibiotic and anaerobic cover with metronidazole for 5–7 days. Flucloxacillin is more appropriate for mastitis or wound infection because the usual pathogen is *Staphylococcus*.

POSTNATAL MENTAL ILLNESS

Incidence

Postnatal depression is one of the most common medical diseases of pregnancy, with 10% of women fulfilling the criteria for a depressive disorder. Psychosis is much rarer, affecting 0.2% of births. These disorders should be distinguished from the 'baby blues', which affects up to 70% of women, with a peak incidence on day 4 to 5. Tearfulness, anxiety and irritability normally settle with reassurance and support from family and friends.

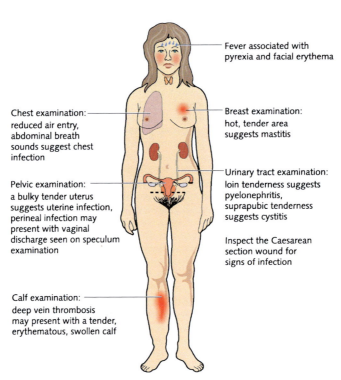

Chest examination: reduced air entry, abdominal breath sounds suggest chest infection

Pelvic examination: a bulky tender uterus suggests uterine infection, perineal infection may present with vaginal discharge seen on speculum examination

Calf examination: deep vein thrombosis may present with a tender, erythematous, swollen calf

Fever associated with pyrexia and facial erythema

Breast examination: hot, tender area suggests mastitis

Urinary tract examination: loin tenderness suggests pyelonephritis, suprapubic tenderness suggests cystitis

Inspect the Caesarean section wound for signs of infection

Fig. 31.3 Examination of the patient with postnatal pyrexia.

Postnatal mental illness has been increasingly given recognition in both the medical and general press as being a serious cause of maternal mortality (see Chapter 32).

History

Chapter 22 lists the risk factors for postnatal depression and some of these should be sought at the time of the antenatal booking, as recommended in the triennial report into maternal death (see Chapter 32). Puerperal psychosis in particular has associated risks: previous psychotic illness gives the woman a 1:2 chance of postnatal disease and a family history a 1:4 chance.

The common symptoms of postnatal depression and puerperal psychosis are shown in Boxes 31.3 and 31.4, respectively. The peak time of onset for postnatal depression is a gradual onset 4–6 weeks postpartum, whereas the onset of psychosis is usually very sudden.

BOX 31.3   SYMPTOMS OF POSTNATAL DEPRESSION

- Anxiety
- Low mood
- Fatigue
- Irritability
- Feelings of inadequacy
- Ambivalence towards the baby
- Reduced or absent libido

BOX 31.4   SYMPTOMS OF PUERPERAL PSYCHOSIS

- Insomnia or early morning wakening
- Lability of mood
- Overactivity
- Disorientation
- Lack of insight
- Hallucinations
- Persecutory beliefs, recurrent thoughts of death

COMMUNICATION

Risk factors for postnatal mental illness include a previous history of mental health disorder either in or outside of pregnancy, as well as a family history of general and perinatal mental illness. Therefore it is essential to enquire about these sensitively in the antenatal period to aid prediction and allow early detection and management of postnatal mental illness.

Management

- Prevention.
- Pharmacological.
- Psychological/social.

The mainstay of management is prevention, which has improved recently as media interest increases public awareness. Early diagnosis and training of professionals to recognize the problems are also vital and has resulted in the development of the Edinburgh Postnatal Depression Scale, which is used successfully by health visitors across the UK.

Psychotherapy may be the first-line treatment for postnatal depression. Drug treatment is described in Chapter 22. As with any drug in pregnancy, use should be considered if the benefits outweigh the risks. The tricyclic antidepressants can be given safely both antenatally and postnatally. The newer selective serotonin reuptake inhibitors are probably safe, but there is less evidence to support this. Lithium may be toxic to the baby and is therefore not recommended with breastfeeding. Electroconvulsive therapy is safe.

Health visitors and support groups all have an important role in helping the mother with postnatal illness.

THROMBOEMBOLIC DISEASE

Thromboembolic disease is the most common cause of pregnancy-related maternal mortality in the UK (see Chapter 32). Chapter 22 describes the risk factors, diagnosis and management in detail. Of particular importance are those women who undergo caesarean section. However, it is vital not to forget that a woman who has had a normal delivery might still have significant risk factors, such as older age, obesity or hypertension, which necessitate thromboprophylaxis in the postpartum period of up to 6 weeks.

Chapter Summary

- Primary postpartum haemorrhage (PPH) is defined as bleeding more than 500 mL within 24 hours of delivery.
- The commonest causes of primary PPH are uterine atony and genital tract trauma.
- Secondary PPH is defined as bleeding more than 500 mL that starts 24 hours after delivery and occurs within 6 weeks.
- The commonest causes of secondary PPH are endometritis and retained products of conception.
- Use the ABC (airways, breathing, circulation) approach when initially assessing a bleeding patient.
- Puerperal infection is defined as a maternal temperature of 38°C maintained for 4–6 hours in the first 14 days after delivery.
- Postnatal depression is one of the most common medical diseases of pregnancy, with 10% of women fulfilling the criteria for a depressive disorder; psychosis is much rarer, affecting 0.2% of births.
- Post-delivery, women should be risk assessed for thromboprophylaxis.

FURTHER READING

Cantwell, R., Clutton-Brock, T., Cooper, G., et al., 2011. Saving mothers' lives: reviewing maternal deaths to make motherhood safer: 2006–2008. The eighth report of the confidential enquiries into maternal deaths in the United Kingdom. BJOG. 118, 1–203. https://doi.org/10.1111/j.1471-0528.2010.02847.x.

National Institute for Health and Care Excellence (NICE), 2007. National evidence-based clinical guideline 37. Postpartum care. NICE, London, UK.

National Institute for Health and Care Excellence (NICE), 2007. National evidence-based clinical guideline 45. Antenatal and postnatal mental health. NICE, London, UK.

Royal College of Obstetricians and Gynaecologists (RCOG), 2009. Reducing the risk of thrombosis and embolism during pregnancy and the puerperium. RCOG green-top guideline no. 37. RCOG, London, UK.

Royal College of Obstetricians and Gynaecologists (RCOG), 2012. Sepsis following pregnancy, bacterial. RCOG green-top guideline no. 64b. RCOG, London, UK.

Royal College of Obstetricians and Gynaecologists (RCOG), 2016. Postpartum haemorrhage, prevention and management. RCOG green-top guideline no 52. RCOG, London, UK.

Maternal collapse and maternal death $\quad$ 32

INTRODUCTION

Maternal collapse is a rare but serious event that requires prompt effective management. The Royal College of Obstetricians and Gynaecologists (RCOG) defines maternal collapse as 'an acute event involving the cardiorespiratory systems and/or brain, resulting in a reduced or absent conscious level (and potentially death), at any stage in pregnancy and up to six weeks after delivery'. In view of the serious nature of a maternal collapse and the importance of prompt management, most units in the UK run training sessions to educate clinicians on how this should be managed. The aim of this chapter is to give an overview of the main causes and initial management. The causes are summarized in Fig. 32.1.

Maternal deaths include any woman who dies antenatally and up to 1 year postnatally. It is a rare but traumatic and distressing experience for all involved. It has wide reaching implications not only for the family of the deceased but also for the medical team, with the lessons that can be learned from the tragedy being important both clinically and personally. This chapter discusses the National Confidential Enquiry that collates patient case details and publishes the lessons that need to be learnt across all units.

THE COLLAPSED PATIENT

The prospect of a collapsed pregnant patient can be very daunting for any clinician. The use of maternity or obstetric early warning charts can help recognize those patients at risk of collapse. As with any patient, the importance of summoning help and following the airway, breathing, circulation (ABC) guide of management is paramount. There are, however, important differences in management of the pregnant patient, compared with a nonpregnant patient:

- Maintenance of a left lateral tilt during resuscitation to prevent aortocaval compression and increase venous return to the heart (Fig. 32.2).
- The mother takes priority over the fetus and unless needed to aid maternal resuscitation, delivery of the fetus should be delayed until the mother is stable.

Fig. 32.3 shows an algorithm for the initial management of the collapse patient.

CAUSES OF MATERNAL COLLAPSE

Haemorrhage

Haemorrhage is the most common cause of collapse in obstetric patients. In many cases, the bleeding will be obvious, or revealed. However, in cases such as concealed placental abruption, after a caesarean or ruptured ectopic pregnancy, it may be concealed and a high index of clinical suspicion is required. Thirteen mothers died from haemorrhage in the last confidential enquiry into causes of maternal death [Mothers and Babies: Reducing Risk through Audit and Confidential Enquiries across the UK (MBRRACE) 2012–2014]. There has been minimal change in these rates over the last three reports (see later).

Major haemorrhage can be due to:

- placenta praevia/accreta
- placental abruption
- uterine rupture or a non-obstetric intra-abdominal bleed (splenic rupture etc.)
- postpartum bleeding (secondary to uterine atony or trauma)

More information on individual causes can be found in Chapter 20 (Antepartum haemorrhage) and Chapter 31 (Postnatal complications). National management guidelines

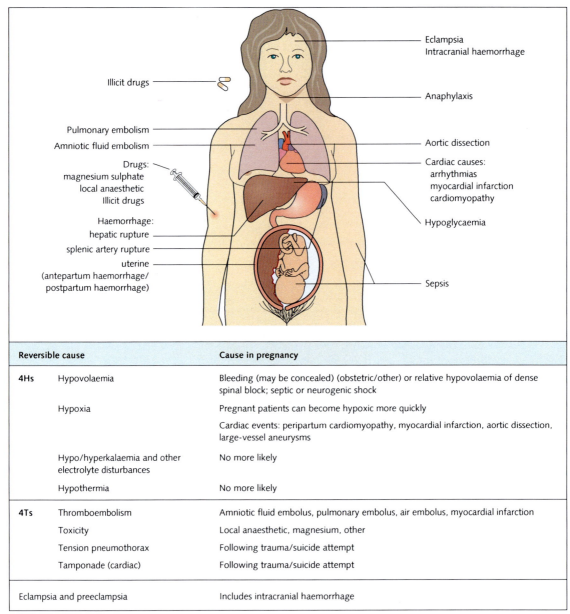

Fig. 32.1 Causes of maternal collapse (RCOG guideline no. 56).

Reversible cause		Cause in pregnancy
4Hs	Hypovolaemia	Bleeding (may be concealed) (obstetric/other) or relative hypovolaemia of dense spinal block; septic or neurogenic shock
	Hypoxia	Pregnant patients can become hypoxic more quickly
		Cardiac events: peripartum cardiomyopathy, myocardial infarction, aortic dissection, large-vessel aneurysms
	Hypo/hyperkalaemia and other electrolyte disturbances	No more likely
	Hypothermia	No more likely
4Ts	Thromboembolism	Amniotic fluid embolus, pulmonary embolus, air embolus, myocardial infarction
	Toxicity	Local anaesthetic, magnesium, other
	Tension pneumothorax	Following trauma/suicide attempt
	Tamponade (cardiac)	Following trauma/suicide attempt
Eclampsia and preeclampsia		Includes intracranial haemorrhage

and training tools have helped the management of haemorrhage including:

- use of maternity early warning charts
- prompt recognition and resuscitation
- involvement of a senior multidisciplinary team (i.e. haematologists, anaesthetists)
- optimization of haemoglobin levels antenatally
- early recourse to methods such as uterine artery embolization or hysterectomy

The latter can be life-saving especially in individuals who decline blood products.

In cases of massive antepartum haemorrhage, prompt delivery of the fetus and placenta should be considered to allow control of bleeding, depending on the gestation of the pregnancy.

Thromboembolism

Thromboembolism is the leading cause of direct maternal death according to the most recent confidential enquiry (MBRRACE 2012–14), although the use of prophylactic measures such as compression stockings and low-molecular-weight heparin are thought to have contributed to a decline in deaths over the last 10 years.

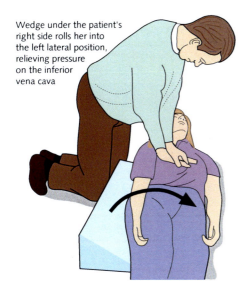

Wedge under the patient's right side rolls her into the left lateral position, relieving pressure on the inferior vena cava

Fig. 32.2 Left tilt in the collapsed patient.

Pregnancy is a prothrombotic state and, therefore, all patients should be educated about signs and symptoms as well as how to seek help. All patients should be risk assessed to identify those who require thromboprophylaxis:

- at booking
- at 28 weeks
- on every antenatal admission
- after delivery

Pulmonary embolism (PE) can present with chest pain, tachycardia, tachypnoea and shortness of breath. Large PEs can, however, cause maternal collapse. Initial management with cardiopulmonary resuscitation, oxygen and anticoagulation should be commenced until the diagnosis can be ruled out. In certain cases thrombolysis may be necessary. See Chapter 22 (Medical disorders in pregnancy) for further details on this topic.

Preeclampsia and eclampsia

Pre-eclampsia and eclampsia are both discussed in detail in Chapter 21: Hypertension in pregnancy. With regard to the collapsed patient, eclampsia should always be considered a cause of maternal collapse. By definition, eclampsia is seizure-like activity associated with hypertension and proteinuria. Patients who are found collapsed may have had an eclamptic fit which may or may not have been witnessed. If an eclamptic fit is suspected, management with magnesium sulphate and antihypertensives should be started. The recognition of the importance of prompt treatment of hypertension, particularly systolic hypertension, is essential to prevent serious complications such as stroke. Therefore patients with headache and visual disturbances who have high blood pressure must have urinalysis and blood tests to exclude pre-eclampsia. It should be emphasized that stabilization of the mother in these cases takes precedence over the fetus.

Rates of maternal deaths from pre-eclampsia and eclampsia have declined as there were only two deaths reported in the last MBRRACE report.

Sepsis

Sepsis is no longer the leading direct cause of maternal death. However, prompt management is still essential when faced with a collapsed patient in whom sepsis is suspected. Septic patients may present with:

- pyrexia/hypothermia
- tachycardia
- tachypnoea
- hypotension
- rigors
- confusion
- collapse

To maximize the patient's chances of survival, prompt treatment with intravenous (IV) antibiotics and IV fluids within an hour of diagnosis is paramount, as stressed in the National Campaign for Sepsis Management, (the 'Golden hour'). Close multidisciplinary liaison with the anaesthetists and microbiologists is essential. Rates of sepsis as a cause for maternal death have fallen following national recommendations.

RED FLAG

Sepsis Six pathway for the immediate management of suspected sepsis:

1. administer oxygen – maintain saturations >94%
2. take blood cultures, consider urine microscopy, culture and sensitivity, vaginal swab, sputum, etc. as indicated
3. give broad-spectrum antibiotics
4. give intravenous fluids
5. check serial lactate, call critical care if >4
6. measure urine output, start fluid balance chart with or without urinary catheter

Amniotic fluid embolism

An amniotic fluid embolism (AFE) is a rare but very serious cause of maternal collapse, which carries a high rate of mortality. An AFE is thought to occur when amniotic fluid enters maternal circulation and travels to distant sites such as the lungs and occludes pulmonary vessels. In addition, an anaphylactic-like reaction is thought to occur. These patients then rapidly develop a coagulopathy and haemorrhage can ensue. Sadly the diagnosis is often made retrospectively at postmortem and in patients who do survive, there can be significant morbidity. Patients may present with:

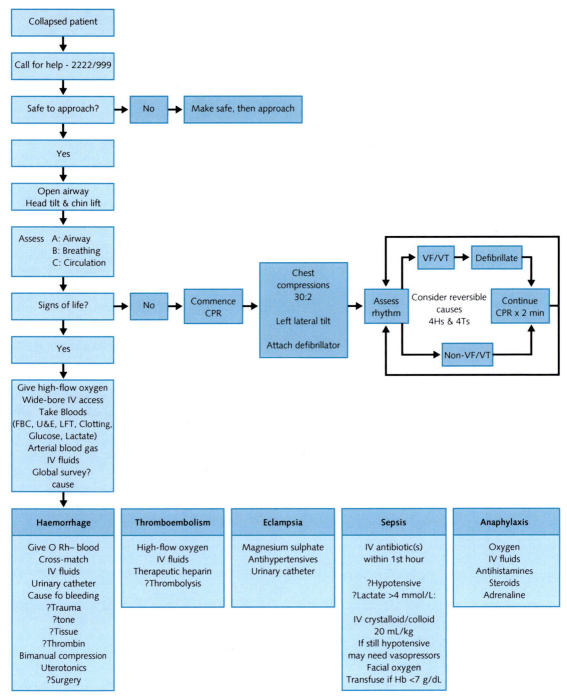

Fig. 32.3 Algorithm for the initial management of the collapsed obstetric patient. *CPR,* Cardiopulmonary resuscitation; *FBC,* full blood count; *IV,* intravenous; *LFT,* liver function test; *U&E,* urea and electrolytes; *VF,* ventricular fibrillation; *VT,* ventricular tachycardia.

- acute hypotension
- hypoxia
- respiratory distress
- seizures
- cardiac arrest

It should be considered as a diagnosis when patients collapse during labour, caesarean section, manual removal of placenta or within 30 minutes of these.

Management of these patients is largely supportive with maintenance of their airway, breathing and circulation. Cardiopulmonary resuscitation may be necessary and regular blood tests, including clotting studies, to identify any possible coagulopathy should be performed. Close liaison with the anaesthetic and haematology teams is vital, with prompt correction of any coagulopathy.

Cardiac disease

Cardiac disease has now become the leading cause of indirect maternal death and in the most recent report was responsible for 51 deaths. The exact causes of death included aortic dissection, myocardial infarction and cardiomyopathy.

Cardiac disease must be considered in patients:

- with a history of congenital heart defects
- with a history of previous cardiac surgery
- with a history of rheumatic fever or infective endocarditis
- who smoke
- who have hypertension
- who have a high body mass index

Patients may present collapsed or give a history of chest pain (central crushing), which radiates to the jaw, left arm and/or back. An electrocardiogram should be performed and medical advice sought as soon as possible.

> **RED FLAG**
>
> Signs and symptoms that warrant further assessment for cardiac causes of collapse:
> - central chest pain
> - interscapular pain
> - wide pulse pressure
> - new cardiac murmur
> - orthopnoea

Ectopic pregnancy

An ectopic pregnancy can be defined as implantation of an embryo outside of the uterine cavity (see Chapter 18). However, pregnancies may implant at the site of a previous caesarean section, also referred to as 'scar ectopics', whilst still technically being in the uterine cavity.

Most commonly the site of implantation is the fallopian tube and if left unnoticed, the pregnancy will eventually rupture. The rupture can lead to massive blood loss and, sadly, even death.

The diagnosis must always be considered in women of childbearing age who present with abdominal pain. A pregnancy test should be performed and if positive, an ectopic pregnancy should be ruled out by ultrasound scan and blood tests. In some cases, an ectopic pregnancy can present as gastrointestinal upset and the patient may not know they are pregnant. A high index of suspicion is required in all patients who present with pain and bleeding in early pregnancy. Education about signs and symptoms of an ectopic should be given to all patients as well as information on how to seek help.

Any patient who presents with a positive pregnancy test with an intrauterine device in-situ (Mirena or copper coil) should be treated as an ectopic until proven otherwise.

Drug toxicity

Drug toxicity can occur due to a number of causes and should be borne in mind when assessing a collapsed patient. Any history of the following should be considered:

- recreational drug use
- epidural analgesia can cause collapse due to a 'high epidural block' or 'total spinal' anaesthetic
- local anaesthetic agents may have had inadvertent IV administration
- magnesium toxicity of pre-eclampsia patients with renal dysfunction
- anaphylaxis

Patients who are thought to have taken illicit drugs can present in a number of ways. Patients taking opiates such as heroine can present with reduced consciousness and respiratory depression. These patients can have pinpoint pupils and will respond rapidly to treatment with naloxone. Ecstasy and cocaine users can present with seizures, hyperthermia, headaches and chest pain. Seizures can be treated with benzodiazepines such as diazepam.

A 'high epidural block' or 'total spinal' is thought to occur when there is excessive intrathecal spread of local anaesthetic drug. In addition, it can also occur if there is inadvertent spinal injection of high doses of local anaesthetic. Depression of cervical nerves follows and the patient may complain of difficulty breathing, light headedness or collapse. Prompt recognition and supportive measures including IV fluids, intubation and vasopressors are essential as these patients can rapidly progress to cardiac arrest.

The treatment for magnesium overdose is 10 mL of 10% calcium gluconate by IV injection over 10 minutes.

Anaphylaxis

Anaphylaxis is a very serious potentially fatal hypersensitivity reaction that needs prompt recognition and management. Anaphylactic reactions affect a number of systems and cardiac arrest can rapidly occur. Any recent administration of drugs should be noted, especially antibiotics, and any known allergies identified, including latex.

Anaphylaxis is said to be likely when there is rapid onset and progression of symptoms with life-threatening airway, breathing or circulation problems and skin or mucosal changes (RCOG). Rapid treatment with oxygen, IV fluids, steroids, antihistamines and adrenaline is required along with removal of any potentially triggering factors. Intensive care may be needed and again, a multidisciplinary approach is advised.

Hypoglycaemia or hyperglycaemia

Hypoglycaemia and hyperglycaemia should be considered in pregnancy as patients may have pre-existing diabetes or gestational diabetes (see Chapter 22). A finger-prick blood glucose level should be taken for every collapsed patient as part of their assessment and acted on promptly.

Hypoglycaemia as a cause of collapse is likely to be severe and should be treated urgently with IV glucose (50 mL of 50% glucose), which should rapidly correct the situation.

Hyperglycaemia when presenting with a collapse can indicate diabetic ketoacidosis. Blood and urinary ketones should be measured. Prompt treatment with IV fluids and sliding scale insulin is important as well as monitoring of potassium levels.

> ### COMMUNICATION
>
>
> A maternal collapse can be traumatic, not only for the woman but also for her birth partners who may have witnessed the event and the medical staff involved in the care. Debriefing the patient and her family will allow them to understand what occurred and also prevent future complications such as post-traumatic stress disorder, postnatal depression and tocophobia.

MATERNAL DEATH

Maternal mortality rates in the UK have fallen dramatically since the early 1900s. Since 1952, triennial reports have been published to report on the deaths and make recommendations about changes in practice. Maternal deaths, however, still continue to happen and the reporting and learning from these events is essential to further reduce the rates of maternal mortality.

Fig. 32.4 shows the falling trend in maternal mortality over time.

Mothers and Babies: Reducing Risk through Audit and Confidential Enquiries

MBRRACE is an organization whose aim is to improve the care given to mothers by carrying out confidential enquiries into maternal and infant deaths.

Every year, a report is published highlighting the main causes of maternal death and trends over the last 3 years. Each report focuses on a particular theme (e.g. mental health or cardiac disease), and then provides recommendations to help reduce the risks. In the most recent report published in December 2017 the maternal mortality rate was 8.8/100,000 maternities.

Definitions

When assessing maternal deaths, various definitions are used to categorize them:

- **Maternal deaths:** Deaths of women while pregnant or within 42 days of the end of the pregnancy from any cause related to or aggravated by the pregnancy or its management, but not from accidental or incidental causes (includes ectopic pregnancy, miscarriage and terminations of pregnancy).

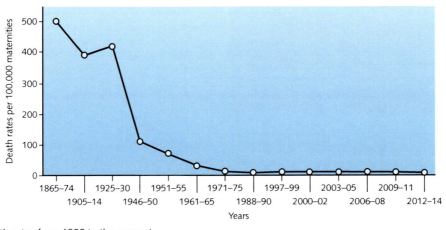

Fig. 32.4 Death rates from 1952 to the present.

- **Direct maternal death:** Deaths resulting from obstetric complications of the pregnant state (pregnancy, labour and puerperium), from interventions, omissions, incorrect treatment or from a chain of events resulting from any of the above.
- **Indirect maternal death:** Deaths resulting from previous existing disease, or disease that developed during pregnancy and which was not the result of direct obstetric causes, but which was aggravated by the physiological effects of pregnancy.
- **Late maternal death:** Deaths occurring between 42 days and 1 year after abortion, miscarriage or delivery that are the result of direct or indirect maternal causes.
- **Coincidental:** Deaths from unrelated causes, which happen to occur in pregnancy or the puerperium.

Causes of maternal death

Table 32.1 displays the maternal death rates for direct and indirect causes from the recent confidential reports. Most of these causes have been described in more detail earlier in the chapter in relation to maternal collapse. Two further causes are discussed in the following sections.

Psychiatric illness

The majority of deaths related to psychiatric illness are due to suicide. Maternal mental health was a highlighted topic in the December 2015 MBRRACE report. It highlighted that good communication with networks between primary care, perinatal mental health services and maternity services is critical to provide the best care for woman with mental health problems.

> **RED FLAG**
>
> The following signs and symptoms should prompt urgent senior psychiatric assessment:
> - recent significant change in mental state
> - new thoughts or acts of violent self-harm
> - new and persistent expression of incompetency as a mother affecting bonding with her infant

Coincidental maternal deaths

This category includes a large number of varied causes of death, with road traffic accidents and murder being the two most common. Domestic violence remains a major cause for concern to all clinicians caring for obstetric patients and should be actively screened for at each contact. Patients suffering from domestic violence are likely to be:

- late bookers
- have a poor attendance record
- have repeated admissions for seemingly trivial matters

Partners may appear to be domineering, constantly present during all visits and those who do not let the patient answer questions should raise concerns about domestic violence. Where indicated, professional interpreters should be used rather than family members and any concerns acted upon.

Table 32.1 Direct and indirect causes of maternal death from the last three confidential reports

	Year				
	2000–2002	2003–2005	2006–2008	2009–2011	2012–2014
Direct deaths					
Sepsis	13	18	26	15	7
Preeclampsia/ eclampsia	14	18	19	10	2
Thrombosis/ thromboembolism	30	41	18	30	20
Amniotic fluid embolism	5	17	13	7	16
Ectopic	11	10	6	4	7
Haemorrhage	17	14	9	14	13
Anaesthesia	6	6	7	3	2
Indirect deaths					
Cardiac disease	44	48	53	51	51
Other indirect causes	50	50	49	72	23
Coincidental	36	55	50	23	41

COMMUNICATION

If there is any disclosure of domestic violence, it is advised to inform the specialist safeguarding team immediately who can provide continuity of care to the woman and also make appropriate referrals to social services to ensure the newborn infant or any existing children are protected.

● Chapter Summary

- Maternal collapse is 'an acute event involving the cardiorespiratory systems and/or brain, resulting in a reduced or absent conscious level (and potentially death), at any stage in pregnancy and up to six weeks after delivery'.
- There are many causes of maternal collapse with haemorrhage being the most common.
- A pregnant woman should be resuscitated in a left lateral position to avoid aortocaval compression.
- A maternal death is defined as the death of a women while pregnant or within 42 days of the end of the pregnancy; it is further categorized into direct, indirect and coincidental causes.

FURTHER READING

MBRRACE-UK Mother and Babies: Saving lives, improving mothers care 2013–15. December 2017. Available at: www.npeu.ox.ac.uk.

Royal College of Obstetricians and Gynaecologists (RCOG), 2011. Maternal collapse in pregnancy and the puerperium. RCOG green-top guideline no. 56. Available at: www.rcog.org.uk.

Sepsis Trust Maternity Guidelines, Available at: www.sepsistrust. org.

UKOSS UK Obstetric Surveillance System, Available at: www.npeu. ox.ac.uk.

Obstetrics & Gynaecology OSCEs

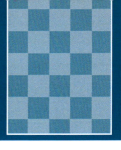

OBSTETRICS OSCES

1. ANTEPARTUM HAEMORRHAGE

Candidate instructions

You have been asked to take a history from Mrs SS who is 36 weeks in her first pregnancy and has presented with vaginal bleeding. After you have completed your history, please summarize your findings and then you will be asked five questions with regard to this case.

Patient details

Name: Samantha Smith

Age: 34 years

Presenting complaint (PC): Vaginal bleeding

History of presenting complaint (HPC): This is your first pregnancy and so far you have attended all your antenatal appointments and scans and have had no problems in the pregnancy. You are rhesus negative and all other booking blood tests were normal. You are a smoker.

Your anomaly ultrasound scan showed that your placenta was not low lying. At 28 weeks you were found to be anaemic and have been commenced on ferrous sulphate.

You are now 36 weeks' pregnant. This morning you woke up with intermittent abdominal pain and noticed some vaginal bleeding. Your abdomen feels tense. You have felt good fetal movements today.

Obstetric history: G1P0

Gynaecology history: Last smear was taken 3.5 years ago and results were normal. Regular menstrual cycle prepregnancy with periods lasting 5 days and occurring every 28 days with normal flow.

Medical history (MH): Nil

Drug history (DH): Ferrous sulphate

Allergies: Nil

Smoking history (SH): Smoker – cut down to five a day in pregnancy

Family history (FH): Mother had preeclampsia in first pregnancy

Checklist

- Introduces self and gains consent to take a history.
- Identifies patient.
- Starts with an open question to establish PC.
- Identifies salient points in the HPC (i.e., vaginal bleeding associated with abdominal pain).
- Enquires about fetal wellbeing by asking about fetal movements.
- Enquires about the history of this pregnancy (i.e., booked at correct gestation, attended all the antenatal ultrasound scans, blood test results).
- Identifies that the patient is rhesus negative.
- Identifies that the placenta was not low lying at the 20-week anomaly ultrasound scan.
- Identifies risk factors for abruption such as SH.
- Enquires about smear history and establishes that she is due a smear test.
- Completes the history by asking about MH, DH, allergies, SH and FH.

Questions

1. What is the most likely diagnosis?
   - Antepartum haemorrhage secondary to placental abruption – because the vaginal bleeding is associated with abdominal pain, as opposed to the painless vaginal bleeding that typically occurs with a placenta praevia.
2. What are the risk factors for placental abruption?
   - Previous abruption.
   - Advanced maternal age.
   - Multiparity.
   - Maternal hypertension or preeclampsia.
   - Abdominal trauma (e.g., assault, road traffic accident).
   - Cigarette smoking.
   - Lower socioeconomic group.
   - External cephalic version.
3. Explain the difference between a concealed and revealed haemorrhage?
   - A revealed haemorrhage is when maternal blood escapes from the placental sinuses and tracks down between the membranes and the uterus and runs through the cervix into the vagina.
   - A concealed haemorrhage is when the blood remains sealed within the uterine cavity; in this case the degree of hypovolemic shock can be out of proportion to the vaginal loss that is visualized.
4. This woman is rhesus negative, what investigations and management are required for this?
   - The patient should receive anti-D as she has had an antepartum haemorrhage, which is a sensitising event.

- A Kleihauer test should be performed to diagnose fetomaternal haemorrhage. This test of maternal blood allows quantification of the degree of haemorrhage and therefore guides the dose of anti-D that is needed.

5. What are the complications of a placental abruption?
   - This depends on the volume of the antepartum haemorrhage, and your assessment of the maternal and fetal health. With major blood loss, maternal observations must be checked and airway, breathing, circulation resuscitation started urgently if necessary. The fetal heart rate must be auscultated and electronic monitoring started as this woman is more than 28 weeks' pregnant.
   - Once the woman is stable, delivery may be indicated if the fetal heart rate monitoring is abnormal. The neonatal team must be informed as well as the rest of the multidisciplinary team, including the anaesthetist, so that delivery can be expedited. The haematology team must also be informed as blood and blood products may be needed. There is a risk of developing disseminated intravascular coagulation and the urine output must be monitored carefully to exclude renal failure.

2. POSTNATAL SEPSIS

Candidate instructions

You have been asked to take a history from Mrs RD. She has presented to hospital 5 days following an emergency caesarean section for delivery of her third child for failure to progress in labour. She attended her GP surgery today complaining of feeling generally unwell. Her temperature at the GP surgery was 38.3°C. Once you have completed your history please summarize your findings. You will then be asked five questions with regard to this case.

Patient details

Name: Rachel Dean
Age: 37 years
Presenting complaint: Generally unwell
History of presenting complaint: This morning you woke up with abdominal pain that was worse than the postoperative pain you have been having. You have noticed that your vaginal loss has increased and you have passed some small clots. The loss is offensive. The wound appears clean and dry. Your temperature was raised at the GP surgery. You do not have any other symptoms.

This was your third pregnancy. This pregnancy has been uncomplicated and you had consultant-led care as you had had a previous caesarean section. At 40^{+10}

weeks' gestation, you had an induction of labour, with artificial rupture of your membranes and intravenous syntocinon was commenced after 4 hours because you had not started contracting. After 12 hours of labour, the doctors recommended a caesarean section as you had not progressed past a cervical dilatation of 4 cm.

The caesarean was complicated by scar tissue from your previous caesarean section. You lost 700 mL of blood and did not require a blood transfusion. Your postoperative recovery was uncomplicated and you were able to go home on day 2.

You are breastfeeding your new baby and that is going well.

Obstetric history: You delivered your first child 8 years ago; the pregnancy was uncomplicated and you had a normal vaginal delivery. Your second child was delivered 5 years ago by elective caesarean section for breech presentation.

Gynaecology history: Your smear tests are up to date and have always been normal. You have had normal regular periods since age 14 years.

Medical history (MH): Mild asthma

Drug history (DH): Blue (salbutamol) and brown (beclomethasone) inhaler

Allergies: Penicillin

Smoking history (SH): Nonsmoker, occasionally drinks alcohol. Lives with husband and three children.

Family history (FH): Nil

During the consultation you get irritated as you need to get home to your children and you are concerned about the new baby as you only left a small amount of expressed milk at home and will need to feed him soon.

Checklist

- Introduces self and gains consent to take a history.
- Explains why it is important to take a clear history and perform an examination, sepsis is an important cause of maternal morbidity and mortality.
- Identifies patient.
- Starts with an open question to establish presenting complaint.
- Performs a systems enquiry to establish the cause of sepsis, including headache, sore throat, breast pain, shortness of breath, chest pain, cough, abdominal pain, gastrointestinal symptoms, nature of vaginal loss, urinary symptoms, calf tenderness.
- Clarifies previous obstetric history.
- Asks about the details of this pregnancy.
- Asks about the details of the labour.
- Enquires about complications at caesarean section.
- Enquires about any postnatal problems.
- Establishes if she is breastfeeding.
- Completes the history by asking about PGH, MH, DH, allergies, SH and FH.
- Addresses the patient's concerns about being away from her newborn baby and two other children.

Questions

1. What are the differential diagnoses in this case?
   - Endometritis.
   - Pelvic collection.
   - Wound infection.
   - Mastitis.
2. What investigations need to be performed?
   - Full blood count to check the white cell count.
   - C-reactive protein level to assess inflammation.
   - Blood cultures to attempt to colonize the causative organism.
   - Lactate level.
   - High vaginal swab.
   - Wound swab.
   - Urine dipstick and midstream urine sample if there are any positive findings.
3. What are the steps in the Sepsis Six pathway for the immediate management of suspected sepsis?
   1. Administer oxygen – maintain saturations >94%.
   2. Take blood cultures, consider urine microscopy, culture and sensitivity; vaginal swab; sputum, etc. as indicated.
   3. Give broad-spectrum antibiotics.
   4. Give intravenous fluids.
   5. Check serial lactate; call critical care if >4.
   6. Measure urine output, start fluid balance chart with or without urinary catheter.
4. What is the most common causative organism of postnatal sepsis?
   - Group A streptococcus.
5. What are the five most common causes of direct maternal deaths in the most recent national confidential enquiry?
   - Thrombosis.
   - Haemorrhage.
   - Sepsis.
   - Ectopic pregnancy.
   - Amniotic fluid embolism.

3. SHOULDER DYSTOCIA AND THIRD-DEGREE PERINEAL TEAR

Candidate instructions

Your fellow medical student was unwell yesterday and missed a tutorial on shoulder dystocia. They have asked you to help, by teaching them about the relevance and management of shoulder dystocia. You may use a doll and model pelvis if available.

Checklist

- Check with the medical student their current knowledge on shoulder dystocia.

- Explain that shoulder dystocia is a problem of the pelvic inlet, preventing the shoulders from delivering once the head is out. It is not a problem of the pelvic outlet.
- Excessive traction on the fetal head to facilitate the delivery of the shoulders can cause damage to the brachial plexus nerve roots in the neck (i.e., Erb palsy).
- There is a risk of increasing hypoxia as the fetus is lodged in the vagina with pressure on the umbilical cord.
- Explain the manoeuvres to aid delivery using the HELPERR pneumonic:
   - *H* – Call for help (i.e., obstetrician, labour ward coordinator, anaesthetist, paediatrician).
   - *E* – Evaluate for episiotomy – this is not to aid delivery of the shoulders but to allow adequate space to perform the internal procedures that help delivery.
   - *L* – Legs into McRoberts position – the hips are flexed in knee–chest position to widen the anteroposterior diameter of the maternal pelvis.
   - *P* – Suprapubic pressure – can be continuous or intermittent and is applied on the maternal abdomen suprapubically on the posterior aspect of the fetal shoulder to enable delivery.
   - *E* – Enter manoeuvres – internal rotation techniques, where the operator puts hands inside the vagina to try and rotate the anterior shoulder from under the pubic symphysis.
   - *R* – Remove (i.e., deliver the posterior arm so that there is more space for the shoulders to deliver).
   - *R* – Roll the patient onto all fours and repeat all the steps above.
- Ask the medical students to demonstrate what they have learnt.

Questions

1. What are the risk factors for a shoulder dystocia? Antenatal and intrapartum:
   - gestational diabetes
   - macrosomia
   - previous shoulder dystocia
   - raised maternal body mass index
   - postdates
   - instrumental delivery
2. What are the common complications following a shoulder dystocia?
   - Postpartum haemorrhage.
   - Third-degree tear.
3. How are third-degree tears classified?
   - Grade 3a tear – Less than 50% of external anal sphincter (EAS) thickness torn.
   - Grade 3b tear – More than 50% of EAS thickness torn.
   - Grade 3c tear – Both EAS and internal anal sphincter (IAS) torn.

- Fourth-degree tear – Injury to the perineum involving the anal sphincter complex (EAS and IAS) and anorectal mucosa.
4. What percentage of patients sustain a third-degree tear?
   - 3%
5. Following a third-degree tear, what information should you provide to the patient?
   - Debrief on extent of their tear and what symptoms to monitor.
   - Antibiotics.
   - Analgesia.
   - Laxatives.
   - Referral to physiotherapy.
   - Discussion on future mode of delivery.
   - Patient information leaflet.

GYNAECOLOGY OSCES

4. EMERGENCY CONTRACEPTION

Candidate instructions

You are working in accident and emergency and a 21-year-old female patient attends requesting emergency contraception.

Please take a relevant history from her, advise her about options for emergency contraception and advise on future contraceptive options.

OSCE patient instructions

Personal details: Rebecca Jones, 21 years old, university student (studying law)

Presenting complaint: You have a new boyfriend of 1 month and during vaginal intercourse last night the condom split. You have no other casual partners and you believe your boyfriend also does not. He is your first sexual partner in over a year and you have had a negative sexually transmitted infection (STI) screen a few months ago.

Medical/surgical history: Nil of note – no migraines, venous thromboembolism (VTE), stroke. No regular medications. No allergies.

Obstetrics and gynaecology history: No pregnancies. No history of STI. Never used hormonal or intrauterine contraception – condoms only. Not yet had a smear. Regular 30-day cycle with heavy flow for 3 days and lighter flow for a further 3. Last menstrual period 3 weeks ago. No intermenstrual bleeding, no postcoital bleeding, no vaginal discharge.

Social history/Family history (FH): Body mass index 24 kg/m^2. Smoker (10/day). Lives in university accommodation. No FH of VTE/stroke/migraine.

Mark scheme

- Introduces self and establishes rapport.
- Identifies patient name and personal details.
- Open questions regarding presenting complaint.
- Addresses patient concern.
- Establishes time of unprotected intercourse and number of occasions.
- Inquires STI risk:
  - regular or casual partners, number of casual partners in the past year, any previous STI
- Obstetrics and gynaecology history including:
  - Last menstrual period, menstrual history, contraceptive history, smear history, any previous pregnancies
  - Medical history including:
  - any history of migraine, VTE, stroke
- Social history and FH.
- Drug history.
- Explains the emergency contraceptive options:
  - Levonorgestrel (Levonelle) – single-dose 1.5-mg tablet which must be used within 72 hours of unprotected sexual intercourse. It can only be used once per cycle.
  - Ulipristal acetate (EllaOne) – single dose 30-mg tablet which must be used within 120 hours of unprotected sexual intercourse. It can be used as many times as needed per cycle.
  - Copper intrauterine device can be inserted up to 120 hours (5 days) following unprotected sexual intercourse or more, if not more than 5 days after the earliest predicted date of ovulation.
- Explains to take the contraception immediately.
- Explains what to do if vomiting or diarrhoea occur after taking contraceptive.
- Explains may have a heavy period.
- Discusses future contraception options.
- Advises STI screening.
- Explores that ideas, concerns and expectations are met.

Questions

1. What are common side-effects of emergency contraception?
   Side-effects include dizziness, nausea, headaches, breast tenderness or abdominal pain. Vomiting is a common side-effect and if within 2 hours of ingestion, the treatment should be repeated.
2. What are absolute contraindications for combined hormonal contraception?
   Contraindications to combined hormonal contraception include:
   - >15 cigarettes a day
   - ischaemic heart disease, atrial fibrillation, stroke or severe hypertension

- previous or current personal history of VTE or known thrombogenic mutations
- migraine with aura
- current breast cancer

All women can use emergency contraception safely and effectively – no medical conditions are contraindicated as it is a one-off dose.

3. How does the copper intrauterine device work?

It is a T-shaped plastic and copper device that works by both spermicidal action and thickening cervical mucus. The copper has a toxic effect on the sperm and ovum, which prevents fertilization. It can remain in place for up to 10 years.

4. If a woman is already taking hormonal contraception but misses a dose, can she still take emergency contraception?

Yes, the additional hormone dose is small and only taken as a one-off.

5. Can emergency contraceptives be used more than once?

Emergency contraception can be repeated safely, even within the same menstrual cycle. However, it is important to counsel women about more suitable long-acting contraceptive options.

5. SMEAR TEST

Candidate instructions

You are working at a genitourinary medicine clinic and a 25-year-old woman attends for her first smear test. She is anxious about the procedure.

Please explain the procedure and then perform a cervical smear.

OSCE patient instructions

Personal details: Phillipa Lake, 25 years old, shop assistant

Presenting complaint: You have attended for your first cervical smear as part of the screening programme. You have had one previous speculum with a sexually transmitted infection (STI) test. You have had three previous regular sexual partners. You feel very nervous because your friend recently had a smear text and said it was very painful.

Medical/surgical history: Nil of note

Obstetrics and gynaecology history: No pregnancies. No history of STI. Regular 30-day menstrual cycle. Last menstrual period 2 weeks ago. No intermenstrual bleeding, no postcoital bleeding, no vaginal discharge.

Social/family history: Maternal aunt has had abnormal smear tests in the past.

Mark scheme

- Introduce self and establish rapport.
- Identify patient name and personal details.
- Address patient concern.
- Explain the basis of screening programme to identify precancerous changes to treat appropriately.
- Explain how smear is performed:
  - Explain the need for chaperone; the procedure may feel uncomfortable but should not hurt. Advise that you can stop if the patient wishes.
  - Ask if the patient would like to empty their bladder first.
  - Explain the position that the patient will need to be in for the smear.
  - Check understanding and gain consent prior to the procedure.
- Perform the smear test:
  - Wash hands and put on gloves.
  - Inspect vulva.
  - Warn the patient you are about to insert the speculum – gently insert the speculum sideways and once inserted rotate 90° so handle is upwards.
  - Open the speculum blades to achieve a full view of the cervix and lock the position of the speculum.
  - Inspect the vaginal tissue and cervix.
  - Insert the endocervical brush into the endocervical canal through the open speculum.
  - Rotate the brush five times a full 360°.
  - Remove the endocervical brush and deposit it in the liquid-based cytology container.
  - Gently remove the speculum and dispose of it.
  - Re-cover the patient and wash hands.
- Label the sample and the cytology form.
- Summarize the findings to the patient.
- Explain how results will be received by the patient.
- Explore that ideas, concerns and expectations are met.

Questions

1. When are cervical smears performed?

As part of the screening programme cervical smears are performed on a 3 yearly basis between the ages of 25 and 49 years and on a 5 yearly basis from the ages of 50 to 64 years.

2. What are known risk factors for cervical cancer?
   - Human papilloma virus.
   - Smoking.
   - Young age/first intercourse/pregnancy.
   - Smoking.
   - Oral contraceptive pill.
   - Human immunodeficiency virus.

3. What types of human papilloma virus (HPV) are associated with development of cervical cancer?

HPV types 16, 18, 6 and 11 are all known to cause cervical cancer with 16 and 18 known as 'high-risk subtypes'.

4. Dyskaryosis is found at the time of cervical smear. What is the next step for investigations and diagnosis?
   Women with abnormal smear test results and positive HPV should be referred for colposcopy. Cervical intraepithelial neoplasia is diagnosed from histology, therefore a biopsy should be performed in order for the diagnosis to be made.

5. An abnormality is noted on the cervix during an examination in pregnancy – what should be done about this?
   Colposcopy procedure can be safely performed in pregnancy if there is any concern about cervical lesions. It will not cause any risk to the pregnancy. However, routine smear tests can be temporarily delayed until after pregnancy.

6. FERTILITY INVESTIGATIONS

Candidate instructions

You are working at a GP surgery and a 34-year-old woman and her partner attends for an appointment. They have been trying to conceive a pregnancy for 18 months without success.

Please take a relevant history from the couple and discuss the first-line investigations that you will request.

OSCE patient instructions

Personal details – female: Emma Bennett, 34 years old, caterer, body mass index (BMI) 23 kg/m^2

Presenting complaint: 18 months of subfertility, no previous pregnancies. She and her partner have regular, unprotected vaginal intercourse without difficulty.

Medical/surgical history: Nil of note, no regular medications, no allergies

Obstetrics and gynaecology history: No known gynaecological diagnosis. Regular 28-day menstrual cycle, last menstrual period 3 weeks ago. Heavy flow for 3 days then light for 2. Associated with moderate pain for the first days of her period. No intermenstrual or postcoital bleeding. No pain on intercourse. Had chlamydia aged 19 years, which was treated. Smears up to date and normal. Previously had Implanon removed 2 years ago.

Social/family history: Nil of note. Smokes 2–3 cigarettes a day. Drinks approximately 8 units a week socially.

Personal details – male: Simon Bennett, 35 years old, builder, BMI 28 kg/m^2

Presenting complaint: Has never fathered any pregnancies.

Medical/surgical history: No regular medications, no allergies. No previous injury or operations on the groin or testicles. No chronic medical conditions or childhood infections. No sexually transmitted infection (STI) history.

Social/family history: Nonsmoker. Drinks approximately 15 units a week socially. Previously used anabolic steroids approximately 2 years ago when working out in the gym.

Mark scheme

- Introduces self and establishes rapport.
- Identifies patient name and personal details of female and male partners.
- Addresses their concerns.
- Establishes time of subfertility and regularity of intercourse.
- Establishes whether either partner have conceived a pregnancy.
- Obstetrics and gynaecology history including:
  - Last menstrual period, menstrual history, contraceptive history, smear history, STI history, signs of polycystic ovarian syndrome
- Medical and surgical history from female including:
  - chronic conditions, regular medications, over-the-counter medication, allergies
- Medical and surgical history from male including:
  - chronic conditions, regular medications, over-the-counter medication, allergies
  - groin or testicular infections or operations
- Social and family history of both:
  - alcohol, smoking and drug history
- Discuss initial investigations to perform:
  - Examination – BMI, abdominal, vaginal and testicular
  - Transvaginal ultrasound – to identify structural abnormalities of the pelvic organs
  - Blood tests – hormone profile
  - Semen analysis – to asses for male factor infertility
- Suggest referral to fertility clinic after results of the investigations are reviewed.
- Explore that ideas, concerns and expectations are met.

Questions

1. What are possible underlying causes for their primary infertility and what highlights this in the history?
   Female factor
   - Previous history of chlamydia – previous STIs can cause tubal pathology.
   - Moderate pain during periods – this could suggest an underlying diagnosis of endometriosis, although her history is otherwise suggestive of this.

Male factor

- Previous use of anabolic steroids – these drugs are known to reduce sperm quality and quantity, which can be permanent.

2. What are the fertility rates amongst the general population trying to conceive?

   Over 80% of couples conceive successfully within 1 year if the woman is aged under 40 years and they are having regular unprotected vaginal sexual intercourse. Of the remaining who do not conceive in the first year, half will go on to conceive within a second year.

3. What conservative measures can Emma and Simon do to help their chances of conception?

   Conservative measures to be suggested include:

   - optimize BMI through diet and exercise
   - stop smoking
   - reduce alcohol intake

4. Their investigation results come back. Emma has a normal ultrasound and hormone profile. Simon has a semen analysis which shows <5 million spermatozoa per mL with 1% normal forms – what do you advise they do next?

   This semen analysis is abnormal showing oligozoospermia and decreased normal forms. A repeat test should be performed in 3 months' time to confirm these results.

   In the meantime, Simon should perform conservative measures to improve semen production, such as male supplements, loose fitting underwear, reduction of alcohol intake to additionally help.

5. Simon's repeat semen analysis shows similar results – what options are available to the couple?

   It would be advisable to refer Simon to see a urologist, in case of any potential reversible pathology, such as a varicocele.

   If this is not successful, options include in-vitro fertilization, intracytoplasmic sperm injection or donor sperm insemination.

SELF-ASSESSMENT QUESTIONS

Single best answer (SBA) questions

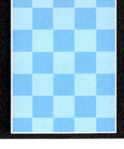

Chapter 1 Basic anatomy and examination

1. A woman has an appointment in the antenatal clinic. She is 34 weeks' pregnant. Which of the following cannot be determined by abdominal palpation alone?
   A. Gestation.
   B. Fetal lie.
   C. Engagement.
   D. Presentation.
   E. Fetal heart rate.

2. You examine a woman who is at 38 weeks' gestation. Which of the following is not used as assessment for the Bishop score?
   A. Consistency.
   B. Dilatation.
   C. Station.
   D. Position.
   E. Colour of liquor.

3. A woman who is at 36 weeks' gestation should have a symphysis-fundal height (SFH) of approximately?
   A. 36 cm.
   B. 33–39 cm.
   C. 34–36 cm.
   D. 33–38 cm.
   E. 33–37 cm.

4. A woman who is at 39 weeks' gestation is being induced for pregnancy-induced hypertension. Which is the most important factor in determining her success?
   A. Cervical dilatation.
   B. Engagement.
   C. Consistency.
   D. Bishop score.
   E. Cervical length.

5. A 50-year-old presents with a lump in the vagina and urinary leakage during coughing. What is the most appropriate initial assessment?
   A. Urodynamics.
   B. Assessment with Cusco's speculum.
   C. Assessment with Sims speculum.
   D. Physiotherapy assessment.
   E. Pelvic ultrasound.

Chapter 3 Common investigations

1. Which of the following cannot be identified with a bedside urine dipstick?

   A. Haematuria.
   B. Proteinuria.
   C. Glucosuria.
   D. Human chorionic gonadotropin.
   E. Bence Jones protein.

2. Regarding the National Cervical Screening Program which of the following is not correct?
   A. Smears are 3 yearly from the age of 25 to 49 years.
   B. Smears are 5 yearly from the age of 50 to 64 years.
   C. No smears required after 65 years of age if all normal.
   D. Smear test 3 yearly from the age of 20 years.
   E. If abnormalities are found, tests may be performed more frequently.

3. A 40-year-old woman presents with a pelvic mass. The most appropriate initial investigation for this is?
   A. Transabdominal ultrasound.
   B. X-ray.
   C. Computed tomography scan.
   D. Transvaginal ultrasound.
   E. Magnetic resonance imaging (MRI).

4. A 25-year-old undergoes a laparoscopy to investigate her pelvic pain. What is not a recognized complication of a laparoscopy?
   A. Bladder injury.
   B. Ureteric injury.
   C. Vascular injury.
   D. Bowel injury.
   E. Hepatic injury.

5. A 65-year-old woman presents with recurrent postmenopausal bleeding. Ultrasound in the past was normal. What is the most appropriate investigation?
   A. General anaesthetic (GA) hysteroscopy.
   B. Outpatient hysteroscopy.
   C. Transvaginal ultrasound.
   D. Full blood count.
   E. Three-dimensional ultrasound.

Chapter 4 Abnormal uterine bleeding

1. Which of the following is not a recognized cause of abnormal menstrual bleeding?
   A. Coagulopathy.
   B. Fibroids.
   C. Malignancy.

D. Systemic lupus erythematosus (SLE).

E. Adenomyosis.

2. A 45-year-old woman presents with heavy regular periods. She requests appropriate management and has tried hormonal treatment in the past with no success. Her husband has had a vasectomy. Which should be offered in the first instance?

A. Tranexamic acid.

B. Mirena coil.

C. Total abdominal hysterectomy.

D. Endometrial ablation.

E. Uterine artery embolization.

3. A 55-year-old woman presents with postmenopausal bleeding. An ultrasound demonstrates an endometrial thickness of 8 mm. What is the most appropriate next form of management?

A. Blind curettage biopsy.

B. Outpatient hysteroscopy and biopsy.

C. Inpatient hysteroscopy and biopsy.

D. Repeat ultrasound in 4 months.

E. Hysterectomy.

4. A 47-year-old woman opts to have a hysterectomy. What complication must she be most warned of?

A. Haemorrhage.

B. Pain.

C. Injury to viscera.

D. Postoperative fever.

E. All of the above.

5. A 65-year-old woman presents with two episodes of postmenopausal bleeding. What is the most likely cause?

A. Atrophic vaginitis.

B. Endometrial fibroid.

C. Anovulatory cycle.

D. Endometrial adenocarcinoma.

E. Endometrial polyp.

Chapter 5 Fibroids

1. What position are fibroids found within the uterus?

A. Submucosal.

B. Subserous.

C. Pedunculated.

D. Intramural.

E. All of the above.

2. With regard to the prevalence of fibroids which is not true?

A. They are more common in Afro-Caribbeans.

B. Can grow in pregnancy.

C. Decrease in the postmenopause period.

D. Can become malignant in 1:100 cases.

E. Can be present in up to 50% of women over 40 years of age.

3. A 48-year-old woman presents with symptoms suggestive of fibroids. An ultrasound confirms the presence of multiple fibroids. Which of the following is not a typical symptom of fibroids?

A. Hydronephrosis.

B. Menorrhagia.

C. Chronic pelvic pain.

D. Urinary frequency.

E. Difficulty conceiving.

4. A 40-year-old woman presents with menorrhagia and a palpable pelvic mass measuring 14 weeks in size. You suspect uterine fibroids. What would be the most appropriate initial investigation in this instance?

A. Magnetic resonance imaging.

B. Computed tomography scan.

C. Hysteroscopy.

D. Pelvic ultrasound.

E. Hysteroscopy and pelvic ultrasound.

5. A 49-year-old woman with heavy periods and a large fibroid uterus does not want surgical intervention, but would like her fibroids to reduce in size and to have less heavy bleeding. What would be the appropriate management for her?

A. Hysterectomy.

B. Endometrial ablation.

C. Uterine artery embolization (UAE).

D. Mirena coil.

E. Long-term iron sulphate.

Chapter 6 Endometriosis

1. Which of the following is the main symptom of endometriosis?

A. Asymptomatic.

B. Pelvic pain.

C. Dyschezia.

D. Dyspareunia.

E. All the above.

2. A 25-year-old patient presents with pelvic pain. Her mother had endometriosis diagnosed many years ago and she suspects she may also have it. How would endometriosis be most accurately diagnosed in her case?

A. Pelvic ultrasound scan.

B. Magnetic resonance imaging.

C. Laparoscopy with biopsy.

D. Laparoscopy alone.

E. Laparotomy.

3. Which of the following is not a theory for endometriosis causation?

A. Genetic.

B. Antegrade menstruation.

C. Immunological.

D. Seeding.
E. Metaplasia.

4. A 30-year-old presents with cyclical pelvic pain and dyspareunia. She is suspected to have endometriosis but does not want surgery and wishes to manage her symptoms conservatively. Which medical management for endometriosis is currently used the least?
   A. Gonadotropin-releasing hormone.
   B. Combined oral contraceptive pill.
   C. Progesterone.
   D. Laparoscopy.
   E. Danazol.

5. You are counselling a 20-year-old about her laparoscopy she is about to undergo to treat her suspected endometriosis. Which of the following statements about laparoscopic management of endometriosis is least true?
   A. Laser ablation can be used.
   B. Excision of endometriosis can be performed.
   C. Once excised endometriosis does not recur.
   D. There is a risk of vascular injury.
   E. There is a risk of bladder injury.

Chapter 7 Pelvic pain and dyspareunia

1. When a woman presents the pelvic pain which of the following should be ruled out?
   A. Pelvic inflammatory disease.
   B. Ectopic pregnancy.
   C. Ovarian torsion.
   D. Ovarian cyst rupture.
   E. All of the above.

2. A 20-year-old woman presents acutely with severe right-sided pelvic pain, with guarding. Her pregnancy test is negative, and her blood tests are normal. Ultrasound reveals a 7-cm simple ovarian cyst. What is the most appropriate next step?
   A. Give analgesia and manage conservatively.
   B. Laparoscopic appendectomy.
   C. Laparoscopic oophorectomy.
   D. Repeat blood tests.
   E. Laparoscopic ovarian cystectomy.

3. A 28-year-old woman presents with deep dyspareunia, pelvic pain and discomfort passing stool around the time of her period. The most likely diagnosis is?
   A. Pelvic inflammatory disease (PID).
   B. Endometriosis.
   C. Nerve entrapment.
   D. Irritable bowel syndrome.
   E. Adenomyosis.

4. A 20-year-old woman attends the emergency department with severe pelvic pain and shoulder tip pain. The most important test to help with the diagnosis is?
   A. Urine β-human chorionic gonadotropin (β-HCG).
   B. High vaginal swab.
   C. Pelvic ultrasound.
   D. Full blood count.
   E. Pelvic magnetic resonance imaging.

5. A 32-year-old woman who has had six laparoscopies in the past for pelvic pain re-presents with generalized pelvic pain. Her last laparoscopy was reported as normal. You rule out an acute cause. Magnetic resonance imaging recently was normal. She is taking regular paracetamol and ibuprofen. What would be the most appropriate management for her?
   A. Investigative laparotomy.
   B. Laparoscopy and proceed.
   C. Repeat magnetic resonance imaging in 4 months.
   D. Offer referral to support groups.
   E. Consider second-line analgesia.

Chapter 8 Vaginal discharge and sexually transmitted infections

1. Which of the following is not a pathological cause of vaginal discharge?
   A. Cervical carcinoma.
   B. Cervical ectropion.
   C. *Candida albicans.*
   D. *Chlamydia trachomatis.*
   E. Fistula.

2. A patient has been diagnosed with candida infection. Which of the following supports this diagnosis?
   A. Grey, fishy-smelling discharge.
   B. Thick, itchy, white discharge.
   C. Dysuria.
   D. Urinary frequency.
   E. Lower abdominal pain.

3. A patient presents with abnormal vaginal discharge. Which aspect of her history is most helpful to rule out an infective cause?
   A. Age.
   B. Weight loss.
   C. Irregular vaginal bleeding.
   D. Anorexia.
   E. Sexual history.

4. Which of the following in a patient's history is known to predispose them to pelvic inflammatory disease (PID)?
   A. Monogamous relationship.
   B. >25 years of age.

C. History of sexually transmitted infection (STI).

D. Later onset of sexual activity.

E. Use of the Mirena intrauterine system.

5. A patient is diagnosed with acute pelvic inflammatory disease (PID). Which of the following signs does NOT support that diagnosis?

A. Raised temperature >37.5°C.

B. Tachycardia.

C. Vulval pruritis.

D. Abdominal tenderness.

E. Adnexal mass.

Chapter 9 Pelvic inflammatory disease

1. Pelvic inflammatory disease is most likely to cause?

A. Subfertility.

B. Fitz-Hugh–Curtis.

C. Chronic pain.

D. Salpingitis.

E. All of the above.

2. Which of the following organisms is not typically known to cause pelvic inflammatory disease (PID)?

A. *Neisseria gonorrhoeae*.

B. *Chlamydia trachomatis*.

C. *Gardnerella vaginalis*.

D. *Mycoplasma genitalium*.

E. *Pseudomonas*.

3. A 26-year-old woman presents with fever, vaginal discharge and pelvic pain. You suspect pelvic inflammatory disease (PID). What is the most important next step?

A. Pelvic ultrasound.

B. Take vaginal swabs.

C. Await full blood count and C-reactive protein blood test results.

D. Computed tomography scan.

E. Commence broad-spectrum antibiotics.

4. Which of these is not an appropriate first-line investigation for pelvic inflammatory disease (PID)?

A. White cell count.

B. C-reactive protein.

C. Erythrocyte sedimentation rate.

D. Laparoscopy.

E. Sexually transmitted disease screen.

5. With respect to pelvic inflammatory disease (PID) which of the following is not correct?

A. Can cause ectopic pregnancy.

B. Can cause long-standing pain.

C. Is sexually transmitted.

D. If treated, it will not cause problems in the future.

E. Can occur in all age groups.

Chapter 10 Contraception and termination of pregnancy

1. A 29-year-old woman enquires about contraception. Which of the following protects the most against sexually transmitted infections (STIs)?

A. Withdrawal method.

B. Female diaphragm.

C. Female condom.

D. Cervical cap.

E. Male condom.

2. A 36-year-old couple have completed their family. Which method has the lowest failure rate?

A. Combined oral contraceptive pill.

B. Barrier.

C. Progestin-only pills.

D. Laparoscopic female tubal ligation.

E. Vasectomy.

3. A 33-year-old woman would like a reliable form of contraception. She has had two children born by normal vaginal delivery. She has a stressful job and travels regularly. Her periods can also be quite heavy and painful. What is the most appropriate form of contraception?

A. Combined oral contraceptive pill.

B. Progestin-only pills.

C. Female sterilization.

D. Intrauterine device.

E. Intrauterine system (IUS).

4. A 28-year-old woman requests emergency contraception 73 hours after unprotected intercourse. She has had some allergy to metal jewellery in the past. What would be the most appropriate form of contraception?

A. Intrauterine system.

B. EllaOne.

C. Mirena coil.

D. Intrauterine device (IUD).

E. Levonelle.

5. A 25-year-old woman opts for a termination of pregnancy. She would like the complications of the procedure explained to her. Which of the following is not a known complication/risk of a surgical procedure?

A. Pain.

B. Infection.

C. Prolonged vaginal bleeding.

D. Cerebral ischaemic event.

E. Uterine perforation.

Chapter 11 Benign gynaecological tumours

1. A 54-year-old woman presents with a suspected ovarian mass. Which of the following is unlikely to increase her risk of an ovarian tumour?
   A. Infertility treatment.
   B. Use of ovulation induction medication.
   C. Tamoxifen.
   D. Smoking.
   E. Hyperthyroidism.

2. A 44-year-old woman presents with abdominal pain and a palpable pelvic mass. Useful initial investigations are performed. Which of the following is not recommended as an initial investigation?
   A. Urine human chorionic gonadotropin (HCG).
   B. Haemoglobin (Hb).
   C. Pelvic ultrasound scan.
   D. White cell count (WCC) and C-reactive protein (CRP).
   E. Ca-125.

3. A woman is diagnosed with a dermoid ovarian cyst. Which of the following statements is most correct?
   A. Are never bilateral.
   B. Mainly present in the 30s age group.
   C. Mainly malignant.
   D. Have an over 50% chance of torting.
   E. Present commonly having ruptured already.

4. Regarding the risk of malignancy index which of the following is not true?
   A. A score <25 indicates an approximately 3% risk of malignancy.
   B. The premenopausal score is 1.
   C. Ca-125 mg/100 mL is used in the score.
   D. The postmenopausal score is 3.
   E. Solid areas on ultrasound are significant and add to the score.

5. What is the most appropriate initial action if a 21-year-old woman presents to the emergency department with a 7-cm left-sided ovarian cyst seen on scan, severe pain and vomiting?
   A. Ca-125 blood test.
   B. Computed tomography scan.
   C. Discussion with an oncology multidisciplinary team.
   D. Laparoscopy with or without ovarian cystectomy.
   E. Magnetic resonance imaging.

Chapter 12 Gynaecological malignancies

1. Which of the following is not a risk factor for cervical cancer?
   A. Human papilloma virus (HPV).
   B. Smoking.

C. Multiple sexual partners.
D. Early age of first intercourse.
E. History of endometriosis.

2. Sarah is a 65-year-old and has not had a period for 14 years. She attended the general practitioner as she has noted abdominal bloating and nausea. An ultrasound scan showed a multiloculated right-sided ovarian cyst, and her Ca-125 is 90. What is her risk of malignancy index?
   A. 270.
   B. 720.
   C. 90.
   D. 810.
   E. 320.

3. A 73-year-old woman noted a few episodes of vaginal spotting and her transvaginal ultrasound showed an endometrial thickness of 9 mm. What is the next most important investigation she should undergo?
   A. Computed tomography scan of the abdomen and pelvis.
   B. Magnetic resonance imaging.
   C. Hysterosalpingogram.
   D. Endometrial biopsy.
   E. Cervical cytology.

4. Which of the below is not a risk factor for developing vulval cancer?
   A. Lichen sclerosis.
   B. Cervical intraepithelial neoplasia.
   C. Lichen planus.
   D. Human papillomavirus.
   E. Paget.

5. Which of the following most accurately confirms endometrial pathology?
   A. Hysteroscopy and biopsy.
   B. Pipelle biopsy.
   C. Magnetic resonance imaging of the pelvis.
   D. Laparoscopy.
   E. Transvaginal ultrasound scan.

Chapter 13 Benign vulval disease

1. A 45-year-old woman presents with pruritus vulvae. Which of the following is suggestive of an infective cause:
   A. Progressively worsening symptoms over 6 months.
   B. Menorrhagia.
   C. A thick creamy white discharge.
   D. Red plaques in the vulval area.
   E. Fused labia.

2. The following are important in the management of a woman with pruritus vulvae:
   A. Administering antibiotics.
   B. A speculum examination of the cervix and smear test.
   C. All women should be seen in colposcopy clinic.
   D. Excision of the area of the discomfort.
   E. An abdominal X-ray.

3. Which of the following is the possible method of investigation of vulval disease?
   A. C-reactive protein (CRP).
   B. Biopsy of the vulva.
   C. Ultrasound scan.
   D. Hysteroscopy.
   E. Endocervical swabs.

4. Which of the following is correct about lichen sclerosis:
   A. The vulval skin always appears white.
   B. Skin biopsy shows thinning of the epidermis.
   C. A biopsy is not necessary as the diagnosis is usually obvious.
   D. Surgical excision is first-line treatment.
   E. A short course of antibiotic treatment is usually required.

5. Which of the following statements about female genital mutilation (FGM) is not correct?
   A. There are four types.
   B. It is illegal to arrange, or assist in arranging, for a UK national or UK resident to be taken overseas for the purpose of FGM.
   C. It is an offence for those with parental responsibility to fail to protect a girl from the risk of FGM.
   D. If FGM is confirmed in a girl under 18 years of age, reporting to the police is mandatory and this must be within 1 month.
   E. De-infibulation is illegal.

Chapter 14 Urogynaecology

1. Which of the following is not a recognized symptom of vaginal prolapse?
   A. Lump appearing at the end of the day.
   B. Increased urinary frequency.
   C. Urinary tract infection (UTI).
   D. Low back pain.
   E. Loin pain.

2. Which of the following muscle does not form part of the pelvic floor?
   A. Coccygeus.
   B. Obturator internus.
   C. Piriformis.

D. Pectineus.
E. Pubococcygeus.

3. What is the most common cause of vaginal prolapse?
   A. Postmenopause.
   B. Pregnancy.
   C. Obesity.
   D. Heavy lifting.
   E. Pelvic mass.

4. In a 45-year-old woman who presents with stress and urge incontinence, the next appropriate management is?
   A. Bladder retaining.
   B. Prescribe an antimuscarinic.
   C. Pelvic floor exercise.
   D. Urodynamics.
   E. Anterior and posterior vaginal wall repair.

5. The most appropriate next step in a woman who presents with recurrent urinary tract infections (UTIs) is?
   A. Renal tract imaging.
   B. Flexible cystoscopy.
   C. Urodynamics.
   D. Prophylactic low-dose antibiotics.
   E. Repeat midstream urinalysis.

Chapter 15 Gynaecological endocrinology

1. Which of the following is a possible cause of precocious puberty?
   A. Congenital adrenal hyperplasia.
   B. Hyperprolactinaemia.
   C. Hypothyroidism.
   D. Turner syndrome.
   E. Cystic fibrosis.

2. A 28-year-old woman presents with facial hair growth. Her body mass index is $30\,kg/m^2$ and she takes regular medication for asthma, gastritis, contraception and is on antibiotics for a urinary tract infection. Which of these drugs can cause hirsutism?
   A. H2 antagonists (e.g., cimetidine).
   B. Prednisolone.
   C. Combined oral contraceptive pill.
   D. Penicillin.
   E. Progestogens.

3. An 18-year-old girl presents with a history of primary amenorrhoea. What is the most likely diagnosis?
   A. Fibroids.
   B. Testicular feminization.
   C. Premature ovarian failure.
   D. Polycystic ovarian syndrome.
   E. Lichen sclerosis.

4. In congenital adrenal hyperplasia, what is the most common enzyme defect?
   A. 20-Hydroxylase deficiency.
   B. 21-Hydroxylase deficiency.
   C. 22-Hydroxylase deficiency.
   D. 19-OH hydroxylase deficiency.
   E. 20-OH hydroxylase deficiency.

5. A 25-year-old woman is diagnosed with polycystic ovarian syndrome (PCOS). Which of the following is considered when diagnosing PCOS?
   A. >12 peripheral follicles seen on the ovaries at ultrasound.
   B. Raised testosterone levels.
   C. Raised luteinizing hormone-to-follicle-stimulating hormone ratio.
   D. Oligomenorrhoea.
   E. Body mass index (BMI) > 30 kg/m².

Chapter 16 Subfertility

1. A woman aged 30 years, who is fit and well, has been trying to conceive for 6 months unsuccessfully. How would you proceed?
   A. Refer for in-vitro fertilization.
   B. Reassure and arrange review if unsuccessful after 2 years.
   C. Reassure and arrange review if unsuccessful after 1 year.
   D. Perform a laparoscopy.
   E. Take a hormone profile blood test.

2. A woman aged 28 years presents with subfertility, weight gain, irregular periods and hirsutism. All blood tests come back normal. Which additional investigation will be most helpful?
   A. Thyroid function tests.
   B. Pelvic/transvaginal ultrasound.
   C. Hysterosalpingogram.
   D. Semen analysis.
   E. Laparoscopy.

3. A 35-year-old couple have been trying to conceive for 2 years. Female factor subfertility investigations are all normal. Semen analysis results were as follows: volume 1 mL, concentration <1 million/mL, motility 5%, normal forms 1%. Which procedure would be advised?
   A. Intrauterine insemination.
   B. In-vitro fertilization (IVF).
   C. Donor sperm.
   D. Donor oocyte.
   E. IVF intracytoplasmic sperm injection (ICSI).

4. A 41-year-old woman undergoes in-vitro fertilization treatment. She presents with bloating, shortness of

breath and abdominal pain. A chest X-ray confirms bilateral pleural effusion. What is the likely diagnosis?
   A. Ovarian hyperstimulation syndrome.
   B. Acute respiratory distress syndrome.
   C. Chest infection.
   D. Ascites.
   E. Acute liver failure.

5. A 43-year-old woman undergoes in-vitro fertilization (IVF) treatment. Which of the following does not negatively affect your chances of successful IVF?
   A. Aged over 40 years.
   B. Never had a pregnancy.
   C. Aged under 30 years.
   D. Drinking >20 units alcohol a week.
   E. Body mass index (BMI) < 19 kg/m².

Chapter 17 Menopause

1. Which of the following statement about menopause is true?
   A. Menopause is defined by an absence of periods for 6 months.
   B. Menopause is defined by the absence of periods for over 1 year above the age of 35 years.
   C. Premature menopause is an absence of periods for over 1 year in a woman over the age of 45 years but under 51 years.
   D. Menopause is defined as cessation of periods for more than 1 year in a woman over the age of 45 years.
   E. Menopause is defined by absence of periods for at least 6 months after the age of 50 years.

2. A 55-year-old woman enquires about commencing hormone replacement therapy (HRT). She is concerned about breast cancer. The risk of breast cancer is increased with which of the following?
   A. Oestrogen only HRT.
   B. Vaginal oestrogen.
   C. Selective serotonin reuptake inhibitor.
   D. HRT containing progesterone.
   E. Serotonin and noradrenaline reuptake inhibitor.

3. A 54-year-old woman experiences symptoms of menopause. Which of the following is not a symptom of menopause?
   A. Joint pains.
   B. Hot flushes.
   C. Fluctuations in mood.
   D. Sweats.
   E. Arrhythmias.

4. A 50-year-old woman commences hormone replacement therapy (HRT) containing oestrogen and progesterone. She experiences some side-effects

and consults her general practitioner. Which of the following is not a side-effect of HRT?
A. Breast tenderness.
B. Leg cramps.
C. Nausea.
D. Bloating.
E. Photophobia.

5. A woman aged 35 years presents to her general practitioner with secondary amenorrhoea for over 1 year. She is concerned about premature menopause. What is the most accurate way of determining this?
A. Elevated follicle-stimulating hormone (FSH) and luteinizing hormone (LH) levels taken 6 weeks apart.
B. Elevated LH levels taken 4 weeks apart.
C. Reduced LH levels taken 4 weeks apart.
D. Elevated FSH levels taken 5 weeks apart.
E. Elevated FSH levels taken 3 weeks apart.

Chapter 18 Early pregnancy complications

1. A 26-year-old woman attends accident and emergency with mild lower abdominal pain and vaginal spotting. Her β-human chorionic gonadotropin is positive and her last menstrual period was 6 weeks ago. Her observations are stable and haemoglobin 134. How would you like to proceed?
A. Admit to hospital and consider laparoscopy.
B. Admit to hospital for observation.
C. Arrange an ultrasound scan (USS) at soonest opportunity.
D. Reassure and discharge without follow-up.
E. Reassure and discharge with USS booked in 2 weeks.

2. A 34-year-old woman attends early pregnancy unit with mild abdominal pain, no bleeding and a positive pregnancy test. She is clinically well and observations are stable. She has transvaginal ultrasound scan but no pregnancy is seen either intrauterine or extrauterine. How can this be described?
A. She has a confirmed ectopic pregnancy.
B. She has a confirmed intrauterine pregnancy.
C. It is possible to rule out ectopic pregnancy.
D. She has had a miscarriage.
E. It is not yet possible to rule out ectopic pregnancy.

3. A 25-year-old woman is being seen in early pregnancy unit with a pregnancy of unknown location. No pregnancy can be seen on scan. Her serial serum β-human chorionic gonadotropin levels are as follows:
Day 1: 258 IU/L
Day 3: 490 IU/L
How can we describe this scenario?

A. Normal rise, conclusive of intrauterine pregnancy.
B. Normal rise, can exclude ectopic pregnancy.
C. Normal rise, cannot exclude ectopic pregnancy.
D. Suboptimal rise suggestive of miscarriage.
E. Suboptimal rise suggestive of ectopic pregnancy.

4. Which of these statements regarding ectopic pregnancy is incorrect?
A. Risk factors for ectopic pregnancy include previous tubal surgery.
B. Ectopic pregnancies can be managed surgically, medically or conservatively.
C. A falling serum β-human chorionic gonadotropin (β-HCG) eliminates risk of ectopic pregnancy rupturing.
D. Ectopic pregnancy can present with nausea and vomiting in early pregnancy.
E. Laparoscopic salpingostomy preserves the fallopian tube.

Chapter 19 Antenatal booking and prenatal diagnosis

1. A 40-year-old primiparous woman attends antenatal clinic at 12 weeks' gestation. She has a history of essential hypertension, with a family history of multiple pregnancy. She is allergic to penicillin. Which factor in her history is the most important in the antenatal risk assessment?
A. Maternal age of 40 years.
B. Primiparity.
C. Essential hypertension.
D. Family history of multiple pregnancy.
E. Allergy to penicillin.

2. Which of the following is not a routine booking investigation?
A. Full blood count.
B. Blood group.
C. Hepatitis B status.
D. High vaginal swab.
E. Urine microscopy, culture and sensitivity.

3. When should an amniocentesis be performed?
A. Before 12 weeks.
B. After 15 weeks but before 19 weeks.
C. After 20 weeks.
D. After 12 weeks but before 13 weeks.
E. After 15 weeks.

4. A 41-year-old woman in her third pregnancy attends for her antenatal booking appointment at 10 weeks. She wishes specialist advice about her risk of Down syndrome, particularly as she already has two children, one of whom suffers from autism. Which

screening test would you recommend as the most informative?
A. Ultrasound scan at 18–20 weeks.
B. Noninvasive prenatal testing at 16 weeks.
C. Chorionic villus sampling at 12 weeks.
D. Quadruple test at 16 weeks.
E. Combined test at 12 weeks.

Chapter 20 Antepartum haemorrhage

1. A 22-year-old woman with a history of drug misuse presents to the labour ward at 26 weeks' gestation with a 6-hour history of constant abdominal pain and some vaginal bleeding. What is the most likely diagnosis?
A. Symphysis pubis dysfunction.
B. Preterm labour.
C. Uterine fibroid degeneration.
D. Placental abruption.
E. Acute fatty liver of pregnancy.

2. A 26-year-old woman who is 28 weeks' pregnant with no medical or gynaecological history of note presents with a history of fresh vaginal bleeding within the last 12 hours. On further questioning, the bleeding started after sexual intercourse. What is the most likely diagnosis?
A. Cervical polyp.
B. Vulval varicosities.
C. Cervical ectropion.
D. Cervical carcinoma.
E. Vaginitis.

3. Ultrasound scan is useful in the diagnosis of which of the following causes of antepartum haemorrhage?
A. Cervical polyp.
B. Vasa praevia.
C. Circumvallate placenta.
D. Placental abruption.
E. Placenta praevia.

4. A 32-year-old woman, who is known to have essential hypertension, attends with a sudden onset of fresh vaginal bleeding and abdominal pain at 29 weeks in her first pregnancy. The doctor suspects a placental abruption. What is the most important initial management?
A. Haemoglobin.
B. Airway, breathing, circulation (ABC) resuscitation.
C. Cardiotocograph.
D. Group-and-save serum.
E. Ultrasound scan.

Chapter 21 Hypertension in pregnancy

1. A 20-year-old patient who is 36 weeks' pregnant attends clinic with a blood pressure of 156/102 mmHg. She has 2+ of protein in her urine. What investigations are required?
A. Electrocardiogram, chest X-ray and V/Q scan.
B. Liver function tests, full blood count, urea and electrolytes, urine protein-to-creatinine ratio and clotting.
C. Thyroid functions tests.
D. Serum cortisol.
E. Renal ultrasound.

2. Which of the following medications is considered as first line for treatment of hypertension in pregnancy in nonasthmatic patients?
A. Enalapril.
B. Nifedipine.
C. Methyldopa.
D. Labetalol.
E. Hydralazine.

3. Which medication should be administered as soon as possible in a patient thought to be having an eclamptic seizure?
A. Diazepam.
B. Methyldopa.
C. Labetalol.
D. Hydralazine.
E. Magnesium sulphate.

4. Which of the following is NOT a common symptom of preeclampsia?
A. Headache.
B. Itching.
C. Epigastric pain.
D. Oedema.
E. Visual disturbance.

5. A 38-year-old woman with a history of essential hypertension attends the antenatal clinic following her booking appointment. Her general practitioner has already changed her regular antihypertensives to labetalol 200 mg twice a day. What would be the most beneficial drug to start?
A. Folic acid 400 mcg.
B. Folic acid 5 mg.
C. Aspirin 75 mg.
D. Vitamin D 10 mcg.
E. Enalapril 5 mg.

Chapter 22 Medical disorders in pregnancy

1. Which of the following is NOT a risk factor for gestational diabetes?
A. Body mass index $> 30 \text{kg/m}^2$.
B. South Asian origin.
C. Family history of type 2 diabetes in a first-degree relative.

D. Previous gestational diabetes.
E. Husband with type 2 diabetes.

2. Which of the following is not a known risk factor for venous thromboembolism in pregnancy?
   A. Thrombophilia (factor V Leiden, protein C deficiency, antiphospholipid syndrome).
   B. Age >35 years.
   C. Body mass index > 30 kg/m^2.
   D. Parity > 3.
   E. Age <20 years.

3. Anaemia in pregnancy should be identified and treated where necessary. What levels of haemoglobin are acceptable at booking and at 28 weeks?
   A. >11.0 g/dL at booking and >10.5 g/dL at 28 weeks.
   B. >11.0 g/dL at booking and >9.5 g/dL at 28 weeks.
   C. >10.0 g/dL at booking and >10.5 g/dL at 28 weeks.
   D. >9.0 g/dL at booking and >11.0 g/dL at 28 weeks.
   E. >7.0 g/dL at booking and >10.5 g/dL at 28 weeks.

4. What three steps have been shown to reduce the vertical transmission of human immunodeficiency virus (HIV) from mother to fetus?
   A. Antibiotics, elective caesarean section and breastfeeding.
   B. Hand washing, vaginal delivery and steroids.
   C. Avoidance of breastfeeding and antiretroviral medication [highly active antiretroviral therapy (HAART)] to the mother and to the baby.
   D. Avoidance of intercourse, breastfeeding and antibiotics.
   E. Steroids, elective caesarean section and antibiotics.

5. A 32-year-old patient who has had type 1 diabetes since her teens comes to see you because she plans to stop the oral contraceptive pill. What advice is the most important?
   A. Start taking folic acid 0.4 mg daily.
   B. Start aspirin 75 mg daily.
   C. Book an oral glucose tolerance test.
   D. Start taking folic acid 5 mg daily.
   E. Plan for midwifery-led care.

6. Which of the following is NOT part of the antenatal care of patients with epilepsy?
   A. Aim to control seizures with monotherapy.
   B. Take folic acid 5 mg daily from preconception until 12 weeks' gestation.
   C. Prescribe vitamin K 10 mg daily from preconception until 12 weeks' gestation.

D. Encourage breastfeeding.
E. Arrange a detailed fetal ultrasound scan to exclude cardiac defects.

7. A 26-year-old primiparous woman presents to the labour ward at 33 weeks' gestation with a 2-day history of feeling increasingly unwell with nausea and vomiting. On admission, she has mildly raised blood pressure. She has blood investigations which show a raised alanine aminotransferase, a very high uric acid level and low blood glucose. What is the most likely diagnosis?
   A. Fulminating preeclampsia.
   B. Acute fatty liver of pregnancy.
   C. Obstetric cholestasis.
   D. Pregnancy-induced hypertension.
   E. Cholelithiasis.

8. About 2 weeks postnatally, a 36-year-old multiparous woman starts to worry that her partner is spying on her as she cares for her baby. She begins to think she can hear someone telling she is doing tasks incorrectly. Her partner calls the health visitor who suspects that the most likely diagnosis is:
   A. Baby blues.
   B. Bipolar disorder.
   C. Schizophrenia.
   D. Postnatal depression.
   E. Puerperal psychosis.

Chapter 23 Common presentations in pregnancy

1. A 34-year-old woman is seen in antenatal clinic complaining of 2 weeks of lower abdominal discomfort. On further questioning, she has no urinary symptoms or vaginal discharge but is passing hard stools. What is the most likely diagnosis?
   A. Peptic ulcer disease.
   B. Ligament pain.
   C. Constipation.
   D. Ovarian cyst rupture.
   E. Cystitis.

2. A 25-year-old Asian woman measures small for dates at 32 weeks' gestation which is confirmed on ultrasound scan. Her Body mass index at booking was 21 kg/m^2. She has normal blood pressure, no proteinuria and has had a normal fetal anomaly ultrasound scan. Which of the following is the most likely cause for being small for dates?
   A. Gestational diabetes.
   B. Gestational trophoblastic disease.
   C. Constitutional.
   D. Preeclampsia.
   E. Fetal chromosomal anomaly.

3. A 36-year-old woman in her third pregnancy at 36 weeks presents with central lower abdominal pain and difficulty walking. She has no urinary or bowel symptoms. What is the likely diagnosis?
   A. Urinary tract infection.
   B. Appendicitis.
   C. Ligament pain.
   D. Symphysis pubis dysfunction.
   E. Gallstones.

4. A woman of Indian origin measures large for dates at her 28th week antenatal appointment and her midwife arranges a growth ultrasound scan. The ultrasound scan shows a macrosomic baby with polyhydramnios. Which is the most important investigation to perform next?
   A. TORCH screen.
   B. Glucose tolerance test.
   C. Rhesus status.
   D. Full blood count.
   E. Amniocentesis.

Chapter 24 Multiple pregnancy

1. A 33-year-old woman has a monochorionic twin pregnancy. Ultrasound scan at 22 weeks shows discrepant growth and liquor volumes. Which is the most likely diagnosis?
   A. Gestational diabetes.
   B. Preeclampsia.
   C. Fetal infection.
   D. Maternal anaemia.
   E. Twin-to-twin transfusion syndrome.

2. A 25-year-old woman in her second pregnancy is induced at 37 weeks with a twin pregnancy. The labour progresses at a normal rate and both babies are delivered normally. However, she has a heavy blood loss after delivery of approximately 900 mL. Which is the most likely cause?
   A. Uterine atony.
   B. Second-degree tear.
   C. Placental abruption.
   D. Retained placenta.
   E. Maternal infection.

3. A 29-year-old woman has an ultrasound scan at 13 weeks which shows she is expecting twins. It is a spontaneous conception. The scan shows a lambda sign looking at the membranes, one placental mass and two male fetuses. Which of the following statements is true?
   A. The pregnancy is a monochorionic pregnancy.
   B. The twins must be identical.
   C. The pregnancy must be dizygotic.

D. The pregnancy is a dichorionic pregnancy.
E. There is a placenta praevia.

Chapter 25 Preterm labour

1. A 19-year-old woman attends the labour ward at 28 weeks' gestation with increasingly regular tightenings every 10 minutes. On cervical assessment, there is cervical effacement and dilatation of 1 cm. Which is your first line of management?
   A. Urinalysis.
   B. Administration of steroids.
   C. Liaising with the paediatric team.
   D. Tocolysis.
   E. Caesarean section.

2. Which of the following is NOT a risk factor for preterm labour?
   A. Bacterial vaginosis.
   B. Previous preterm delivery.
   C. Previous caesarean section.
   D. Multiple pregnancy.
   E. Lack of social support.

3. A 31-year-old woman in her first pregnancy has been diagnosed with preterm prelabour rupture of membranes at 33 weeks. You are called to assess her on the antenatal ward. Which feature of your history and examination makes you most concerned for the wellbeing of the woman and her baby?
   A. Maternal tachypnoea.
   B. Vaginal swab confirms candida infection.
   C. Small amount of mucoid vaginal bleeding.
   D. White blood cell count of 15×10^9/L.
   E. Pain on passing urine (dysuria).

Chapter 26 Labour

1. During the course of labour, abdominal palpation is the most appropriate method of assessing which of the following parameters?
   A. Position of the presenting part.
   B. Strength of uterine contractions.
   C. Station of the presenting part.
   D. Presence of caput.
   E. Baseline variability of the fetal heart rate.

2. Which of the following terms does NOT describe the mechanism for delivery of the fetal head?
   A. Flexion.
   B. External rotation.
   C. Extension.
   D. Abduction.
   E. Internal rotation.

3. In obstetric palpation, which factor is the most important for assessing progress in labour?

A. Symphysis-fundal height.
B. Fetal presentation.
C. Engagement.
D. Fetal position.
E. Liquor volume.

4. In vaginal examination, which factor is the most important for assessing progress in labour?
A. Presence of caput.
B. Presence of moulding.
C. Fetal position.
D. Cervical dilatation.
E. Station.

Chapter 27 Fetal monitoring in labour

1. In a low-risk primiparous woman, which of the following indications necessitate continuous fetal monitoring in labour?
A. Irregular contractions.
B. Mucoid show.
C. Second stage of labour.
D. Pethidine analgesia.
E. Meconium-stained liquor.

2. A 39-year-old primiparous woman has progressed spontaneously in labour to 6 cm. She is having continuous electronic fetal monitoring because she had a small antepartum haemorrhage in the latent phase of labour. The monitoring appears to have been pathological for 50 minutes. What is the most appropriate course of action?
A. Fetal blood sampling.
B. Intravenous fluids.
C. Epidural anaesthesia.
D. Check maternal blood pressure.
E. Caesarean section.

3. With regard to cardiotocograph monitoring, what is the definition of an acceleration?
A. Increase in the fetal heart rate (FHR) of 5 bpm above the baseline rate lasting for 15 seconds.
B. Increase in the FHR of 15 bpm above the baseline rate lasting for 15 seconds.
C. Decrease in the FHR of 15 bpm below the baseline for 15 seconds.
D. Increase in the FHR of 5 bpm above the baseline rate lasting for 5 seconds.
E. Increase in the FHR of 15 bpm above the baseline rate lasting for 5 seconds.

Chapter 28 Operative interventions in labour

1. A 31-year-old primiparous woman has a forceps delivery and perineal trauma involving the perineal

muscles and external anal sphincter muscle? What is the correct classification for the perineal trauma described?
A. Midline episiotomy.
B. First-degree perineal tear.
C. Fourth-degree perineal tear.
D. Third-degree perineal tear.
E. Second-degree perineal tear.

2. Which of the following is NOT indicated in the care of a woman having a vaginal delivery after caesarean section?
A. Continuous fetal monitoring.
B. Intravenous cannula.
C. Blood sent for group and save.
D. Epidural anaesthesia.
E. Amniotomy.

3. A woman has been started on syntocinon for augmentation of labour as meconium-stained liquor was noted when her membranes ruptured spontaneously. She is 4 cm dilated and is contracting 6 in 10 and the cardiotocograph shows atypical decelerations. What is the immediate management?
A. Deliver the baby by caesarean section.
B. Reduce/stop the syntocinon infusion.
C. Start oxygen therapy.
D. Start intravenous fluids.
E. Give terbutaline.

Chapter 29 Complications of labour

1. A 33-year-old low-risk Caucasian woman in her first pregnancy is in spontaneous labour but has not progressed from 5 cm in the last 4 hours. What should be assessed as the most likely cause for this failure to progress in labour?
A. Incoordinate uterine activity.
B. Female circumcision.
C. Left ovarian cyst.
D. Fetal goitre.
E. Opiate analgesia.

2. A 38-year-old African woman is in her fifth pregnancy with a diagnosis of preterm labour at 35 weeks. The membranes rupture while she is being assessed for signs of labour. There is a prolonged fetal bradycardia which is not recovering. Which is the most likely diagnosis?
A. Fetal infection.
B. Uterine rupture.
C. Amniotic fluid embolism.
D. Umbilical cord prolapse.
E. Hyperstimulation of the uterus.

3. Which of the following is NOT a contraindication to external cephalic version (ECV)?
   A. Ruptured membranes.
   B. Multiparity.
   C. Placenta praevia.
   D. Severe preeclampsia.
   E. Multiple pregnancy.

Chapter 30 Stillbirth

1. The definition of a stillbirth is …
   A. A baby born with no signs of life at or after 20 completed weeks of pregnancy.
   B. A fetus in-utero greater than 24 completed weeks of pregnancy found to have no cardiac activity.
   C. A baby born with no signs of life at or after 28 completed weeks of pregnancy.
   D. A fetus in-utero greater than 22 completed weeks of pregnancy found to have no cardiac activity.
   E. A baby that is born with no signs of life at or after 24 completed weeks of pregnancy.

2. As part of the investigations of a stillbirth a TORCH screen for infections is performed. Which of the following infections is NOT tested for?
   A. Toxoplasmosis.
   B. Parvovirus B19.
   C. Malaria.
   D. Cytomegalovirus.
   E. Rubella.

Chapter 31 Postnatal complications

1. Management of postpartum haemorrhage must start with:
   A. Identifying the cause of bleeding.
   B. Multidisciplinary team approach.
   C. Basic resuscitation [airway, breathing, circulation (ABC)].
   D. Contacting haematology and anaesthetic specialists.
   E. Making an accurate estimation of the blood loss.

2. The definition of secondary postpartum haemorrhage (PPH) is as follows:
   A. >500-mL vaginal bleeding 24 hours after delivery, within 6 weeks.
   B. >1000-mL vaginal bleeding after delivery up to 6 weeks.
   C. >2000-mL vaginal bleeding postdelivery.
   D. >500-mL vaginal bleeding within 24 hours of delivery.
   E. <2000-mL vaginal bleeding within 24 hours of delivery.

3. A 29-year-old primiparous woman, known to have fibroids, has just delivered a baby weighing 4.1 kg, after being induced and having a long first stage of labour. As the placenta delivers, she suddenly feels faint and passes 700 mL of blood and clot vaginally. What is the most likely cause of the postpartum haemorrhage?
   A. Genital tract trauma.
   B. Retained placental cotyledon.
   C. Cervical ectropion.
   D. Placenta accreta.
   E. Uterine atony.

4. A 33-year-old woman who delivered 3 days previously by normal vaginal delivery has called her community midwife as she feels increasingly unwell with lower abdominal pain and a fever. Her 7-year-old son is off school with a sore throat. The most likely possible cause of sepsis in this patient is:
   A. Urinary tract infection.
   B. Mastitis.
   C. Pneumonia.
   D. Endometritis.
   E. Group A streptococcus.

Chapter 32 Maternal collapse and maternal death

1. A 19-year-old girl attends accident and emergency with abdominal pain and vaginal spotting. She gives a urine sample which reveals she is pregnant. Her last period was around 7 weeks ago. She is surprised by the news and then collapses. What is the most likely cause of her collapse which must be urgently excluded?
   A. Appendicitis.
   B. Urinary tract infection.
   C. Ectopic pregnancy.
   D. Vasovagal syncope.
   E. Gastroenteritis.

2. A 34-year-old solicitor who is 35 weeks' pregnant in her first pregnancy is at her office when she begins to feel unwell. She complains of abdominal pain and then collapses. On arrival at the hospital her blood pressure in 76/44 mmHg and her pulse is 132 bpm. Her uterus is 'woody hard' and tender on palpation. What is the most likely cause of collapse?
   A. Sepsis.
   B. Placental abruption.
   C. Uterine rupture.
   D. Vasovagal syncope.
   E. Acute myocardial infarction.

3. You are alone assessing a 40-year-old lady who has just arrived from Uganda at 36 weeks and is feeling unwell. You palpate her abdomen and find she

measures small for dates and has a blood pressure of 182/122 mmHg. She then appears to have a seizure and is unconscious. What is the most appropriate next line of action?

A. Start cardiopulmonary resuscitation.
B. Put the patient in recovery position and wait until she wakes up.
C. Call for help, position the patient with a left lateral tilt and protect airway until help arrives.
D. Organize an electrocardiogram once she wakes up.
E. Take an arterial blood gas.

4. In the latest MBRRACE-UK report, 2012–14, what was found to be the leading cause of indirect maternal death?

A. Ectopic.
B. Haemorrhage.
C. Anaesthesia.
D. Cardiac disease.
E. Murder.

Extended-matching questions (EMQs)

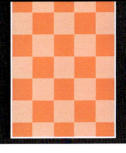

Each answer can be used once, more than once or not at all.

Chapter 1 Basic anatomy and examination

Symptoms related to anatomy

A. 20 Weeks' gestation
B. Cystocele
C. Ovarian cyst
D. Deep infiltrating endometriosis
E. Fibroid uterus
F. Vaginal atrophy
G. Stress incontinence
H. Pelvic inflammatory disease
I. Scarring
J. Adhesions

With regard to the following scenarios using your knowledge of anatomy, please indicate what the likely diagnosis is?

1. A 35-year-old woman presents with increased urinary frequency, heavy periods and a palpable pelvic lump up to the umbilicus.
2. A 30-year-old woman presents with pelvic pain. On examination you palpate tender and scarred uterosacral ligaments bilaterally.
3. A 55-year-old woman presents with vaginal soreness. On examination the labia are friable and appear white.

Chapter 3 Common investigations

A. Urine human chorionic gonadotropin (HCG)
B. Hysteroscopy
C. Laparoscopy
D. Transabdominal ultrasound
E. Transvaginal ultrasound
F. Cystoscopy
G. Midstream urine
H. High vaginal swab
I. Hysterosalpingogram
J. Cervical smear
K. 3D ultrasound
L. Ca-125

For each scenario below, choose the most likely investigation that will help with management from the corresponding option list given above.

1. A 25-year-old woman with left-sided pelvic pain and PV spotting.
2. A 27-year-old woman who is brought in to the emergency department unstable with severe pelvic pain and free fluid seen on ultrasound in the department.
3. A 45-year-old with recurrent haematuria, previous urinalysis has been normal.
4. A 60-year-old woman with postmenopausal bleeding and ultrasound which has demonstrated an endometrial thickness of 8 mm.
5. A 40-year-old presents with a pelvic mass.

Chapter 4 Abnormal uterine bleeding

Management of abnormal uterine bleeding

A. Tranexamic acid
B. Mefenamic acid
C. Laparoscopic hysterectomy
D. Abdominal hysterectomy
E. Endometrial ablation
F. Transcervical resection of endometrium
G. Copper coil
H. Mirena coil
I. Uterine artery embolization (UAE)
J. Myomectomy
K. Hysteroscopy with resection of endometrial polyp
L. Hysteroscopy with resection of endometrial fibroid

For each scenario below, choose the most likely corresponding option from the list given above.

1. A 45-year-old woman presents with heavy menstrual bleeding. She has tried medical therapy and ablation, but it has been unsuccessful. She would like definitive management.
2. A 21-year-old woman presents with heavy painful menstrual bleeding. She has had one termination of pregnancy (TOP) in the past.
3. A 47-year-old woman with heavy regular periods who has tried medical therapy. She has been sterilized in the past.
4. A 21-year-old who would like to conceive but has heavy periods.
5. A 35-year-old with intermenstrual bleeding. Ultrasound identified a 2 × 1 cm endometrial mass with feeding vessel.

Chapter 5 Fibroids

Management of fibroids

A. Repeat ultrasound in 6 months
B. Repeat magnetic resonance imaging (MRI) in 6 months
C. Transcervical resection of fibroids
D. Transcervical resection of polyp
E. Focussed ultrasound
F. Myomectomy
G. Focussed MRI-guided ultrasound
H. Tranexamic acid
I. Hysterectomy
J. Hysteroscopy + biopsy
K. Endometrial ablation
L. Uterine artery embolization

For each scenario below, choose the most likely corresponding option from the list given above

1. A 28-year-old woman with subfertility has heavy periods.
2. A 40-year-old has known fibroids approximately 30 weeks in size, with hydronephrosis diagnosed on scan. She would like to conceive.
3. A 50-year-old postmenopausal woman with 28-week fibroid uterus has hydronephrosis diagnosed on scan.
4. A 47-year-old woman has heavy periods, increased urinary frequency and a large fibroid uterus diagnosed on scan. She declines to have surgery.
5. A 35-year-old woman has a pedunculated fibroid diagnosed incidentally on scan measuring 3 cm.

Chapter 6 Endometriosis

Patient with endometriosis

A. Combined oral contraceptive pill
B. Progesterone pill
C. Nonsteroidal antiinflammatory drugs (NSAIDs)
D. NSAIDs + Tranexamic acid
E. Gonadotropin-releasing hormone
F. Danazol
G. Laparotomy with total abdominal hysterectomy and bilateral salpingo-oophorectomy
H. Laparoscopy with treatment of endometriosis
I. Laparoscopy + excision of endometriosis
J. Mirena coil
K. Mirena coil + NSAIDs
L. Laparoscopy with treatment of endometriosis + Mirena coil

For each patient with endometriosis, select the most appropriate management.

1. A 25-year-old who has tried analgesia to help with painful periods but continues to be symptomatic. She does not want hormones.
2. A 17-year-old with irregular painful periods.
3. A 21-year-old who has heavy painful periods and does not like taking tablets. She has had a laparoscopy in the past which confirmed endometriosis.
4. A 27-year-old who had laser treatment to endometriosis but now after 1 year the pain has recurred.
5. A 35-year-old with pelvic pain has tried analgesia which has been unsuccessful and is trying to conceive.

Pelvic pain

A. Pelvic inflammatory disease
B. Ovarian torsion
C. Irritable bowel syndrome
D. Ovarian cyst rupture
E. Ruptured ectopic pregnancy
F. Haemorrhagic ovarian cyst
G. Endometriosis
H. Adenomyosis
I. Adhesions
J. Appendicitis
K. Ureteric colic
L. Inflammatory bowel syndrome

For each scenario below, choose the most likely diagnosis from the list given above.

1. A 19-year-old woman presents with chronic pelvic pain, deep dyspareunia and dyschezia.
2. A 25-year-old presents with acute right-sided pelvic pain, a palpable mass on vaginal examination and haemoglobin of 80. Urine β-human chorionic gonadotropin is negative.
3. A 36-year-old who has had multiple operations presents with chronic generalized pelvic pain.
4. A 40-year-old woman presents with regular painful, heavy periods.
5. A 20-year-old presents with acute right-sided pelvic pain, she feels faint. She has had a previous appendectomy.

Chapter 8 Vaginal discharge and Sexually Transmitted Infections

Vaginal discharge

A. Bacterial vaginosis
B. *Candida albicans*
C. *Trichomonas vaginalis*
D. *Chlamydia trachomatis*
E. *Neisseria gonorrhoea*
F. Cervical carcinoma
G. Retained tampon
H. Toxic shock syndrome
I. Foreign body

For each scenario described below, choose the single most likely diagnosis from the list of options given above.

1. A 20-year-old woman who is 8 weeks' pregnant presents with a 2-week history of fishy-smelling PV discharge. It is nonitchy and creamy coloured. She has had previous episodes outside of pregnancy which resolved spontaneously. She is in a monogamous relationship with the same partner for 5 years. On speculum examination there is a small amount of smooth grey discharge seen coating the vaginal walls.
2. A 14-year-old girl presented to the accident and emergency department with her mother. She has been feeling unwell with abdominal pain, high temperature, rigors, nausea and vomiting and an offensive PV discharge. She has been busy and stressed with examinations at school. Her period started 4 days ago and she has been using tampons.
3. A 35-year-old lady has been referred from her GP to colposcopy clinic. She has recently arrived in the UK from Sub-Saharan Africa and the GP is concerned that she has never had a smear and has been complaining of an offensive blood-stained PV discharge. On speculum examination there is a fungating, bleeding cervical mass that was biopsied.
4. A 26-year-old woman presents to gynaecology clinic with a history of postcoital PVB mixed with discharge. She is up to date with her cervical smears, which have been normal. She is in a new relationship and is using the combined oral contraceptive pill (COCP) for contraception. She recalls feeling unwell 3 days ago with right upper quadrant discomfort which has now resolved. Speculum examination showed an inflamed 'strawberry appearance' of the cervix, consistent with cervicitis. An endocervical swab was taken.
5. A 6-year-old girl is seen in general outpatient department with her parents. She has been having persistent vaginal discharge on her underwear and the GP has not found a cause. An abdominal ultrasound scan has been unremarkable. She is an only child and has a good relationship with both her parents and is especially close to her mother who she wants to be like 'when she grows up'. There is no suspicion of abuse. The parents comment that she is usually very talkative and inquisitive and likes exploring around the house. However, she recently has not been herself and appears to be in intermittent discomfort in the suprapubic region. She has been booked on an elective list for an examination under anaesthetic.

Chapter 9 Pelvic Inflammatory Disease

Pelvic pain and dyspareunia

A. Adenomyosis
B. Bacterial vaginosis
C. *Candida* infection
D. Cervical cancer
E. Endometriosis
F. Urinary tract infection
G. *Chlamydia*
H. Gonococcal infection
I. Cervical ectopy

For each scenario described below, choose the single most likely diagnosis from the list of options given above.

1. A 37-year-old woman presents with deep dyspareunia, menorrhagia and dysmenorrhoea. The uterus is fixed and tender on bimanual examination. At laparoscopy, 'powder burn' areas were seen in the pouch of Douglas.
2. At laparoscopy on a 24-year-old woman with pelvic pain and dyspareunia, adhesions around the liver are seen.
3. A 38-year-old woman, para 3 + 1, presents with secondary dysmenorrhoea. She reports increase in pelvic pain midcycle with climax at the onset of menses. She also complains of lower back 'dragging' pain. On examination she has a bulky, anteverted mobile uterus with a doughy consistency. No discrete masses can be felt. Pelvic ultrasound scan confirms the diagnosis.
4. A 26-year-old diabetic woman complains of a 2-week history of superficial dyspareunia. She has noticed that this has been associated with increasing amounts of PV discharge and itching. She has just recovered from a chest infection for which she was on antibiotics. On speculum examination there is a copious amount of thick vaginal discharge with a 'cottage cheese' consistency.
5. A 31-year-old woman, 19 weeks' pregnant, presents to her GP with a 3-day history of pelvic pain. On direct questioning she has noticed increased urinary frequency which she attributed to the pregnancy and dysuria. No PV bleeding or constitutional symptoms were seen. Urine analysis is nitrate positive and showed some haematuria.

Chapter 10 Contraception and termination of pregnancy

Method of contraception

A. Natural method
B. Barrier method
C. Combined oral contraceptive pill (COCP)
D. Depo-Provera
E. Intrauterine system (IUS)
F. Intrauterine device (IUD)
G. Laparoscopic female sterilization
H. Male sterilization
I. Ulipristal acetate (EllaOne)
J. Termination of pregnancy

For the following scenarios, which contraceptive method would be most appropriate in the first instance?

1. A 41-year-old woman enquires about contraception. She has a body mass index (BMI) of 32 kg/m^2. She does not get regular periods, but they are heavy when they come on.
2. A 25-year-old woman with a BMI of 20 kg/m^2 would like contraception. She occasionally gets midcycle pain which can be quite uncomfortable.
3. A 28-year-old woman would like a reliable form of contraception. She had the IUD previously, but it had to be removed due to discomfort.

Chapter 11 Benign gynaecological tumours

Investigations and management of gynaecology pathology

A. Ca-125
B. Emergency laparotomy
C. Emergency laparoscopy
D. Transvaginal/transabdominal ultrasound
E. Laparoscopy + bilateral salpingo-oophorectomy
F. White blood cells and C-reactive protein
G. Urine human chorionic gonadotropin test
H. Computed tomography abdomen/pelvis
I. Magnetic resonance imaging abdomen/pelvis
J. Haemoglobin

For each scenario below, choose the most appropriate course of management from the list given above.

1. A 23-year-old woman who presents with right-sided pelvic pain. BHG is negative.
2. A 55-year-old woman with a right-sided 6-cm ovarian cyst presents with acute pelvic pain and vomiting.
3. A 30-year-old woman presents with right pelvic pain. Ultrasound reveals an 8-cm ovarian cyst with free fluid. She feels faint and is slightly tachycardic.
4. A 55-year-old postmenopausal woman presents with left iliac fossa pain that is troublesome for her. Ultrasound revealed a 3-cm simple cyst. Her risk of malignancy index is very low.
5. A 60-year-old woman had an incidental finding of a 4-cm ovarian cyst identified on ultrasound.

Chapter 12 Gynaecological malignancies

Two-week wait gynaecology referrals

A. Cervical ectropion
B. Endometrial hyperplasia
C. Endometrial cancer
D. Haemorrhagic ovarian cyst
E. Endometriosis
F. Ovarian cancer
G. Cervical intraepithelial neoplasia
H. Leiomyosarcoma
I. Vulval intraepithelial neoplasia
J. Human papillomavirus (HPV)
K. Paget disease
L. Polycystic ovarian syndrome (PCOS)

For each scenario below, choose the most likely diagnosis from the list given above.

1. A 46-year-old premenopausal woman presents with abdominal bloating and a unilateral loculated ovarian cyst. Her Ca-125 is 29.
2. A 65-year old woman has a pipelle biopsy result showing 'proliferation of endometrial glands with an increase in the gland-to-stroma ratio compared to proliferative endometrium'.
3. A 25 year-old-woman presents with heavy irregular bleeding patterns since menarche and weight gain. She has no family history of endometrial cancer.
4. A 93-year-old is noted to have a vaginal lesion. She is known to have breast cancer.
5. A 32-year-old woman presents with intermenstrual and postcoital bleeding. Her last smear was HPV negative. On examination there was an abnormal appearance to her cervix, but colposcopy was subsequently normal.

Chapter 13 Benign vulval disease

Pruritus vulvae

A. *Candida* infection
B. Contact dermatitis
C. Lichen sclerosus
D. Carcinoma of the vulva
E. Herpetic lesion
F. Psoriasis
G. Vulval intraepithelial neoplasia
H. Enterobius
I. *Trichomonas vaginalis*
J. Behçet syndrome

For each scenario described below, choose the single most likely diagnosis from the list of options given above.

1. A 65-year-old presents with pruritus vulvae. She has noticed a lump growing on the vulva for the last 6 months. Examination confirms an ulcerated, hard, raised lesion 1 cm in diameter.
2. A 16-year-old has recently become sexually active. She complains of intense pruritus vulvae associated with an offensive discharge with a fishy odour. On examination she has a marked vulvovaginitis and a frothy greenish vaginal discharge.

3. A 60-year-old presents with intermittent episodes of pruritus vulvae. On examination the labia have fused, the tissues are thin and leukoplakia is present.
4. A 35-year-old has developed pruritus vulvae since changing her soap and bubble bath. Examination reveals vulvitis with no discrete lesion visible.
5. A 42-year-old develops an itchy lesion of the left vulva. Examination reveals an erythematous plaque on the left labium majora and scaly plaques on her elbows.

Chapter 14 Urogynaecology

Genital prolapse

A. Vaginal hysterectomy
B. Vaginal hysterectomy + pelvic floor repair
C. Anterior and posterior vaginal wall repair
D. Sacrospinous fixation
E. Colposuspension
F. Tension-free vaginal tape (TVT)
G. Augmentation cystoplasty
H. Pelvic floor repair, then commence antimuscarinic
I. Antimuscarinic agents, then schedule pelvic floor repair
J. Sacrocolpopexy

For each woman with prolapse select the most appropriate management.

1. A 70-year-old woman previously had a complicated hysterectomy for fibroids. She now presents with vault prolapse.
2. A 50-year-old woman presents with cystocele and stress incontinence.
3. A 40-year-old woman who has completed her family presents with abnormal uterine bleeding as well as a prolapse (second-degree uterine descent, second-degree rectocele and cystocele).

Chapter 15 Gynaecological endocrinology

Primary amenorrhoea

A. Haematocolpos
B. Androgen-insensitivity syndrome
C. Hypothalamic hypogonadism
D. Constitutional amenorrhoea
E. Late-onset congenital adrenal hyperplasia
F. Anorexia nervosa
G. Premature ovarian failure
H. Polycystic ovarian syndrome
I. Pregnancy
J. Turner syndrome

For each scenario described below, choose the single most likely diagnosis from the list of options given above.

1. A 16-year-old presents with primary amenorrhoea. On examination she has hirsutism, acne and a body mass index (BMI) of $36\,kg/m^2$.
2. A 17-year-old presents with primary amenorrhoea. On examination she has short stature and an increased carrying angle.
3. A 16-year-old presents with primary amenorrhoea. She is training to be a ballerina and has a BMI of $16\,kg/m^2$.
4. A 17-year-old presents with primary amenorrhoea. On examination she is obese, has male pattern balding and signs of virilism.
5. A 16-year-old presents with primary amenorrhoea. On examination she has normal secondary sexual characteristics, a BMI of $23\,kg/m^2$ and a normal hormone profile.

Chapter 16 Subfertility

Women with subfertility

A. Ovarian hyperstimulation syndrome
B. In-vitro fertilization (IVF)
C. IVF intracytoplasmic sperm injection
D. Intrauterine insemination (IUI)
E. Clomiphene
F. Metformin
G. Antiprogesterone
H. Oocyte retrieval
I. Donor oocyte with IVF
J. Donor sperm with IVF

For each scenario below, choose the treatment option best suited to the following couples with subfertility from the list given above.

1. A couple have been trying to conceive for 1 year. The woman is having irregular periods. Investigations reveal enlarged ovaries with multiple follicles.
2. A female couple in a same sex relationship want to conceive. All investigations are normal.
3. A couple have been trying to conceive for 1 year. Blood tests for her are normal and she has a body mass index of $25\,kg/m^2$. Hysterosalpingogram revealed bilateral fill and spill. His semen analysis is normal.

Chapter 17 Menopause

Patient with menopause

A. Topical oestrogen
B. Combined oral continuous hormone replacement therapy (HRT)
C. Transdermal oestrogen-only HRT
D. Transdermal combined HRT
E. Oral combined HRT
F. Oral oestrogen-only HRT + Mirena coil

G. Oral combined HRT + Mirena coil
H. Alternative options to HRT
I. Oral progesterone-only HRT
J. Transdermal HRT only

For each patient with menopause select the most suitable preparation of HRT they should consider from the list given above.

1. A 50-year-old woman undergoes laparoscopic hysterectomy and bilateral salpingo-oophorectomy for abnormal bleeding. She requests HRT postoperatively. She is concerned about the risk of deep vein thrombosis (DVT).
2. A 60-year-old woman presents with postmenopausal vaginal spotting. Examination does not reveal anything sinister, only vaginal atrophy.
3. A 35-year-old woman is diagnosed with premature ovarian failure. She has quite sensitive skin. She had tried the Mirena coil many years ago as contraception and found it very uncomfortable.

Chapter 18 Early pregnancy complications

Early pregnancy complications

A. Ectopic pregnancy
B. Inevitable miscarriage
C. Complete molar pregnancy
D. Complete miscarriage
E. Placenta praevia
F. Partial molar pregnancy
G. Salpingectomy
H. Incomplete miscarriage
I. Hyperemesis gravidarum
J. Salpingostomy

For each patient in early pregnancy select the most likely diagnosis or management from the list given above.

1. A 35-year-old woman presents with pelvic pain in early pregnancy. Ultrasound diagnoses a right-sided ectopic pregnancy. At laparoscopy her left fallopian tube appears entirely normal. What procedure would you perform to manage the ectopic pregnancy?
2. A 26-year-old woman presents in early pregnancy with pain and PV bleeding. She is 8 weeks' pregnant by dates. Speculum examination reveals an open cervical os. What is the outcome of this pregnancy?
3. A 25-year-old woman presents with pelvic pain and some PV spotting. She is 9 weeks by dates and human chorionic gonadotrophin level 2000. Ultrasound reveals an empty uterus, with a mass measuring 2 × 3 cm adjacent to the left ovary. What is the likely diagnosis?

Chapter 19 Antenatal booking

Antenatal investigations

A. Serum electrophoresis
B. Serum antibody screen
C. Group and screen
D. Toxoplasmosis
E. Hepatitis B
F. Glycosylated haemoglobin
G. Blood glucose level
H. Human immunodeficiency virus (HIV)
I. Hepatitis C
J. Urea and electrolytes

For each scenario described below, choose the single most likely test from the list of options given above. Each option may be used once, more than once or not at all.

1. Check the result of this test if a patient appears to have a microcytic anaemia.
2. This test should be performed at booking in a patient with established diabetes because it is associated with the risk of congenital malformations.
3. A routine test performed on every pregnant women that identifies woman who require anti-D prophylaxis.
4. A good example of a screening test, because intervention can reduce the risk of vertical transmission from 25% to <1%.
5. This test is not part of the routine first-trimester screening and would only be performed in a patient with a history of drug use.

Interventions in the antenatal period

A. Umbilical artery Doppler
B. Cardiotocograph
C. Membrane sweep
D. Speculum examination
E. Cervical cerclage
F. Amniocentesis
G. Chorionic villus sampling
H. Amniodrainage
I. External cephalic version
J. Fetocide

For each scenario described below, choose the single most appropriate intervention from the list of options given above. Each option may be used once, more than once or not at all.

1. At 40 weeks' gestation, a multiparous woman is seen in antenatal clinic. Her pregnancy has been straightforward and she is keen to avoid induction of labour.

2. At 30 weeks' gestation, a primiparous woman complains of a 4-hour history of a clear watery vaginal loss. She has no abdominal pain.
3. A multiparous woman is diagnosed with a breech presentation at 37 weeks. Her pregnancy is uncomplicated.
4. A 38-year-old woman has an increased risk of trisomy 21 on serum screening testing at 16 weeks.
5. At 34 weeks' gestation, ultrasound scan shows a slowing of the fetal growth rate with a reduction in the liquor volume.

Antenatal care

A. Serum ferritin, vitamin B12 and folate
B. Glucose tolerance test
C. Hepatitis B, C and human immunodeficiency virus (HIV) test
D. Varicella zoster immunoglobulin G (IgG)
E. Detailed cardiac ultrasound
F. Amniocentesis
G. Chorionic villous sampling
H. Routine booking investigations
I. Toxoplasmosis IgG
J. Varicella zoster IgM

For each scenario described below, choose the single most appropriate investigations from the list of options given above. Each option may be used once, more than once or not at all.

1. A 21-year-old who works as a nursery nurse presents for antenatal booking at 8 weeks and has never had chicken pox. She is currently clinically well.
2. A 43-year-old presents to antenatal clinic at 16 weeks to discuss her combined screening result which shows a risk of 1:90.
3. A 25-year-old with a history of intravenous drug use attends at 11 weeks for booking.
4. A 37-year-old solicitor in her first pregnancy attends for booking at 9 weeks, she has a normal body mass index and no past medical history of note.
5. A 32-year-old Indian lady with a body mass index of 36 kg/m^2 and a strong family history of type II diabetes.

Chapter 20 Antepartum haemorrhage

Bleeding in the second and third trimesters of pregnancy

A. Molar pregnancy
B. Vasa praevia
C. Ectopic pregnancy
D. Placenta praevia
E. Placental abruption

F. Cervical ectropion
G. Retained placenta
H. Vaginal tear
I. Uterine atony
J. Cervical tear

For each scenario described below, choose the single most likely diagnosis from the list of options given above. Each option may be used once, more than once or not at all.

1. A 35-year-old woman, who has had two previous caesarean sections, presents with vaginal spotting and a transverse lie at 35 weeks.
2. A 22-year-old woman has artificial rupture of membranes during labour and there is heavy vaginal bleeding in association with an abnormal cardiotocography (CTG). The uterus is soft and nontender.
3. A 28-year-old woman has a history of 16 weeks' amenorrhoea. She has severe nausea and vomiting. On abdominal palpation the uterus is 24 weeks in size. No intrauterine sac can be seen on ultrasound scan.
4. A 32-year-old woman is 28 weeks' pregnant. She has a 2-hour history of vaginal bleeding. She also complains of a headache and constant abdominal pain. On examination, the uterus is firm and tender.
5. A 30-year-old woman presents with a postcoital bleed at 22 weeks' gestation.

Chapter 21 Hypertension in pregnancy

Hypertensive diagnoses

A. Pregnancy-induced hypertension
B. Preeclampsia
C. Hypertension secondary to renal disease
D. Essential hypertension
E. Essential hypertension with superimposed preeclampsia
F. Malignant hypertension
G. Phaeochromocytoma
H. Postural supine hypotensive syndrome
I. Severe fulminating preeclampsia
J. HELLP syndrome (*h*aemolysis, *e*levated *l*iver enzymes and *l*ow *p*latelets)

For each scenario described below, choose the single most likely diagnosis from the list of options given above. Each option may be used once, more than once or not at all.

1. A 19-year-old primigravida booked with a blood pressure of 90/60 mmHg at 12 weeks. She had an uneventful pregnancy until 38 weeks' gestation, when she presented with swelling of the lower legs. Her

blood pressure (BP) was noted to be 160/95 mmHg and urinalysis revealed ++ proteinuria.

2. A 39-year-old primigravida books at 13 weeks' gestation. Her blood pressure was 150/90 mmHg at booking and there was no proteinuria. She was started on methyldopa 500 mg t.d.s. which maintained her BP within the normal range for the rest of the pregnancy.

3. A 25-year-old primigravida books at 16 weeks' gestation with a BP of 155/95 mmHg. She has a history or ureteric reflux and recurrent urinary tract infections as a child requiring ureteric reimplantation surgery. Her creatinine was slightly raised.

4. A 41-year-old primigravida booked with a BP of 140/95 mmHg at 10 weeks' gestation. She was commenced on methyldopa and had a normal pregnancy until 34 weeks when she was noted to have developed proteinuria, oedema and a raised serum urate concentration.

5. A 37-year-old woman booked at 12 weeks' gestation with a BP of 95/60 mmHg. She had an uneventful pregnancy until 24 weeks' gestation when she was found to be hypertensive with oedema but normal biochemistry. She was managed conservatively with methyldopa. At 29 weeks she felt unwell and blood tests revealed a haemoglobin concentration of 8.5 g/dL with evidence of haemolysis on blood film. Her platelet concentration was 85×10^9 and her alanine aminotransferase concentration was raised.

Hypertension in pregnancy

A. Postural hypotension
B. Epileptic seizure
C. Eclampsia
D. Preeclampsia
E. Essential hypertension
F. Pregnancy-induced hypertension or gestational hypertension
G. HELLP syndrome (*h*aemolysis, *e*levated *l*iver enzymes and *l*ow *p*latelets)
H. Amniotic fluid embolism
I. Hyperthyroidism
J. Stroke

For each scenario described below, choose the single most likely diagnosis from the list of options given above. Each option may be used once, more than once or not at all.

1. A 31-year-old patient presents at 8 weeks for a booking visit and is found to have blood pressure (BP) of 153/92 mmHg.

2. A 41-year-old patient presents at 29 weeks with proteinuria and a BP of 168/103 mmHg.

3. A 22-year-old patient presents at 38 weeks with a BP of 144/96 mmHg with no proteinuria and no symptoms.

4. A 29-year-old patient who is 35 weeks' pregnant presents with alanine aminotransferase of 213, platelets of 76 with a BP of 180/110 mmHg complaining of a headache and epigastric pain.

5. An 18-year-old patient who is 33 weeks' pregnant is brought in by ambulance fitting with a BP of 205/120 mmHg.

6. A 23-year-old epileptic who is in labour has a BP of 132/84 mmHg has a seizure whilst pushing.

Chapter 22 Medical disorders in pregnancy

Complications of the antenatal period

A. Obstetric cholestasis
B. Gestational diabetes
C. Recurrent antepartum haemorrhage
D. Symphysis pubis dysfunction
E. Iron-deficiency anaemia
F. Intrauterine growth restriction
G. Pyelonephritis
H. Preterm labour
I. Preterm ruptured membranes
J. Deep vein thrombosis

For each scenario described below, choose the single most likely diagnosis from the list of options given above. Each option may be used once, more than once or not at all.

1. A 40-year-old woman with a body mass index (BMI) of 36 kg/m^2 presents to A&E at 18 weeks' gestation with unilateral calf swelling.

2. Ultrasound scan shows a macrosomic fetus with polyhydramnios.

3. At 32 weeks' gestation, a primiparous patient complains of itchy palms and soles. Her liver function tests are abnormal.

4. At 28 weeks' gestation, a multiparous patient presents with severe abdominal pain. On examination, she is pyrexial with nitrites on urinalysis.

5. At 28 weeks' gestation, a multiparous patient presents with severe abdominal pain. On abdominal examination, there are palpable uterine contractions; vaginal examination shows cervical effacement.

Management of medical disorders in pregnancy

A. Take folic acid 5 mg daily
B. Organize leg venous Doppler scan
C. Check serum bile acids
D. Book a glucose tolerance test
E. Organize a chest X-ray
F. Check the peak expiratory flow rate

G. Document any known drug allergies
H. Start aspirin 75 mg daily
I. Check the body mass index
J. Arrange urgent investigations including coagulation screen and glucose level

For each scenario described below, choose the single most appropriate management plan from the list of options given above. Each option may be used once, more than once or not at all.

1. A 32-year-old patient is referred to the obstetrician at 16 weeks' gestation because of a history of previous gestational diabetes.
2. A 25-year-old woman with a 10-year history of epilepsy sees her GP because she is planning to stop the oral contraceptive pill.
3. A primiparous patient presents to the labour ward at 34 weeks' gestation with a 24-hour history of nausea, vomiting and abdominal pain.
4. A 40-year-old multiparous woman with a body mass index of 38 kg/m² at booking attends A&E at 18 weeks' gestation with a 48-hour history of breathlessness and chest pain.
5. A 38-year-old woman with diabetes is planning her first pregnancy. Her blood sugar levels are well-controlled and she has a family history of hypertension.

Investigations for medical disorders in pregnancy

A. Echocardiogram
B. Antenatal and postnatal low-molecular-weight heparin
C. Liver function tests and bile acids
D. Folic acid supplementation and detailed cardiac scan
E. Haemoglobinopathy screen
F. Glucose tolerance test
G. Thyroid function tests
H. Cardiotocography
I. Amniocentesis
J. Fetal blood sampling

For each scenario described below, choose the single most appropriate investigation from the list of options given above. Each option may be used once, more than once or not at all.

1. A 28-year-old Bangladeshi patient presents after an ultrasound showing polyhydramnios, fetal macrosomia and has three +++ of glucose in her urine.
2. A 19-year-old epileptic patient attends at 12 weeks for a plan of care.
3. A 27-year-old attends at 12 weeks and has a family history of pulmonary embolism and had an unprovoked deep vein thrombosis 3 years ago.

4. A 39-year-old attends at 34 weeks with itchy palms and soles but no rash.
5. A 21-year-old patient from Cyprus attends after her booking visit and is found to have a haemoglobin level of 9.1 g/dL.

Chapter 23 Common presentations in pregnancy

Abdominal pain in the second and third trimester

A. Fibroid degeneration
B. Gastroenteritis
C. Symphysis pubis dysfunction
D. Placental abruption
E. Acute appendicitis
F. Ovarian torsion
G. Preeclampsia [preeclamptic toxaemia (PET)]
H. Urinary tract infection (UTI)
I. Gallstones
J. Labour

For each of the clinical findings below, select the pathological process most likely to account for them from the list of options given above. Each option may be used once, more than once or not at all.

1. On abdominal palpation, hard tender uterus, difficulty defining the fetal parts.
2. Nitrites on urinalysis.
3. Regular contractions palpated on abdominal examination, cervical change on vaginal examination.
4. The uterus palpates large for dates, with tenderness elicited over a specific site.
5. The patient is hypertensive and hyperreflexic, with tenderness over the right hypochondrium.

Large for dates and small for dates

A. Gestational diabetes
B. Gestational trophoblastic disease
C. Placental insufficiency
D. Twin pregnancy
E. Oesophageal atresia
F. Renal agenesis
G. Uterine fibroid
H. Trisomy 18
I. Cytomegalovirus infection
J. Maternal ovarian cyst

For each scenario described below, choose the single most likely diagnosis from the list of options given above. Each option may be used once, more than once or not at all.

1. Fetal ultrasound scan at 20 weeks shows anhydramnios.

2. Persistent glycosuria with a macrosomic fetus on ultrasound scan.
3. In-vitro fertilization pregnancy with a symphysis–fundal height at the umbilicus at 14 weeks' gestation.
4. Maternal history of chronic hypertension measuring small for dates at 30 weeks' gestation.
5. An Afro-Caribbean woman who measures large for dates at 20 weeks' gestation.

Chapter 24 Multiple pregnancy

Antenatal care of multiple pregnancies

A. Consultant-led hospital care
B. Chorionicity
C. Homebirth
D. Intrauterine growth restriction
E. Postpartum haemorrhage
F. Zygosity
G. Selective fetal reduction
H. Primiparity
I. Maternal age >40 years
J. Twin-to-twin transfusion syndrome

For each statement below, choose the single most appropriate option from the list given above. Each option may be used once, more than once or not at all.

1. The most important factor in defining the risks associated with different types of twin pregnancy.
2. An essential part of counselling a couple with higher-order multiple pregnancies such as triplets, in order for making informed decisions regarding possible birth outcomes.
3. A complication of 15% of monochorionic pregnancies.
4. The appropriate location for care of any multiple pregnancy.
5. A risk factor in any multiple pregnancy which must be monitored by regular growth scans.

Chapter 26 Labour

Obstetric definitions

A. Fetal presentation
B. Fetal lie
C. Position of the presenting part of the fetus
D. Station of the presenting part of the fetus
E. Perinatal mortality rate
F. Neonatal mortality rate
G. Maternal mortality rate
H. Antepartum haemorrhage
I. Labour
J. Primary postpartum haemorrhage

For each description below, choose the single most likely definition from the list of options given above. Each option may be used once, more than once or not at all.

1. The relationship between the denominator of the presenting part and the maternal pelvis.
2. Any amount of vaginal bleeding after 24 weeks' gestation until delivery of the fetus.
3. The number of maternal deaths per 100,000 live births.
4. Regular, painful uterine contractions in the presence of cervical dilatation and effacement.
5. The relationship between the presenting part of the fetus and the maternal ischial spines.

Interventions in labour

A. Ventouse delivery
B. Lower segment caesarean section
C. External cephalic version
D. Fetal scalp electrode
E. Fetal blood sample
F. Epidural anaesthesia
G. Artificial rupture of membranes
H. Episiotomy
I. Simpson forceps delivery
J. Intravenous syntocinon

For each scenario described below, choose the single most appropriate intervention from the list of options given above. Each option may be used once, more than once or not at all.

1. During labour, there is difficulty monitoring the fetal heart rate in a woman with a body mass index of 40 kg/m^2.
2. In a patient with suspected intrauterine growth restriction, there is a pathological cardiotocography (CTG) in labour. Vaginal examination shows that the cervix is 7-cm dilated.
3. A primiparous patient is contracting irregularly with intact membranes. The CTG is normal and the cervix has been 4-cm dilated for the last 4 hours.
4. There is a prolonged fetal bradycardia lasting 8 minutes. The cervix is 6-cm dilated.
5. A primiparous patient has been actively pushing in the second stage of labour for more than 1 hour. On examination, the fetal head is not palpable abdominally, the vertex is at +1 below the ischial spines in the right occipitotransverse position with no caput or moulding. The CTG is normal.

Terminology in labour

A. Caput
B. Extended breech

C. Shoulder dystocia
D. Meconium
E. Fetal tachycardia
F. Malpresentation
G. Malposition
H. Variability
I. Fetal bradycardia
J. Moulding

For each description below, choose the single most likely term from the list of options given above. Each option may be used once, more than once or not at all.

1. The fetal heart rate is at a baseline level of 170 bpm.
2. The fetal shoulder is over the pelvic inlet in the first stage of labour.
3. The fetal occiput is palpated adjacent to the maternal sacrum at full dilatation.
4. The fetal skull bones can be felt to overlap at 6-cm dilatation.
5. The fetal heart rate differs by 5–10 bpm.

Chapter 29 Complications in labour

Failure to progress

A. Cervical fibroid
B. Persistent occipitoposterior position
C. Previous pelvic fracture
D. Fetal macrosomia
E. Irregular contractions
F. Breech presentation
G. Occipitotransverse position
H. Rickets
I. Transverse lie
J. Brow presentation

For each scenario described below, choose the single most likely diagnosis from the list of options given above. Each option may be used once, more than once or not at all.

1. A 26-year-old woman who has been an insulin-dependent diabetic since the age of 10 years.
2. A primiparous patient with a term pregnancy and a cephalic presentation. Over the past 4 hours, she has remained at 4-cm dilatation on vaginal examination. She is not yet requiring analgesia.
3. A 35-year-old Nigerian woman who is in spontaneous labour. She has a history of having had a previous myomectomy for menorrhagia.
4. A 40-year-old grand multiparous woman who has attended labour ward at term with a 3-hour history of regular contractions and no PV loss. On abdominal palpation, there is nothing in the maternal pelvis.

5. On examination of a multiparous patient, the midwife is able to palpate the fetal orbital ridges and the anterior fontanelle.

Intrapartum complications

A. Failure to progress
B. Meconium-stained liquor
C. Placental abruption
D. Postpartum haemorrhage
E. Cord prolapse
F. Ruptured uterus
G. Uterine hyperstimulation
H. Shoulder dystocia
I. Face presentation
J. Fetal bradycardia

For each scenario described below, choose the single most likely diagnosis from the list of options given above. Each option may be used once, more than once or not at all.

1. A patient who has previously had a caesarean section is having a vaginal delivery in this pregnancy. At 8-cm dilatation, the cardiotocography (CTG) suddenly shows a prolonged fetal bradycardia.
2. After a long labour, a primiparous patient with a body mass index of 35 kg/m² has a ventouse delivery for a prolonged second stage. The fetal head shows the turtle-neck sign as it delivers and there is difficulty delivering the baby.
3. In established labour with a breech presentation, the CTG suddenly shows a prolonged fetal bradycardia.
4. A patient who has been diagnosed with severe preeclampsia is having labour induced at 37 weeks. She starts to complain of constant sharp abdominal pain. The uterus is tender and hard on palpation. The CTG has become suspicious.
5. A patient on intravenous syntocinon is contracting 6 in 10. The CTG shows variable decelerations with a rise in the baseline heart rate.

Chapter 30 Stillbirth

Causes of stillbirth

A. Maternal alanine aminotransferase = 60 IU/L
B. Maternal HbA1c = 15%
C. Fetal haemoglobin = 3 g/dL, positive Coombs test
D. Parvovirus immunoglobulin M (IgM) positive, IgG negative
E. Maternal rubella IgG positive
F. 24-Hour urinary protein 2.1 g/L
G. Fetal karyotype 47XY
H. Fetal karyotype 45XO
I. 24-Hour urinary protein 0.35 g/L

The conditions below are the underlying diagnoses of causes of stillbirth, made on the basis of investigations performed soon after delivery. For each of the diagnoses below, match the test result from the list of options given above. Each option may be used once, more than once or not at all.

1. Fetus with Down syndrome
2. Preeclampsia
3. Intrauterine fetal infection
4. Obstetric cholestasis
5. Rhesus isoimmunization
6. Maternal diabetes

Chapter 31 Postnatal complications

Complications of the postnatal period

A. Puerperal psychosis
B. Postnatal depression
C. Endometritis
D. Deep vein thrombosis
E. Postpartum haemorrhage (PPH)
F. Mastitis
G. Urinary tract infection
H. Pulmonary embolus
I. Dural puncture headache
J. Cerebral vein thrombosis

For each scenario described below, choose the single most likely diagnosis from the list of options given above. Each option may be used once, more than once or not at all.

1. Vaginal bleeding more than 500 mL from 24 hours postdelivery up to 6 weeks.
2. Two weeks after delivery, a primiparous patient complains of low mood and feeling unable to cope with caring for her baby.
3. Two weeks after delivery, a primiparous patient complains that she cannot sleep because she is worried a neighbour is trying to take her baby. On further questioning with her partner, the neighbour has simply been offering to help with babysitting.
4. Six days after emergency caesarean section, a patient complains of increasingly constant severe lower abdominal pain. The lochia is offensive-smelling. On examination, the patient is pyrexial and the uterus is tender.
5. After a prolonged labour and delivery with epidural anaesthesia, a patient complains of being unable to sit upright because of a severe headache.

Postpartum haemorrhage

A. Primary postpartum haemorrhage (PPH)
B. Secondary PPH

C. Second-degree tear
D. Third-degree tear
E. Uterine atony
F. Uterine rupture
G. Retained products of conception
H. Endometritis
I. Placenta accreta
J. Uterine inversion

For each scenario described below, choose the single most likely diagnosis from the list of options given above. Each option may be used once, more than once or not at all.

1. The patient has had a forceps delivery with an episiotomy after a prolonged labour. On examination, the episiotomy has extended into the external anal sphincter and the patient is bleeding heavily from the area.
2. The patient has just had a normal vaginal delivery of a twin pregnancy. She is bleeding heavily. On examination, the uterine fundus is above the umbilicus and poorly contracted.
3. A woman has previously had two caesarean sections. At the time of caesarean section in this pregnancy, the placenta was morbidly adherent to the uterine wall.
4. Bleeding more than 500 mL within the first 24 hours of delivery of the baby.
5. At the time of controlled cord traction in the third stage of labour, the patient suddenly complains of severe abdominal pain and bleeding. The uterine fundus cannot be palpated on abdominal examination.

Chapter 32 Maternal collapse

Causes of maternal collapse

A. Uterine atony
B. Amniotic fluid embolism
C. Postural hypotension
D. Opiate use
E. Pulmonary embolism
F. Epileptic seizure
G. Eclampsia
H. Sepsis
I. Myocardial infarction
J. Uterine rupture

For each scenario described below, choose the single most likely diagnosis from the list of options given above. Each option may be used once, more than once or not at all.

1. This 18-year-old had a forceps delivery of a 4.3-kg baby about 1 hour ago after a long labour that was augmented

with syntocinon. She had syntometrine for the third stage. Her pulse is 100bpm, her blood pressure is 90/45mmHg. Her uterus is palpable above the umbilicus and feels 'boggy'. She is lying in a pool of blood.

2. This woman had her fourth caesarean section yesterday. She was kept on the labour ward overnight as the estimated blood loss at delivery was 800mL. Her husband helped her get up to go to the shower, but then she collapsed by the side of her bed. Her pulse is 94bpm, her blood pressure is 110/55mmHg and her lochia is normal. There is no respiratory distress.

3. This 35-year-old, whose body mass index is 38kg/m^2, has had frequent admissions in her pregnancy, early on with hyperemesis, now, in the third trimester, with symphysis pubis pain. When found she is tachycardic but normotensive, with cyanosis and dyspnoea.

4. This primigravid woman was aiming for home delivery, and wanted to avoid contact with the hospital if at all possible. Her membranes ruptured 3 days ago, at term, and she has had irregular contractions ever since, but labour has not established. She came in because she started to feel unwell, and because fetal movements had reduced over the previous 12 hours. On examination she is tachycardic and pyrexial, and the liquor is yellowish in colour.

5. At 32 weeks, this woman had been referred in by her community midwife who found her blood pressure to be elevated and some proteinuria at a routine antenatal check. She is generally fit and well with no medical history. On arrival she is asked to provide another urine specimen. When she fails to emerge from the toilet the midwife goes in and finds her having a generalized tonic–clonic seizure.

Causes of maternal collapse

A. Placental abruption
B. Postpartum haemorrhage
C. Uterine rupture
D. Amniotic fluid embolism
E. Eclampsia
F. Epileptiform seizure
G. Diabetic ketoacidosis
H. Puerperal septic shock
I. Pulmonary embolism
J. Myocardial infarction

For each scenario described below, choose the single most likely diagnosis from the list of options given above. Each option may be used once, more than once or not at all.

1. A 25-year-old woman was found collapsed at home at 8 weeks' gestation. Her history includes a deep vein thrombosis at the age of 18 years following which she was found to carry the factor V Leiden mutation.

2. A 26-year-old woman underwent a caesarean section in her first pregnancy for fetal distress. This current pregnancy was uneventful and she went into spontaneous labour. She requested an epidural for analgesia. At 7-cm dilatation she felt unwell and collapsed at the same time that the fetal heart rate pattern became bradycardic.

3. A 34-year-old grand multiparous woman presented to the labour ward at 34 weeks' gestation having experienced a small antepartum haemorrhage at home. By the time she arrived she was experiencing severe abdominal pain. Abdominal examination revealed a tender, hard uterus and the fetal heart could not be heard with the Sonicaid. During the examination she collapsed and was unresponsive.

4. An unbooked woman was admitted via ambulance unconscious. The only history available is that she was feeling unwell for the previous few days with headaches and had collapsed at home 'shaking'. On examination, she was unconscious, her blood pressure was 180/110mmHg and urinalysis revealed proteinuria.

5. A 35-year-old multiparous woman spontaneously ruptured her membranes at term in her third pregnancy; 48 hours later she went into labour and had a normal delivery. She went home after 6 hours; 72 hours later she started feeling unwell and feverish. She collapsed at home and was brought into hospital by ambulance. On examination she was unconscious with central cyanosis. Her temperature was 39°C, pulse 120bpm and she was profoundly hypotensive.

Maternal collapse

A. Pulmonary embolism
B. Acute myocardial infarction
C. Amniotic fluid embolism
D. Anaphylactic shock
E. Postural hypotension
F. Placental abruption
G. Eclampsia
H. Hypovolaemic shock

For each scenario described below, choose the single most likely cause of collapse from the list of options given above. Each option may be used once, more than once or not at all.

1. A 41-year-old smoker who is 34 weeks' pregnant brought in by ambulance with fresh vaginal bleeding and a 'woody hard' uterus.

2. A 19-year-old, who is being induced as she is Group B streptococcus positive and has ruptured her membranes at 40 weeks without any contractions, collapses 5 minutes after being given benzylpenicillin prophylactically.

3. A 24-year-old who had a caesarean section 3 hours ago for failure to progress is found collapsed in her bed with a large pool of blood between her legs and a boggy uterus.

4. A 26-year-old who is in labour collapses just after delivery and is noted to be hypoxic and hypotensive; she then begins to bleed heavily and is found to have a raised international normalized ratio 2.5.

5. A 36-year-old Sri Lankan patient who is in labour collapses after complaining of central chest pain which radiates to her jaw. She has a body mass index of 41 kg/m^2 and has gestational diabetes.

Maternal death

A. Sepsis
B. Pulmonary embolism
C. Ruptured ectopic pregnancy
D. Postpartum haemorrhage
E. Puerperal psychosis
F. Intracranial haemorrhage
G. Amniotic fluid embolism
H. Acute myocardial infarction

For each scenario described below, choose the single most likely cause of death from the list of options given above. Each option may be used once, more than once or not at all.

1. A 17-year-old girl who is around 6 weeks' pregnant is seen by her GP complaining of lower abdominal pain and diarrhoea. She is told this may be a viral illness and is sent home. Later she is brought in collapsed by ambulance with a distended abdomen and her urine sample is β-human chorionic gonadotropin positive.

2. A 36-year-old patient attends A&E with a history of fevers and rigors 3 days after a normal vaginal delivery. She is tachycardic and hypotensive and despite resuscitation has a cardiac arrest.

3. A 36-year-old patient who is 34 weeks' pregnant collapses in clinic and is unresponsive. Her blood pressure prior to the collapse was 192/104 mmHg and she was complaining of a headache. She is rapidly intubated and an urgent CT scan shows a large left-sided intracranial bleed with midline shift.

4. A 38-year-old patient who is 37 weeks' pregnant is out walking her dog and complains to her husband of severe right-sided chest pain. He calls an ambulance but she rapidly declines and her lips turn blue. Despite the best attempts, the team is unable to resuscitate her.

5. A 34-year-old who delivered 12 days ago was found collapsed at home next to an empty container of paracetamol. She was noted to be acting strangely the day before by her neighbour, saying that she was a bad mother and everybody hates her.

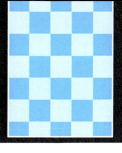
Chapter 1 Basic anatomy and examination

1. E. Fetal heart rate. A–D are commonly determined by good palpation. Fetal heart rate requires the use of a Sonicaid or a Pinard stethoscope.

2. E. Colour of liquor. A–D are used as part of the calculation for Bishop score, whereas the colour of the liquor is not.

3. B. 33–39 cm. Whilst you would expect 36 cm to be the exact measurement, there is always a range and this is SFH ± 3 cm. Hence 33–39 cm is the most correct.

4. D. Bishop score. All factors are important, but the Bishop score encompasses all of these.

5. C. Assessment with Sims speculum. All may be required, but the history suggests a cystocele with stress incontinence. The best assessment for prolapse is an examination with a Sims speculum.

Chapter 3 Common investigations

1. E. Bence Jones protein. All are tested in the urine with A–D by simple urine dipstick; however, Bence Jones requires a 24-hour sample of urine to be collected.

2. D. Smear test 3 yearly from the age of 20 years. Smear tests are performed from the age of 25 years if a woman is sexually active. It was 20 years in the past however. All other statements are true.

3. D. Transvaginal ultrasound. All tests can provide some information, but initially ultrasound is the most appropriate. Transvaginal is more sensitive than transabdominal ultrasound due to the higher frequency used allowing for higher-resolution images. MRI is also very useful, but reserved as a second-line investigation.

4. E. Hepatic injury. Whilst any injury is possible, bladder and ureteric injury can occur during side wall dissection, vascular injury during Veress needle insertion.

5. B. Outpatient hysteroscopy. Ideally this patient requires hysteroscopy and biopsy as her symptoms are recurrent and cancer must be ruled out. An outpatient hysteroscopy is safer than a GA. She has already had an ultrasound so no need to repeat it.

Chapter 4 Abnormal uterine bleeding

1. D. SLE. Abnormal uterine bleeding has multiple causative factors, but lupus is not known to be one of them.

2. D. Endometrial ablation. A and B are not appropriate as although it was not stated, tranexamic acid is likely to have been tried. C and E are still options but the quickest and least invasive will be an endometrial ablation which can be performed as an outpatient procedure. Permanent contraception is advised for this (which is fine as her husband has had a vasectomy).

3. B. Outpatient hysteroscopy and biopsy. The next appropriate form of management is to obtain an endometrial biopsy. This can be performed with blind biopsy but if there is a polyp for instance, this may be missed. A hysteroscopy is more appropriate. This is more safely and quickly performed as an outpatient.

4. E. All of the above. There are several risks of a hysterectomy which need to be explained to women before they consent to a procedure. All the above are important as well as others.

5. A. Atrophic vaginitis. Initially an ultrasound and hysteroscopy with biopsy is likely to be required (if the endometrial thickness is enlarged). However, statistically atrophic vaginitis is the most likely cause.

Chapter 5 Fibroids

1. E. All of the above. Fibroids can be present in many positions throughout the uterus, so all are true.

2. D. Can become malignant in 1:100 cases. Malignant change is only in 1:1000 cases or less.

3. C. Chronic pelvic pain. Fibroids cause many symptoms but not typically pain. They can cause pain in red degeneration or if a pedunculated fibroid becomes torted, but this is not common.

4. E. Hysteroscopy and pelvic ultrasound. All can provide information for fibroids. But inevitably a pelvic ultrasound and hysteroscopy are likely. An ultrasound can measure the size and location of the fibroid and a hysteroscopy is used to assess if there is a submucosal fibroid causing bleeding and whether it can be resected via hysteroscopy (if so, it can also be performed at the same time).

5. C. UAE. A and B are both surgical options so not appropriate. The Mirena coil will not shrink the size of the fibroids. She may require iron, but UAE is likely to improve her symptoms and hopefully reduce the size of the fibroids.

Chapter 6 Endometriosis

1. E. All the above. Endometriosis can cause all the symptoms above, and it is completely variable from patient to patient. Some women may have endometriosis and demonstrate no symptoms at all.

2. C. Laparoscopy with biopsy. Whilst all investigations may suggest endometriosis, it can only be definitively diagnosed with histological confirmation once a biopsy has been taken.

3. B. Antegrade menstruation. Several theories exist as to what causes endometriosis. It is likely that the cause is multifactorial. However, it is retrograde (Sampson theory) menstruation not antegrade that is likely to cause it.

4. E. Danazol. All are management options for endometriosis, but danazol is the least used currently due to its side-effects.

5. C. Once excised endometriosis does not recur. There is a chance that once endometriosis is excised it will not recur; however, because it is a chronic condition, recurrence can still occur.

Chapter 7 Pelvic pain and dyspareunia

1. E. All of the above. All are possible causes of acute pelvic pain. The differential diagnosis can be quite varied, therefore all of the above must be ruled out. Some like ectopic pregnancy or ovarian torsion will require urgent attention.

2. E. Laparoscopic ovarian cystectomy. It is likely that the diagnosis here is an ovarian torsion, which requires urgent attention. Once detorted the cyst can be removed to prevent a recurrence of the torsion.

3. B. Endometriosis. The symptoms most fit with endometriosis. PID would have produced pain most of the time, not just with the period. This is the same for nerve entrapment and irritable bowel.

4. A. Urine β-HCG. Whilst all tests may be necessary, a woman who presents with acute severe pelvic pain has an ectopic pregnancy until proven otherwise. Hence β-HCG is vital to determine if she is pregnant, and if so an ectopic pregnancy becomes the most likely diagnosis.

5. D. Offer referral to support groups. Pain is a very complex phenomenon. As the laparoscopies have been normal, there is no need for repeat surgery. Imaging again is not likely to alter management. In this instance referral for support is the most appropriate action.

Chapter 8 Vaginal discharge and sexually transmitted infections

1. B. Cervical ectropion. An ectropion is not pathological. It is simply an extension of endocervical columnar epithelium, which bleeds easily, onto the ectocervix and is common in pregnancy due to the influence of oestrogen. No treatment is necessary unless a coexisting infection is proven.

2. B. Thick, itchy, white discharge. The thick, white discharge of candida infection has a typical appearance of cottage cheese noted on speculum examination. It is treated easily with clotrimazole pessary or cream.

3. E. Sexual history. A detailed sexual history is imperative to exclude sexually transmitted infections.

4. C. History of STI. Most common organisms held responsible for PID are *Chlamydia* and *Neisseria gonorrhoeae*, both sexually transmitted infections. Hence any history of previous STI would predispose a patient to PID.

5. C. Vulval pruritis. Vulval pruritis is not characteristically associated with PID.

Chapter 9 Pelvic inflammatory disease

1. E. All of the above. Pelvic inflammatory disease has very significant sequelae and can cause all of the above. Therefore it is important to treat it if suspected.

2. E. *Pseudomonas*. This is the only organism not typically known to cause PID.

3. E. Commence broad-spectrum antibiotics. As PID has such severe consequences if not treated, such as chronic pelvic pain and subfertility, treating before any delay in investigations is the most important step.

4. D. Laparoscopy. Although described as a gold-standard investigation for making the diagnosis of PID, it is not the first-line investigation in view of surgical risks. There are less invasive, effective alternatives available as listed above. The aim should be to effectively diagnose and treat PID without going into the operating theatre, unless it is absolutely necessary

[e.g., diagnosis not clearly defined (possibility of ectopic pregnancy/appendicitis), clinical condition deteriorating, failed initial medical management].

5. D. If treated, it will not cause problems in the future. If treated, PID can still cause ectopic pregnancy and subfertility as a result of adhesions that may have formed following the infection.

Chapter 10 Contraception and termination of pregnancy

1. E. Male condom. All provide contraception, but the most effective for reduction in risk of STIs is the male condom.

2. E. Vasectomy. Of all the methods provided vasectomy has the lowest failure rate (1/2000). A laparoscopic female tubal ligation has a failure rate in the order of 1/200, whereas the others will depend on how well they are used, but irrespective will have a higher failure rate than vasectomy.

3. E. IUS. All will provide a contraception to a variable degree, but the IUS has a very low failure rate (1/200) and will also help with heavy periods (please refer to Table 4.2), so is the preferred choice in this scenario.

4. B. EllaOne. For emergency contraception the options are levonelle, but it is only reliable for up to 72 hours. Alternatively the copper coil or EllaOne can be used beyond 72 hours. EllaOne is effective for up to 5 days. As she may have an allergy to the metal in the IUD, EllaOne is the preferred choice.

5. D. Cerebral ischaemic event. All are risks of a surgical termination except for a cerebral event, which may still occur for other reasons but is not directly known to be related to the procedure.

Chapter 11 Benign gynaecological tumours

1. E. Hyperthyroidism. A–D increase the likelihood of ovarian tumours. Hypothyroidism increases the risk not hyperthyroidism.

2. E. Ca-125. Urine HCG is important to rule out pregnancy. Hb can indicate if there has been an ovarian cyst accident, such as a haemorrhagic ovarian cyst. WCC and CRP are useful to rule out an inflammatory/infective process and ultrasound to diagnose an ovarian cyst. Ca-125 should only be reserved if a malignancy is suspected with other investigations, otherwise it may lead to false positives.

3. B. Mainly present in the 30s age group. Dermoid cysts can present bilaterally, malignancy can occur but is rare. Only a small percentage tort (10%), and although some can rupture at presentation, this is uncommon.

4. C. Ca-125 mg/100 mL is used in the score. A, B, D and E are correct as can be seen in the box present in the chapter. Ca-125 is used in the score but must be in IU/mL (not in mg/100 mL) – Hence C is true.

5. D. Laparoscopy with or without ovarian cystectomy. This is clearly an acute ovarian torsion and so the answer is to immediately detort the ovary and remove the ovarian cyst if feasible. Performing investigations in this instance will lead to delay and the ovary possibly becoming necrotic.

Chapter 12 Gynaecological malignancies

1. E. History of endometriosis. There is no known link between endometriosis and cervical cancer. HPV has been shown to be present in up 100% of cases of cervical cancer.

2. A. 270. With a unilateral located cyst her ultrasound score is 1 × postmenopausal score 3 × Ca-125.

3. D. Endometrial biopsy. This patient requires endometrial sampling to assess for endometrial hyperplasia or endometrial cancer as the underlying cause for her postmenopausal bleeding. This can now be done as an outpatient with hysteroscopy. She may go on to require further imaging.

4. C. Lichen planus. All the other options increase risk of developing vulval cancer

5. A. Hysteroscopy and biopsy. A biopsy must be taken to confirm endometrial pathology. Conditions such as endometrial hyperplasia would not be seen on imaging. Biopsy at hysteroscopy has a higher specificity than a pipelle biopsy.

Chapter 13 Benign vulval disease

1. C. A thick creamy white discharge. A thick creamy white discharge supports a diagnosis of infection, possibly candida. An acute onset, rather than progressively worsening symptoms over 6 months suggests infection. There is no association between menorrhagia and pruritus vulvae. Red plaques in the vulval areas suggest psoriasis or eczema. Fused labia suggest lichen sclerosis.

2. B. A speculum examination of the cervix and smear test. Cervical intraepithelial neoplasia is often

associated with vulval intraepithelial neoplasia. Antibiotics should only be prescribed where infection is found. Women should be referred to colposcopy only where clinically indicated. Surgical intervention is not common practice. Abdominal X-ray is not a usual part of the routine work-up for pruritus vulvae.

3. B. Biopsy of the vulva. Biopsy of the vulva for histological diagnosis. CRP does not identify a cause, but provides a marker for infective causes only. Ultrasound is not commonly used to investigate vulval disease; computed tomography and magnetic resonance imaging are more sensitive when considering vulval malignancy. Hysteroscopy alone does not identify vulval pathology, but an examination under anaesthetic may. Endocervical swabs will exclude endocervical infection only.

4. B. Skin biopsy shows thinning of the epidermis. The epidermis is usually thin and hyalinized. Lichen sclerosis can appear as white or reddish plaques. A skin biopsy is mandatory to exclude malignant change. About 50% of symptoms of pruritus vulvae can recur following surgical excision. A long course of steroids is often required.

5. E. De-infibulation is illegal. FGM is illegal practice. However, we may come across patients who have had FGM in other countries in the past. Especially in pregnancy it can cause difficulties during childbirth. Therefore, de-infibulation may be carried out electively or during childbirth. It is illegal to re-infibulate (put back the FGM). Instead only haemostatic sutures should be placed to stop bleeding (not to re-oppose the edges to put back the FGM).

Chapter 14 Urogynaecology

1. E. Loin pain. Loin pain is not a direct symptom of prolapse. Prolapse may not become apparent at the beginning of the day, but as one is on their feet, this may get worse due to gravity. If there is a cystocele, women may need to go to empty their bladder more often or have difficulty emptying it. Any stasis of urine predisposes to UTI. Any prolapse of the genital organs may cause nerve irritation and lower back pain as the ligaments stretch.

2. D. Pectineus. All other muscles contribute to the pelvic floor, with the puborectalis, pubococcygeus, and iliococcygeus forming the levator ani.

3. B. Pregnancy. All will cause a prolapse but as pregnancy is common, it is also the most common cause.

4. D. Urodynamics. When there are symptoms suggestive of stress and urge incontinence, urodynamic investigations are imperative so that it can be confirmed and management tailored.

5. A. Renal tract imaging. All these steps may be required, but in recurrent UTIs there may be urinary tract pathology causing the infections or the kidneys may have been affected due to all the infections. Therefore renal tract imaging is the most important.

Chapter 15 Gynaecological endocrinology

1. A. Congenital adrenal hyperplasia. Congenital adrenal hyperplasia is due to adrenal hyperandrogenism. Hyperprolactinaemia causes amenorrhoea. Hypothyroidism, Turner syndrome and cystic fibrosis cause delayed puberty.

2. E. Progestogens. Most synthetic progestogens can have androgenic side-effects due to stimulation of androgen receptors. H2 antagonists can cause gynaecomastia in men. Prednisolone, although a steroid, is not associated with hirsutism. The combination of oestrogen and progesterone in the combined oral contraceptive pill counteracts the androgenic side-effects of progesterone alone.

3. B. Testicular feminization. The genotype for testicular feminization is XY, therefore by definition there is primary amenorrhoea. Fibroids cause menorrhagia. Premature ovarian failure can occur at this age, but it usually presents as secondary amenorrhoea. Polycystic ovary syndrome usually presents as secondary amenorrhoea. Lichen sclerosis is a vulval skin condition, which does not cause primary amenorrhoea.

4. B. 21-Hydroxylase deficiency. Whilst other enzyme deficiencies are possible, 21-hydroxylase deficiency is the most common currently known.

5. E. BMI $> 30 \text{kg/m}^2$. A–D are used as part of the Rotterdam criteria. Whilst a patient with PCOS may have a BMI $> 30 \text{kg/m}^2$, this is not used as part of the diagnostic criteria.

Chapter 16 Subfertility

1. C. Reassure and arrange review if unsuccessful after 1 year. It can take up to 2 years to conceive spontaneously. Therefore if there is no known abnormality, further investigations should not be undertaken until this time subsides.

2. B. Pelvic/transvaginal ultrasound. It is likely to be a case of polycystic ovarian syndrome. Together with

her symptoms if multiple ovarian peripheral follicles are seen on ultrasound scan, it would confirm the diagnosis. Initially clomiphene citrate can be tried in this instance as anovulatory cycles will be occurring.

3. E. IVF ICSI. There is male factor affecting fertility in this instance, therefore IVF with ICSI is likely to give the best results.

4. A. Ovarian hyperstimulation syndrome. Ovarian hyperstimulation can cause fluid to accumulate in all pleural and peritoneal cavities, which accounts for the symptoms experienced in this case.

5. C. Aged under 30 years. If your age is over 40 years, you have never had a pregnancy, drinking excessive alcohol or having a high or low BMI can negatively affect your chances of having a successful IVF. The older a woman is, the fewer eggs she is likely to have, which can negatively affect IVF. Therefore if a woman is younger, her chances of successful IVF are increased.

Chapter 17 Menopause

1. D. Menopause is defined as cessation of periods for more than 1 year in a woman over the age of 45 years. Menopause is confirmed by absence of periods for >1 year over the age of 45 years, not with blood tests.

2. D. HRT containing progesterone. HRT containing synthetic progesterone carries a risk of breast cancer in the order of 1/1000.

3. E. Arrhythmias. All A–D are symptoms of menopause, but arrhythmias are not a recognized symptom.

4. E. Photophobia. Photophobia is not a recognized side-effect of HRT, whereas A–D can be.

5. D. Elevated FSH levels taken 5 weeks apart. As she is under 45 years, in this instance blood tests of FSH are taken for the diagnosis 5 weeks apart.

Chapter 18 Early pregnancy complications

1. C. Arrange an USS at soonest opportunity. Spotting may be normal in early pregnancy, but an ectopic pregnancy cannot be ruled out until an ultrasound is performed.

2. E. It is not yet possible to rule out ectopic pregnancy. This patient is in early pregnancy and has a pregnancy of unknown location. From the above stems an ectopic pregnancy cannot be ruled out and that is the most correct answer.

3. C. Normal rise, cannot exclude ectopic pregnancy. Until an ultrasound confirms an intrauterine pregnancy, ectopic cannot be ruled out. An ultrasound should therefore be performed in a week's time to see if an intrauterine pregnancy is visible.

4. C. A falling serum β-HCG eliminates risk of ectopic pregnancy rupturing. An ectopic pregnancy can rupture at any time and patients must be informed of this. A falling HCG is indicative of a failing pregnancy only.

Chapter 19 Antenatal booking and prenatal diagnosis

1. C. Essential hypertension. A history of essential hypertension is the most important factor because this, in conjunction with A and B, increases the risk of developing preeclampsia.

2. D. High vaginal swab. There is currently no recommendation by the National Screening Committee to perform a high vaginal swab at booking. However, it is currently being considered, to diagnose group B streptococcus infection.

3. E. After 15 weeks. Amniocentesis can be performed from 15 to 22 weeks, or possibly later in the pregnancy after 32 weeks. There is a 1% risk of miscarriage associated with the procedure. Before 15 weeks, the loss rate is higher, and fetal limb abnormalities have been reported. After 22 weeks, there is a risk of extreme preterm birth.

4. B. Noninvasive prenatal testing at 16 weeks. The noninvasive prenatal test can be done from 10 weeks' gestation, and involves taking a sample of maternal blood from which fetal DNA is extracted for chromosome testing. It is more than 99% accurate, but is not yet currently available on the NHS.

Chapter 20 Antepartum haemorrhage

1. D. Placental abruption. A placental abruption classically presents with vaginal bleeding associated with abdominal pain. It can occur at any stage in pregnancy. It is associated with cigarette smoking and cocaine use.

2. C. Cervical ectropion. During pregnancy, the normal tube-like shape of the cervix everts to expose the columnar epithelium within the cervical canal. This type of epithelium is prone to bleeding from pressure during intercourse.

3. E. Placenta praevia. Placental abruption and vasa praevia are more commonly clinical diagnoses which

necessitate urgent delivery rather than awaiting scans. A scan for placental location will diagnose placenta praevia and determine the grading, either major or minor.

4. B. ABC resuscitation. For any patient with bleeding, either antenatal or postnatal, basic assessment of ABC is essential including checking maternal pulse, blood pressure and respiratory rate.

Chapter 21 Hypertension in pregnancy

1. B. Liver function tests, full blood count, urea and electrolytes, urine protein-to-creatinine ratio and clotting. The history and examination findings suggest that this patient may have preeclampsia. This must be urgently investigated further with liver function tests, a platelet count, clotting studies and urine protein quantification

2. D. Labetalol. Labetalol is recommended by National Institute for Health and Care Excellence (NICE) guidelines as first-line treatment for hypertension in pregnant nonasthmatic patients.

3. E. Magnesium sulphate. An international multicentre study (MAGPIE trial) recommended that magnesium sulphate should be used in the immediate management of an eclamptic seizure.

4. B. Itching. Itching is a common presentation in patients with obstetric cholestasis. Patients with preeclampsia can present with headaches, epigastric pain, oedema and visual disturbances.

5. C. Aspirin 75 mg. Starting low-dose aspirin is the most beneficial at reducing the risk of developing preeclampsia. Folic acid and vitamin D supplementation is recommended for all women antenatally. Angiotensin-converting enzyme inhibitors such as enalapril are contraindicated in pregnancy.

Chapter 22 Medical disorders in pregnancy

1. E. Husband with type 2 diabetes. The husband's medical history is not relevant to his partner's risk of gestational diabetes.

2. E. Age <20 years. Older age, rather than younger age, is associated with an increased risk of venous thromboembolism in pregnancy.

3. A. >11.0 g/dL at booking and >10.5 g/dL at 28 weeks. These indices are generally agreed as appropriate normal values for these gestations.

4. C. Avoidance of breastfeeding and antiretroviral medication (HAART) to the mother and to the baby. These three factors have been proven to reduce HIV vertical transmission. With an undetectable viral load, there is increasing evidence that vaginal delivery has a similar risk of vertical transmission to caesarean section.

5. D. Start taking folic acid 5 mg daily. Folic acid 5 mg is recommended from preconception until 12 weeks' gestation to reduce the incidence of neural tube defects. Overall, fetal anomalies are increased in patients with diabetes, particularly if there is poor glucose control at the time of conception.

6. C. Prescribe vitamin K 10 mg daily from preconception until 12 weeks' gestation. Vitamin K should be prescribed in the third trimester of pregnancy, usually from 36 weeks' gestation and should be advised for the neonate.

7. B. Acute fatty liver of pregnancy. The history and the investigations, with the very high uric acid and hypoglycaemia, are in keeping with a diagnosis of acute fatty liver of pregnancy.

8. E. Puerperal psychosis. The history fits with a diagnosis of puerperal psychosis. Treatment should involve admission to a mother and baby unit and antipsychotic medication, as well as social support.

Chapter 23 Common presentations in pregnancy

1. C. Constipation. The effect of increasing serum progesterone in pregnancy causes a slowing of gastrointestinal motility, commonly resulting in symptoms such as heartburn and constipation.

2. C. Constitutional. Although a fetal chromosomal anomaly can be associated with low birth weight, the more common reason for being small for dates in an Asian woman is constitutional. The standard growth charts used in the UK are based on a Caucasian population.

3. D. Symphysis pubis dysfunction. Symphysis pubis dysfunction can progressively get worse throughout the pregnancy causing increasing difficulty with mobility, as progesterone affects bony joints. Women can be referred to physiotherapy where they can be assessed for crutches or even a wheelchair. Appendicitis usually presents with localized tenderness in the right iliac fossa and pyrexia. Gallstones present with right upper quadrant pain. Ligament pain is bilateral and worse on movement.

4. B. Glucose tolerance test. As the woman has risk factors for diabetes, this needs to be ruled out first as it is the most likely cause of fetal macrosomia and polyhydramnios. If the glucose tolerance test was negative, then infection would have to be ruled out with TORCH screen testing for toxoplasmosis, cytomegalovirus and rubella.

Chapter 24 Multiple pregnancy

1. E. Twin-to-twin transfusion syndrome. Twin-to-twin transfusion syndrome complicates 15% of monochorionic twin pregnancies. Therefore scans should be performed every 2 weeks from 16 weeks. Stage 1 disease presents with discrepant liquor volumes.

2. A. Uterine atony. Because of the larger placental site in a multiple pregnancy, postpartum haemorrhage is more common and therefore a prophylactic syntocinon infusion should be used for the third stage, regardless of the mode of delivery.

3. D. The pregnancy is a dichorionic pregnancy. A lambda sign seen on scan at 11–14 weeks indicates that this pregnancy must be dichorionic, and not monochorionic. Determining zygosity is not important clinically – however, a dichorionic pregnancy could be dizygotic or it could be a monozygotic pregnancy that splits before day 3 after fertilization.

Chapter 25 Preterm labour

1. B. Administration of steroids. Although A–D are all part of the management plan, steroids should be given first because the woman already appears to be in labour.

2. C. Previous caesarean section. Having had a previous caesarean section does not predispose to an early delivery in the current pregnancy. All the other options are correct.

3. A. Maternal tachypnoea. With preterm prelabour ruptured membranes, infection must be excluded, and the most sensitive sign for this is maternal tachypnoea. Candida infection is common in pregnancy and is of no concern to the fetus. Mucoid vaginal bleeding may simply be the show, or mucus plug coming from the cervix. This can be passed if contractions commence. In pregnancy, the white blood cell count shown is within the normal range.

Chapter 26 Labour

1. B. Strength of uterine contractions. Strength of contractions is best determined by abdominal palpation rather than electronic monitoring. The latter can be used to assess the frequency of contractions, as well as the fetal heart rate. The position, station and presence of caput on the presenting part are part of the vaginal examination.

2. D. Abduction. Abduction of the mother's legs is usually necessary to allow delivery of the baby. This is not part of the mechanism that occurs as the head descends within the maternal pelvis to facilitate delivery.

3. C. Engagement. Assessment of whether the widest diameter of the presenting part has entered the pelvic brim is essential in monitoring the progress of labour (i.e., assessing the engagement of the head).

4. E. Station. All answers A–E are important in assessing progress in labour, but station is the most important – even at full dilatation, vaginal delivery is not possible if the presenting part does not descend past the ischial spines.

Chapter 27 Fetal monitoring in labour

1. E. Meconium-stained liquor. Provided the course of the pregnancy antenatally and during delivery has been normal, meconium-stained liquor is the only indication given for continuous fetal monitoring. It can occur postterm as the fetus is more mature, or it can be associated with fetal hypoxia.

2. A. Fetal blood sampling. In the absence of contraindications such as maternal hepatitis or human immunodeficiency virus infection, or prematurity, a fetal blood sample should be performed if the pattern of the fetal monitoring is diagnosed as pathological.

3. B. Increase in the FHR of 15 bpm above the baseline rate lasting for 15 seconds. An acceleration is an increase in the FHR of 15 bpm above the baseline rate lasting for 15 seconds. This is a feature of a normal cardiotocograph.

Chapter 28 Operative interventions in labour

1. D. Third-degree perineal tear. A third-degree tear involves the anal sphincter and may also involve the internal anal sphincter. It is further classified as 3A, 3B or 3C, depending on how much of the external anal sphincter is torn, and whether the internal anal sphincter is involved as well. A fourth-degree tear goes through to the anal mucosa.

2. E. Amniotomy. Any intervention in labour, including amniotomy, has been shown to increase the risk of scar rupture. Answers A–C are all indicated, whilst D is optional depending on the woman's choice.

4. B. Reduce/stop the syntocinon infusion. The immediate management is to stop the syntocinon infusion as there is evidence of hyperstimulation. This should reduce the frequency of contractions, which may in turn correct the cardiotocograph. You may want to start intravenous fluids and give terbutaline, but these would be second-line management options.

Chapter 29 Complications of labour

1. A. Incoordinate uterine activity. It is not uncommon for uterine contractions to be incoordinate in a primiparous labour resulting in the need for augmentation with intravenous syntocinon.

2. D. Umbilical cord prolapse. An abnormal lie is more common in a grand multiparous woman, and also in preterm labour, with either an oblique lie or a transverse lie. Therefore at the time of ruptured membranes, there is a risk of cord prolapse because the head is not engaged in the maternal pelvis. If it occurs, it results in a fetal bradycardia as the blood vessels in the cord spasm.

3. B. Multiparity. External cephalic version is more likely to be successful in a multiparous patient because the maternal abdominal wall muscles are usually more relaxed. The other factors are all considered contraindications for ECV.

Chapter 30 Stillbirth

1. E. A baby that is born with no signs of life at or after 24 completed weeks of pregnancy.

2. C. Malaria. TORCH is an acronym of the five infections covered in the screening:
   - *t*oxoplasmosis
   - *o*ther diseases, including human immunodeficiency virus, syphilis and measles
   - *r*ubella (German measles)
   - *c*ytomegalovirus
   - *h*erpes simplex
   If the patient has a history of recent travel to a country affected by malaria, then investigations with blood films are required.

Chapter 31 Postnatal complications

1. C. Basic resuscitation ABC. Although all the options are required to manage postpartum haemorrhage, the first, most important step is to ensure that the woman's airway (A), breathing (B) and circulation (C) are intact and maintained. Make sure you are well acquainted with the ABC of basic resuscitation – the essential first response in every emergency situation.

2. A. >500-mL vaginal bleeding 24 hours after delivery, within 6 weeks. Secondary PPH occurs from 24 hours after delivery until 6 weeks. Maintain a high index of clinical suspicion for secondary PPH if a woman presents several weeks postpartum with heavy prolonged vaginal bleeding. Causes include retained products of conception or endometritis.

3. E. Uterine atony. The history is in keeping with uterine atony with the risk factors including a fibroid uterus, prolonged labour and a large baby. This primary postpartum haemorrhage needs urgent assessment of airway, breathing, circulation and then treatment to improve the uterine contractility.

4. E. Group A streptococcus. The key to diagnosis in this patient is the history of her unwell son – the patient should have a throat swab sent to exclude group A streptococcus infection and appropriate antibiotics. Depending on her clinical signs, she may be advised admission to hospital for treatment and monitoring. Sepsis, including postnatally, remains a leading cause of maternal mortality.

Chapter 32 Maternal collapse and maternal death

1. C. Ectopic pregnancy. The history, in conjunction with the positive pregnancy test, is strongly suggestive of an ectopic pregnancy. The patient must be resuscitated (airway, breathing, circulation) and taken to theatre urgently as the pregnancy may have ruptured requiring urgent salpingectomy.

2. B. Placental abruption. The history and examination indicate a likely placental abruption. The examination suggests severe internal (concealed) bleeding – the patient needs resuscitation (airway, breathing, circulation) and urgent delivery.

3. C. Call for help, position patient with a left lateral tilt and protect airway until help arrives. The patient is likely to be having an eclamptic seizure. You must call for help urgently and then protect her airway. Left lateral tilt position will prevent aortocaval compression and increase venous return. She needs urgent stabilization when help arrives.

4. D. Cardiac disease. Cardiac disease, a combination of congenital and acquired, was the leading cause of indirect maternal death.

EMQ answers

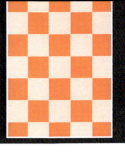

Chapter 1 Basic anatomy and examination

Symptoms related to anatomy

1. E   The large fibroid uterus is likely to cause heavy bleeding and as the bladder cannot expand sufficiently, it is likely to be accounting for the increased urinary frequency.

2. D   Of course you cannot be entirely sure of this diagnosis but pelvic pain with uterosacral involvement is suggestive of endometriosis.

3. F   It is common for postmenopausal women to have vaginal atrophy giving soreness and appearing friable.

Chapter 3 Common investigations

1. A   Any woman with pelvic pain and spotting may be pregnant, hence the simplest and easiest test is a urine HCG.

2. C   If a woman of childbearing age is unstable with pain and free fluid, the diagnosis may be a ruptured ectopic, ovarian cyst rupture or bleeding from another source. However, in any case once resuscitated surgery should be performed without delay.

3. F   This necessitates a cystoscopy to look for stones, cancers or masses, especially if no infections have been identified.

4. B   A hysteroscopy must performed in this instance when the endometrial thickness is above 5 mm to rule out cancer.

5. E   The best investigation initially to delineate pelvic masses is a pelvic ultrasound.

Chapter 4 Abnormal uterine bleeding

Management of abnormal uterine bleeding

1. C   If medical therapy and ablation have failed, the other options include UAE or hysterectomy. As she would like definitive treatment, hysterectomy is the only option and laparoscopic is less invasive than open.

2. H   As she has had a TOP, she would benefit from long-term contraception. Therefore the Mirena coil would help her symptoms and act as contraception.

3. E   As she has been sterilized, she would be a candidate for endometrial ablation. Other options such as UAE or hysterectomy are possible, but ablation is the safest and least invasive. If it does not work, she can try the other options.

4. A   If someone is trying to conceive and has heavy periods, only tranexamic acid or conservative measures are appropriate.

5. K   It is likely that this woman has an endometria polyp. So removal of the polyp via hysteroscopy should alleviate her symptoms.

Chapter 5 Fibroids

Management of fibroids

1. C   It is likely that she has a submucosal fibroid which should be resected. This will help with conceiving and improve her symptoms.

2. F   As she would like to conceive, a myomectomy is the most appropriate to immediately improve her hydronephrosis.

3. I   As childbearing is not an option in this example, hysterectomy would be preferred to myomectomy.

4. L   Uterine artery embolization will help her symptoms if she does not want surgery.

5. A   If no symptoms are present, the fibroid can be monitored to ensure it does not rapidly increase in size. Ultrasound is more appropriate to monitor the size compared with MRI which is more expensive.

Chapter 6 Endometriosis

Patient with endometriosis

1. H   A laparoscopy is indicated when conservative treatment has failed or if the patient declines other methods of management such as hormonal medication.

2. A   If a young woman presents with such symptoms, it is not unreasonable to consider conservative measures in the first instance.

3. L   Laparoscopy + treatment is the appropriate response here as she has endometriosis confirmed from before. In addition, the Mirena coil will help with heavy periods.

4. I   As she has had laser treatment before which was unsuccessful, excision during laparoscopy will now be the treatment of choice.

5. H   Treatment for endometriosis by laparoscopy will not only help with pelvic pain but also help with pregnancy rates. In addition, a tubal dye test could be performed to evaluate tubal patency.

Pelvic pain

1. G   The symptoms described here are characteristic of endometriosis.
2. F   The low haemoglobin and palpable mass are likely to be an ovarian cyst that is haemorrhagic and bleeding. Women can lose significant amounts of blood from an ovarian cyst.
3. I   As she has had several operations, she is likely to have adhesions.
4. H   Painful heavy periods may also be endometriosis but that would also likely give pelvic pain specific to one side or bilaterally where the deposits of endometriosis are likely to be. Painful periods in isolation fits more with an adenomyosis.
5. E   As she has had a previous appendectomy and the pain is severe, the most likely diagnosis unless proven otherwise is an ectopic pregnancy.

Chapter 8 Vaginal discharge and Sexually Transmitted Infections

Vaginal discharge

1. A   Bacterial vaginosis. Bacterial vaginosis is not a sexually transmitted infection. There is a change in the natural flora of the vagina. Its clinical significance is that it has been linked to second-trimester miscarriage.
2. H   Toxic shock syndrome. This girl has been distracted with examinations and has forgotten to change her tampon. Her symptoms and clinical signs are in keeping with toxic shock syndrome.
3. F   Cervical carcinoma. There is no cervical screening programme in this lady's country of origin. It would be prudent to check her human immunodeficiency virus status which is a known risk factor for cervical cancer.
4. D   *Chlamydia trachomatis*. The COCP does not protect against sexually transmitted infections.
5. I   Foreign body. This is the most likely option in this scenario. Foreign body insertion into the vagina is not uncommon in this age group and should be suspected if child abuse has been ruled out.

Chapter 9 Pelvic Inflammatory Disease

Pelvic pain and dyspareunia

1. E   Endometriosis. These are characteristic signs and symptoms of endometriosis.
2. G   *Chlamydia*. Perihepatic adhesions, also known as 'Fitz–Hugh–Curtis syndrome', are a sign of previous *Chlamydia* infection.
3. A   Adenomyosis. This condition typically affects older, parous women. The infiltration of the endometrium into the myometrial layer causes the uterus to become enlarged, globular and have a distinct consistency often reported as 'doughy'.
4. C   *Candida* infection. Typically, *Candida* occurs at times of immunosuppression such as pregnancy, steroid therapy or in women with medical conditions such as diabetes. The normal vaginal flora can also be altered by antibiotic therapy causing overgrowth of *Candida*.
5. F   Urinary tract infection. This is a cause of acute pelvic pain, particularly in pregnant women when it can be responsible for uterine tightenings.

Chapter 10 Contraception and termination of pregnancy

Method of contraception

1. E   The IUS is an excellent contraception and likely to thin the endometrium to reduce the risk of endometrial hyperplasia which this woman is at risk of if she has irregular periods and a raised BMI.
2. C   The COCP as well as providing contraception may reduce the risk of ovulation and hence potentially help with her pain symptoms also.
3. D   The depo is a reliable reversible form of long-term contraception. This would be a good alternative to the IUD.

Chapter 11 Benign gynaecological tumours

Investigations and management of gynaecology pathology

1. D   It is important that a pelvic scan is performed to identify if an ovarian cyst exists, as the other alternative diagnosis is appendicitis.
2. E   This scenario is likely to represent an acute torsion. In a likely postmenopausal woman the most appropriate management would be a bilateral salpingo-oophorectomy.

3. J This is likely to represent a ruptured haemorrhagic cyst. This may resolve spontaneously but one must check the haemoglobin and ensure that a blood transfusion is not required.

4. E Even though this is not likely to be malignant, as she is having symptoms she would benefit from both her ovaries and tubes being removed. If she was premenopausal, she would only require the symptomatic side to be removed.

5. A Any ovarian cyst in a postmenopausal woman must have a risk of malignancy index calculated. A Ca-125 blood test is required to calculate this.

Chapter 12 Gynaecological malignancies

Two-week wait gynaecology referrals

1. D This woman has a low risk of malignancy index score so the pathology is most likely benign.

2. B This is consistent with a diagnosis of endometrial hyperplasia.

3. L As the patient is premenopausal and has had this pattern of her periods since menarche, it is unlikely to be due to malignant pathology. A diagnosis of PCOS is more likely and can be confirmed with a transvaginal ultrasound scan and hormone profile blood tests.

4. K Paget disease of the vulva is associated with primary cancers in 25% of cases. It is possible, however, that this lesion could be benign.

5. A The appearance of a cervical ectropion can commonly be mistaken for a cervical pathology. In this case the patient was HPV negative and had a normal colposcopy.

Chapter 13 Benign vulval disease

Pruritus vulvae

1. D Any lesion that is raised, growing in size and ulcerated is suspicious of carcinoma.

2. I An offensive fishy green discharge is characteristic of *Trichomonas*.

3. C Fused labia in this age group with leukoplakia is characteristic of lichen sclerosus. The treatment being steroids.

4. B The clue is in the history as in a lot of these cases where changes in cleansing products can result in contact dermatitis.

5. F Erythema with plaques in other areas, particularly flexor surfaces, are characteristic of psoriasis, which is quite common. Treatment is usually topical steroids.

Chapter 14 Urogynaecology

Genital prolapse

1. D As she has had a complicated operation, there may be pelvic adhesions, hence a further pelvic operation would pose risk. A sacrospinous fixation is an extraperitoneal approach performed transvaginally.

2. E A TVT and separate cystocele can be performed in this instance but a single colposuspension if performed in an appropriate centre will correct the cystocele and stress incontinence.

3. B As there is uterine pathology also causing bleeding, a vaginal hysterectomy together with a pelvic floor repair is the most logical management. If there was no uterine pathology, organ-sparing surgery can be considered.

Chapter 15 Gynaecological endocrinology

Primary amenorrhoea

1. H Polycystic ovarian syndrome. It is one of the most common causes of amenorrhoea.

2. J Turner syndrome. The features are characteristic of Turner.

3. C Hypothalamic hypogonadism.

4. E Late-onset congenital adrenal hyperplasia.

5. D Constitutional amenorrhoea.

Chapter 16 Subfertility

Women with subfertility

1. E Clomiphene. It is likely that this patient has polycystic ovarian syndrome (PCOS) and is not ovulating due to her irregular periods. As a first course of action clomiphene may be successful by stimulating follicles, which may lead to successful ovulation.

2. J Donor sperm with IVF. As the couple are in a same sex relationship, donor sperm with IVF is the only feasible option.

3. D IUI. This seems like unexplained subfertility. So as an initial course, IUI should be considered, as it is the more similar of assisted fertility techniques.

Chapter 17 Menopause

Patient with menopause

1. C As she has had a hysterectomy, she requires only oestrogen as HRT (progesterone is only required in women who have a uterus

to prevent unopposed oestrogen causing hyperplasia or even cancer). Transdermal oestrogen will not significantly increase her risk of DVT, like oral oestrogens.

2. A — This can be treated simply with topical oestrogens locally. Again, the systemic absorption is low and so for a limited period no significant side-effects have been reported. In addition, as it is local therapy, no progesterone is required if used for a short duration.

3. B — She requires combined oral preparation as she found the Mirena uncomfortable. The oestrogen is essential to reduce the risk of osteoporosis forming in premature ovarian failure.

Chapter 18 Early pregnancy complications

Early pregnancy complications

1. G — An ectopic pregnancy requires treatment; if the contralateral tube appears normal, the best course of action is a salpingectomy.

2. B — An open cervical os is inevitable of miscarriage.

3. A — An empty uterus with an adnexal mass is generally an ectopic pregnancy until proven otherwise.

Chapter 19 Antenatal booking

Antenatal investigations

1. A — Serum electrophoresis to rule out beta-thalassaemia as a cause.

2. F — Glycosylated haemoglobin. The HbA1C level indicates how well controlled the diabetes has been.

3. C — Group and screen. Women who are rhesus negative will require anti-D prophylaxis at 28 weeks and if there are any other sensitizing events.

4. H — HIV. Vertical transmission of HIV is reduced with the use of highly active antiretroviral therapy, planning the mode of delivery based on the viral load and by not breastfeeding.

5. I — Hepatitis C. Intravenous drug users are at higher risk of having hepatitis C.

Interventions in the antenatal period

1. C — Membrane sweep. This encourages spontaneous labour as examining the cervix releases labour inducing prostaglandins.

2. D — Speculum examination. To assess if she has ruptured her membranes. If the watery loss is identified as liquor, then steroids and antibiotics should be administered.

3. I — External cephalic version should be offered to try and turn the baby to a cephalic position so that a vaginal delivery can be achieved.

4. F — Amniocentesis. Fetal cells from the amniotic fluid can be karyotyped to determine if the fetus has trisomy 21.

5. A — Umbilical artery Dopplers. Allows the resistance within the umbilical cord to be assessed and help in planning the timing and mode of delivery.

Antenatal care

1. D — Varicella zoster IgG. To assess if she has had a past exposure and hence immunity to chicken pox.

2. F — Amniocentesis. As the risk is <1 in 150, further confirmatory testing should be offered.

3. C — Hepatitis B, C and HIV test. Intravenous drug users are at higher risk of having these diseases and they may present a risk to the unborn fetus that would need to managed during the pregnancy.

4. H — Routine booking investigations. No additional risk factors have been identified and this is a routine investigation performed at the booking appointment.

5. B — Glucose tolerance test. Risk factors for developing gestational diabetes have been identified: these are Indian origin, raised body mass index and family history. Therefore gestational diabetes mellitus screening should be performed in pregnancy with a glucose tolerance test.

Chapter 20 Antepartum haemorrhage

Bleeding in the second and third trimesters of pregnancy

1. D — Placenta praevia. A low-lying placenta can cause fetal malpresentation as it blocks the cervical os and does not allow the fetal head to engage.

2. B — Vasa praevia. Bleeding comes from the fetal circulation and therefore is associated with CTG abnormalities. The treatment is prompt delivery with the neonatal team present for assessment of fetal blood transfusion after delivery.

3. A — Molar pregnancy. In a molar pregnancy there are elevated human chorionic gonadotropin levels causing the symptoms of nausea and vomiting.

4. E — Placental abruption. This woman has preeclampsia which is associated with placental abruption.

5. F — Cervical ectropion. Can cause bleeding on contact.

Chapter 21 Hypertension in pregnancy

Hypertensive diagnoses

1. B Preeclampsia is defined as hypertension (>140/90 mmHg) and proteinuria (>0.3 g in 24 hours) that develops after 20 weeks' gestation.

2. D Essential hypertension. Diagnosed at booking with a raised booking BP (>140/90 mmHg) and no proteinuria. Blood pressure is usually low in the first trimester due to the physiological changes of pregnancy.

3. C Hypertension secondary to renal disease is the likely diagnosis in view of her previous renal history. There is likely to have been damage to the renal tract causing raised blood pressure.

4. E Essential hypertension with superimposed preeclampsia. Women with essential hypertension are at increased risk of developing preeclampsia and therefore should be started on aspirin 75 mg in the first trimester and continue until 36 weeks' gestation.

5. J HELLP syndrome is defined by evidence of haemolysis, elevated liver enzymes and a low platelet count.

Hypertension in pregnancy

1. E Essential hypertension, as it has been diagnosed at booking. In the first trimester the blood pressure is lowered due to the physiological changes of pregnancy.

2. D Preeclampsia. Raised BP (>140/90 mmHg) after 20 weeks associated with significant proteinuria (>0.3 g in 24 hours).

3. F Pregnancy-induced hypertension or gestational hypertension is diagnosed with raised BP (>140/90 mmHg) after 20 weeks without proteinuria.

4. G HELLP syndrome is a variant of preeclampsia which includes haemolysis, elevated liver enzymes and low platelets.

5. C Eclampsia. A seizure in a pregnant woman should be treated as eclampsia until proven otherwise and as her blood pressure is significantly raised it is the likely cause. Treatment with magnesium sulphate should be commenced.

6. B Epileptic seizure, as she is a known epileptic and does not have raised BP.

Chapter 22 Medical disorders in pregnancy

Complications of the antenatal period

1. J Deep vein thrombosis. Pregnancy is a prothrombotic state and so there is an increased risk of thrombosis.

2. B Gestational diabetes. If not controlled, can cause fetal macrosomia and polyhydramnios.

3. A Obstetric cholestasis. Presents with itching over the palms of the hands and sole of the feet. No associated rash. Excoriation marks may be present. Liver function tests and bile acids will be deranged.

4. G Pyelonephritis. Nitrites in the urine suggest an infection within the renal tract. Treatment with admission and antibiotics is required.

5. H Preterm labour. Labour is defined as regular uterine contractions associated with cervical change, in this case the woman is also preterm.

Management of medical disorders in pregnancy

1. D Book a glucose tolerance test. A previous history of gestational diabetes mellitus (GDM) is a risk factor for developing GDM in the current pregnancy.

2. A Take folic acid 5 mg daily. Neural tube defects are increased in those taking antiepileptic medications; high-dose folic acid can reduce this risk.

3. J Arrange urgent investigations including coagulation screen and glucose level as a diagnosis of acute fatty liver needs to be excluded.

4. E Organize a chest X-ray in the first instance. If this is normal, then further investigations to rule out a pulmonary embolism are needed.

5. H Start aspirin 75 mg daily. This can reduce her risk of developing preeclampsia.

Investigations for medical disorders in pregnancy

1. F Glucose tolerance test. Poorly controlled diabetes can cause fetal macrosomia and polyhydramnios.

2. D Folic acid supplementation and detailed cardiac scan. Antiepileptic medication is associated with neural tube defects and cardiac anomalies.

3. B Antenatal and postnatal low-molecular-weight heparin. At prophylactic dose to reduce the risk of venous thromboembolism in pregnancy.

4. C Liver function tests and bile acids. If abnormal alanine aminotransferase and raised bile acids, then the likely diagnosis is obstetric cholestasis.

5. E Haemoglobinopathy screen to rule out beta-thalassaemia as a cause of her anaemia.

Chapter 23 Common presentations in pregnancy

Abdominal pain in the second and third trimester

1. D Placental abruption. Bleeding from a placental abruption causes the uterus to become tense,

this is different from the tightenings/contractions that occur during labour as it is continuous and the uterus does not relax. The woman will complain of abdominal pain with or without bleeding.

2. H   UTI. Nitrites on a urine analysis indicate the presence of an infection and the woman should be treated for a UTI with antibiotics. A midstream urine sample should be sent to the microbiology laboratory for microscopy, culture and sensitivities so that the antibiotics can be tailored to the identified organism.

3. J   Labour. Labour is defined as regular uterine contractions associated with cervical change.

4. A   Fibroid degeneration. Fibroids can enlarge during pregnancy due to the hormonal changes that occur. They can become so large that they outgrow their blood supply, which causes degeneration of the fibroid and this is painful for the woman.

5. G   Preeclampsia. PET is a multiorgan disease defined as hypertension with proteinuria presenting after 20 weeks' gestation. RUQ in preeclampsia is due to perihepatic oedema.

Large for dates and small for dates

1. F   Renal agenesis. Liquor is produced by the renal kidneys. If the kidneys do not develop, then the fetus cannot produce liquor.

2. A   Gestational diabetes. High levels of glucose in the bloodstream cross through the placenta and cause fetal macrosomia.

3. D   Twin pregnancy. The symphysis–fundal height (SFH) with be increased as the uterus expands to accommodate the two growing fetuses.

4. C   Placental insufficiency. An ultrasound scan needs to be performed when the woman measures small for dates.

5. G   Uterine fibroid. Uterine fibroids can increase the SFH as the uterus and fibroids are measured. An ultrasound scan will reveal if the fetus is growing appropriately.

Chapter 24 Multiple pregnancy

Antenatal care of multiple pregnancies

1. B   Chorionicity. This relates to the placentation. If the placentae are separate, with separate amnions and chorions (dichorionic diamniotic), the blood supply to each fetus during the pregnancy is independent. If there are blood vessel anastomoses between the placentae (monochorionic diamniotic/monochorionic monoamniotic), then there is a risk of uneven distribution of blood.

2. G   Selective fetal reduction. This involved terminating a fetus to reduce the risks of the pregnancy to give the remaining fetus/fetuses a better outcome.

3. J   Twin-to-twin transfusion syndrome. In monochorionic pregnancies there are blood vessel anastomoses between the placenta causing uneven distribution of blood. This can lead to one twin being the donor and one the recipient. The donor twin will be growth restricted and have oligohydramnios whilst the recipient twin will be larger and have polyhydramnios.

4. A   Consultant-led hospital care. A multiple pregnancy is a high-risk pregnancy, so women should receive consultant-led care in a hospital.

5. D   Intrauterine growth restriction. Symphysis–fundal height is not accurate in multiple pregnancies.

Chapter 26 Labour

Obstetric definitions

1. C   Position of the presenting part of the fetus.
2. H   Antepartum haemorrhage.
3. G   Maternal mortality rate.
4. I   Labour.
5. D   Station of the presenting part of the fetus.

Interventions in labour

1. D   Fetal scalp electrode. This will attach to the baby's head and detect the fetal heart rate by direct contact. This should not be applied if the mother has human immunodeficiency virus or hepatitis B.

2. E   Fetal blood sample. The result will allow the doctors to interpret if the baby is becoming acidotic and will aid the timing and mode of delivery.

3. G   Artificial rupture of membranes. This can increase the contract regularity, frequency and intensity and should be done in the first instance before commencing a syntocinon infusion.

4. B   Lower segment caesarean section. As the woman is not fully dilated and the fetal bradycardia is not recovering, this baby needs urgent delivery.

5. A   Ventouse delivery. As all criteria for an instrumental delivery have been met, the forceps cannot be used on an occipitotransverse position.

Terminology in labour

1. E   Fetal tachycardia. A fetal heart rate above 160 bpm is a fetal tachycardia.

2. F   Malpresentation. This is an oblique lie and there is a risk of cord prolapse.

3. G   Malposition. This is an occipitoposterior position.

4. J   Moulding. Fetal skull bones overlap in labour to allow the fetal head to pass through the pelvis.

5. H   Variability. The beat-to-beat variation of the fetal heart rate.

Chapter 29 Complications in labour

Failure to progress

1. D   Fetal macrosomia. Poorly controlled diabetes in pregnancy can cause fetal macrosomia as the excess sugar in the maternal bloodstream crosses to the fetus.

2. E   Irregular contractions. The three Ps needed for successful delivery are passage, passenger and powers. Strong, regular uterine contractions are required for labour to progress.

3. A   Cervical fibroid. Fibroids are more common in Afro-Caribbean women.

4. I   Transverse lie. Multiparity can be a cause for a malpresentation or unstable lie.

5. J   Brow presentation. This represents the largest diameter of the fetal head (mentovertical) at 13.5 cm.

Intrapartum complications

1. F   Ruptured uterus. One of the first signs of scar rupture is fetal distress. Other signs and symptoms include tachycardia, pain along the scar, haematuria and vaginal bleeding.

2. H   Shoulder dystocia. Shoulder dystocia occurs when the anterior shoulder does not deliver due to being lodged behind the symphysis pubis. The baby can become hypoxic and various manoeuvres are applied to attempt delivery of the baby. See Box 29.12.

3. E   Cord prolapse. More likely to occur when there is a malpresentation or the presenting part remains high.

4. C   Placental abruption. Preeclampsia is associated with placental abruption. This can present with vaginal bleeding in a revealed abruption and no bleeding in a concealed abruption. The examination findings include a 'woody' hard uterus that does not relax and it can be associated with fetal distress.

5. G   Uterine hyperstimulation. Occurs when there are more than 5 in 10 contractions and is associated with fetal distress. This is different from tachysystole where there are more than 5 in 10 contractions and no fetal distress.

Chapter 30 Stillbirth

Causes of stillbirth

1. G   A normal karyotype is 46XX or 46XY. This analysis shows 47XY, indicating that the fetus is male and has an extra chromosome – trisomy 21 is seen in Down syndrome.

2. F   Proteinuria of greater than 0.3 g/L is significant and can point to a diagnosis of preeclampsia.

3. D   Parvovirus infection can pass across the placenta and cause fetal anaemia, leading to cardiac failure and fetal death. Positive IgM and negative IgG confirms recent infection.

4. A   Transaminases are often raised in cholestasis, as are bile acids. However, the levels of liver function tests alone do not make the diagnosis, which must also be based on the clinical picture and the absence of hepatitis.

5. C   Rhesus disease causes fetal haemolysis, and therefore anaemia. Coombs test proves the presence of antibodies.

6. B   This level of glycosylated haemoglobin indicates poor control, which predisposes to congenital anomalies and intrauterine death.

Chapter 31 Postnatal complications

Complications of the postnatal period

1. E   PPH. A primary PPH is defined as bleeding more than 500 mL within 24 hours of delivery. In this case this would be a secondary PPH which is defined as bleeding more than 500 mL that starts 24 hours after delivery and occurs within 6 weeks. The commonest cause would be endometritis or retained products of conception.

2. B   Postnatal depression. The timing of these symptoms suggests a diagnosis of postnatal depression; other symptoms that could be present include anxiety, fatigue or irritability.

3. A   Puerperal psychosis. This woman is having persecutory beliefs other symptoms of psychosis including lability of mood, overactivity, disorientation, lack of insight and hallucinations.

4. C   Endometritis. Treatment is with antibiotics.

5. I   Dural puncture headache. Cerebrospinal fluid leaks from the puncture into the dura mater; treatment is with a 'blood patch' to seal the puncture.

Postpartum haemorrhage

1. D   Third-degree tear. Perineal tears involving the anal sphincter complex are classified as a third-degree tears. It is a fourth-degree tear if the anal mucosa has been involved.

2. E Uterine atony. Occurs is when the uterus does not contract after delivery. There can be ongoing bleeding. Treatment is with uterotonic drugs including syntocinon, ergometrine, misoprostol.

3. I Placenta accrete. An abnormal attachment of the placenta to the uterine myometrium. A history of previous caesarean sections increases the risk.

4. A Primary PPH. The commonest causes are uterine atony and genital tract trauma.

5. J Uterine inversion. During the third stage of labour if controlled cord traction is applied before the placenta has delivered, uterine inversion can occur. This causes severe pain if the woman does not have any anaesthesia and brisk bleeding. The treatment is to replace the uterus manually.

Chapter 32 Maternal collapse

Causes of maternal collapse

1. A A long labour, the need for syntocinon augmentation and a big baby all predispose to poor uterine contraction after delivery leading to postpartum haemorrhage.

2. C This multipara is predisposed to anaemia, which will have been exacerbated by her blood loss at caesarean section. The standing up has led to her fainting.

3. E Pregnancy, obesity and immobility are all risk factors for thromboembolic disease.

4. H This woman has developed chorioamnionitis, with infection ascending up and around the baby, producing a systemic illness. She needs antibiotic treatment and delivery.

5. G Hypertension and proteinuria raise suspicion of preeclampsia, which can rapidly deteriorate into an eclamptic episode. Fits in pregnancy, even in those previously labelled epileptic, should always be suspected of being related to preeclampsia.

Causes of maternal collapse

1. I Pulmonary embolism. History of a previous deep vein thrombosis and having the factor V Leiden mutation put this woman at high risk of a thromboembolism and she should have been advised to commence prophylactic low-molecular-weight heparin as soon as she knew she was pregnant.

2. C Uterine rupture. One of the first signs of uterine scar rupture is fetal distress. Other signs and symptoms include tachycardia, pain over the scar, haematuria and vaginal bleeding.

3. A Placental abruption can present with or without vaginal bleeding. The uterus is continuously hard on palpation with no relaxation. It can be associated with preeclampsia.

4. E Eclampsia. Preeclampsia is defined as hypertension and proteinuria that develops after 20 weeks' gestation. It is a multiorgan disease that can involve the liver, kidneys and fetoplacental circulation. It can lead to eclampsia when the blood pressure is not controlled.

5. H Puerperal septic shock. Postnatal/genital tract sepsis is one of the leading cause of maternal death. One of the first signs of sepsis can be tachypnoea.

Maternal collapse

1. F Placental abruption. Smoking increases the risk of placental abruption. A woody hard uterus is a common examination finding during an abruption.

2. D Anaphylactic shock. Allergies to medications should always be documented along with the reaction that occurs.

3. H Hypovolaemic shock secondary to unrecognized postpartum haemorrhage due to uterine atony.

4. C Amniotic fluid embolism occurs at or within 30 minutes of delivery and can lead to disseminated intravascular coagulopathy.

5. B Acute myocardial infarction. Classical symptoms of myocardial infarction with central chest pain radiating to the jaw.

Maternal death

1. C Ruptured ectopic pregnancy. Any woman who complains of abdominal pain in early pregnancy should be referred to the local early pregnancy department for an ultrasound scan to locate the pregnancy. Ectopic pregnancies can present with diarrhoea due to the intraabdominal bleeding irritating the bowel.

2. A Sepsis. Prompt treatment following the Sepsis Six pathway is required for any pyrexia in labour or postpartum.

3. F Intracranial haemorrhage. Uncontrolled raised blood pressure can cause intracranial haemorrhage.

4. B Pulmonary embolism. Pregnancy is a coagulopathic state and therefore the risk of thromboembolism is increased.

5. E Puerperal psychosis.

Alanine transaminase A blood test that measures the amount of a liver enzyme.

Alkaline phosphatase A liver enzyme, normal to have raised level in pregnancy as it is produced by the placenta.

Amenorrhoea Absence of menstrual period in a woman of reproductive age.

Amniotic fluid The fluid that surrounds a fetus in the uterus.

Antepartum haemorrhage Bleeding in pregnancy after 24 weeks.

Artificial rupture of membranes Midwife or doctor breaks the bag of waters around the baby.

Body mass index (BMI) Measure of height and weight; BMI greater than $30\,kg/m^2$ is a risk factor for a more complicated pregnancy.

Blood pressure Measure of the pressure needed to pump blood around the body.

Booking bloods Routine standard blood tests performed when a woman books for antenatal care. These include screening for human immunodeficiency virus, haemoglobinopathies, hepatitis B, syphilis, and full blood count, group and save and random blood glucose level.

Breech The baby is presenting bottom first.

Cardiotocograph Recording on paper of the baby's heartbeat.

Cephalic/ceph The head of the baby is presenting into the maternal pelvis.

Cervix The opening to the uterus.

Clonus An examination for cerebral irritability. A clonus of three beats or over is considered significant.

Colposcopy A diagnostic procedure to examine a magnified view of the cervix.

C-reactive protein Blood test done to see if there is inflammation or infection in the body.

Cryoprecipitate A source of fibrinogen, vital to blood clotting.

Cusco's A bivalve speculum.

Cystocele Prolapse of the bladder into the anterior vaginal wall.

Cystoscopy Endoscopy (camera investigation) of the urinary bladder via the urethra.

Dyschezia Pain and difficulty in defecating.

Dyskaryosis Abnormal cytological changes of the cervical cells.

Dysmenorrhoea Pain during the menstrual period.

Dyspareunia Pain during sexual intercourse – can be deep or superficial.

Dysuria Pain during urination.

Fetal blood sample Blood test from baby's scalp taken during labour to check on baby's condition.

Fetal fibronectin test A swab taken to see if preterm delivery is likely to happen.

Fetal heart rate Baby's heart rate.

Fetal lie The direction of the long axis of the fetus compared with the mother.

Fetal scalp electrode Clip put on baby's head to allow the heart beat to be checked.

Fitz–Hugh–Curtis syndrome Liver capsule adhesion as a complication of pelvic inflammatory disease.

Fresh frozen plasma Liquid portion of the blood that has been frozen and preserved.

Full blood count Measure of the white blood cell, red blood cell and platelet levels in the blood.

General anaesthetic Giving medication to induce a controlled state of unconsciousness.

Gravid A pregnant uterus.

Group and save To find out the blood group and save a sample.

Haematuria The presence of blood in the urine.

Haemoglobin Measure of the oxygen-carrying protein in the red blood cells.

Haemolysis Rupture of the red blood cells, elevated liver enzymes (showing damage to the liver) and low platelets (cells vital to help the blood to clot).

Hysteroscopy Endoscopy (camera investigation) of the uterus via the cervical canal.

Intensive therapy unit Specialized ward that provides care for severe and life-threatening illnesses.

Intramuscular An injection of medication into a muscle.

Intravenous An injection of medication into a vein.

Laparoscopy Minimally invasive laparoscopic camera investigation of the abdomen or pelvis.

Leiomyoma Uterine fibroid.

Leucocytes White cells found in blood or urine.

Linea nigra Pigmented vertical line that appears on the abdomen during pregnancy.

Liver function test A blood test to measure how the liver is working.

Major obstetric haemorrhage Bleeding during pregnancy or after delivery of more than 1.5 L.

Maternity triage An assessment area for pregnant women.

Meconium Baby's first bowel motion, green in colour (sometimes seen when the bag of waters around the baby breaks before birth).

Menarche The first menstrual period.

Menopause When menstrual periods cease (defined as for over 1 year).

Menorrhagia Menstrual prior with excessively heavy flow.

Midstream urine A urine sample sent to laboratory to look for infection.

Miscarriage Spontaneous abortion or pregnancy loss before 24 weeks' gestation.

Multidisciplinary team Doctors, anaesthetists and midwives working together.

Neonatal unit A specialized unit for looking after babies.

Obstetric cholestasis Liver problem in pregnancy that causes itching.

Postpartum haemorrhage Bleeding of more than 500 mL after delivery of the baby.

Preeclampsia A disorder of pregnancy with high blood pressure and protein in the urine.

Procidentia Complete prolapse of the uterus beyond the level of the introitus.

Protein creatinine ratio A urine specimen to measure the amount of protein in the urine.

Rectocele Prolapse of the bowel into the posterior vaginal wall.

Sims A U-shaped speculum.

Spontaneous rupture of membranes When the bag of waters around the baby breaks.

Striae gravidarum Atrophic linear stretch marks of pregnancy.

Urea and electrolytes A blood test to look at the function of the kidneys.

Vaginal examination An internal examination of the vagina.

Virgo intacta A person who has never had sexual intercourse.